Organ Donation and Transplantation

Organ Donation and Transplantation

Edited by Rebecca Owen

STATES
ACADEMIC PRESS
www.statesacademicpress.com

States Academic Press,
109 South 5th Street,
Brooklyn, NY 11249, USA

Visit us on the World Wide Web at:
www.statesacademicpress.com

ISBN: 978-1-63989-399-7

Cataloging-in-Publication Data

Organ donation and transplantation / edited by Rebecca Owen.
p. cm.
Includes bibliographical references and index.
ISBN 978-1-63989-399-7
1. Donation of organs, tissues, etc. 2. Transplantation of organs, tissues, etc. 3. Organs (Anatomy).
4. Surgery. I. Owen, Rebecca.

RD129.5 .O74 2022
362.178 3--dc23

Table of Contents

Preface

This book has been a concerted effort by a group of academicians, researchers and scientists, who have contributed their research works for the realization of the book. This book has materialized in the wake of emerging advancements and innovations in this field. Therefore, the need of the hour was to compile all the required researches and disseminate the knowledge to a broad spectrum of people comprising of students, researchers and specialists of the field.

The medical procedure wherein an organ is transferred from one person to another, in order to replace a missing or injured organ, is termed as organ transplantation. The organs or tissues can also be transplanted within a person's own body. These are known as autografts. The transplants between two individuals of the same species are referred to as allografts. There are numerous organs which can be transferred from one person to another such as kidneys, liver, pancreas, heart, uterus and intestine. The donors can be alive or dead. Tissues can also be taken from donors who die of circulatory death. Transplant rejection is one of the most important challenges to organ transplantation. This book unravels the recent studies in the field of organ donation and transplantation. It outlines the clinical aspects of organ donation in detail. This book will prove to be immensely beneficial to students and researchers in this field.

At the end of the preface, I would like to thank the authors for their brilliant chapters and the publisher for guiding us all-through the making of the book till its final stage. Also, I would like to thank my family for providing the support and encouragement throughout my academic career and research projects.

Editor

1

The Society, the Barriers to Organ Donation and Alternatives for a Change

Félix Cantarovich

Abstract

Objectives: To evaluate the current possibilities that transplantation offers to the patients on waiting lists, and to propose alternatives to modify this medical and social crisis.

Introduction: Persistent organ shortage remains a problem. Put simply, patients are dying because people have not understood that donation means to prolong lives. Ignorance and prejudice and mainly fear of dead and mutilation are major causes for inadequate society's response.

Conclusion: The stagnant shortage of organs shows that current educational strategy has not improved people's behavior. Renovate the current message might be a way for a change. New catch phrases like: "After death, our body is a unique source of health"; "Organ donation is not a gift. It is to sharing of a new life for one and all". "Throughout life, we are all potential recipients of a transplant"; could be included in educational programs; in addition, instructive action on this subject addressed to the youth, starting in the schools, could be another positive contribution for a solution to this crucial crisis for the possibilities of welfare of the Society.

Keywords: modifying educational programs, organ donation, organ transplantation, dying in waiting lists, social behavior, school curricula

1. Introduction

Transplantation of organs and tissues has succeeds to associate life and death for the benefits of society. Current evidence suggests that transplantation medicine might be a crucial health guarantee for society. However, the paradoxical shortage of donated organs limits this possibility.

This extraordinary progress of medical sciences offered to the people by health care organization, has generated the need for novels methods and State actions to be able to implement it without any restrictions for the benefit of society.

Certainly, this advance in medical practice should generate new health programs different from those recognized until now. The vital requirement to transform death into life, which is what organ transplants symbolize, requires the end of somebody life. Therefore, the knowledge and acceptance of the metaphor, "transforming death into life", should be recognized by the State and by the people.

It is important that society knows the benefits that organ transplants mean for the security systems. This reality is evidenced in the significant budgets differences of a kidney transplant compared to a same period of patient in hemodialysis.

To achieve this goal, it is essential that people should understand currently the essential solution to solve the inexorable evolution of patients suffering from a terminal organ failure and that our body after death is a unique and irreplaceable source of health.

This possibility depends of people's legal organ donation either during their lives or that at the time of death of their loved ones. Unfortunately, this people's option remained for decades in a partial response.

Organ shortage is a social, psychological, ethical, moral and political problem, causing unjustifiable damage to public health.

As a consequence of organ shortage, patients on waiting lists are "unfairly" dying everyday. In a way, the unjustifiable truth of today is that society is denying another human the chance to live.

Regarding the notion of people "unfairly" dying while waiting for an organ, it is also true that thousands of people are dying everyday because of socio-economic inequalities [1]. However, the reality of this is that such deaths are a consequence of multiple and complex problems, including economic, political, social inequality and corruption. All of these problems are extremely difficult to take care of. In contrast, organ shortage solution fundamentally depends on the change in the current social behavior toward organ donation. This alternative could be achieved if the strategies to modify frequent people's attitude toward organ donation are evaluated and revised.

This social paradox urges a rational response. The puzzle to answer is what is the motive of this crime of "lese majesty" that humanity is committing against itself?

The reasons most responsible for this negative behavior toward organ donation are basically ignorance and misinformation [2–6].

Worldwide, approximately 47% of people who are asked to donate organs and tissues gave their consent despite the fact that in opinion polls, between 75 and 90% of the population is in favor of the donation.

At this moment, more than 125,000 people in the United States are in need of a life-saving organ transplant. And 64% of them are currently on a waiting list—to which roughly one person is added every 10 min—unfortunately, only about half of them will actually receive, the transplant they need this year [7].

A critical analysis of the reasons for the uncertain people behavior toward donation suggests as a valid alternative, that the current message to society has not been able to develop a positive change in this current social conduct [2].

As a proposal, we have suggested a change of the classic slogan "Donate is a gift of life" for "Donate is to share life". In addition, we have proposed the following ideas as useful supplements to modify current behaviors toward donation:

"During life we are all potential recipients of a transplant".

"All monotheistic religions accept organ donation and transplantation".

A social education that allows a real knowledge of this problem will be a challenge to facilitate people understand a human right acquired by the Society: to give or receive donation of organs and tissues during life.

We suggest the aforementioned slogan: "Our body after death is a unique and irreplaceable source of health" as a valid challenge in search of a social change.

It is interesting to note that current people's feelings regarding organ donation does not fully agree with the concepts stated by UNESCO emphasizing that attitudes of society toward organ donation do not conform to the principles of social behavior [8].

It would be important to make people aware, as the main protagonist of the lack of organs, of these significant notions required today by society.

At present, time should ensure the possibility that anyone who requires a transplant can receive it in necessary time. The social security of modern states should use maximum resources in the achievement of educational programs that have analyzed and proposed solutions to the real barriers that generally inhibit the will to donate, in the search of achieving a positive change in the current indefinite social behavior.

In addition, the training of young people through the incorporation of topics on donation and transplants in curricular programs, periodically carried out in schools, colleges and universities, may be another way to develop a change in people's attitudes toward organ donation.

2. The underlying reasons for organ shortage

Ignorance and prejudice continue to be the general causes of society's lack of response to the social need of organ donation; particularly with respect to the deceased donor [3]. Several possible explanations for this behavior have been suggested:

1. People are only partially aware of how accepted, organized and frequent transplantation of organs and tissues is today.
2. People do not consider that they themselves may need a transplant during their life.
3. Society is not cognizant that the body after death offers a unique source of life.

4. Medical teams are largely untrained in organ donation because of insufficient education on this matter [4–7].

5. The decision about organ donor after death, or the response of relatives to donation requests, awakens primal fears such as:

   a. The instinct of self-preservation [9].

   b. The Freudian notion that nobody thinks about his or her own death until a loved one dies [10].

   c. The ancient idea that the integrity of the body is mandatory for the pathway to eternity [11].

   d. The fears concerning a diagnosis of brain death [12, 13].

   e. Beliefs that the organs will first go to the rich and only then to the poor [14–16].

People are not informed about the beneficial impact of transplantation on health budgets, that is, transplantation can reduce the cost of diseases, which would otherwise have to be treated by expensive long-term therapy [17, 18].

The media has featured stories about criminal "organ commerce" [19].

These myths, misinformation and prejudices are barriers that weaken the instincts of solidarity and altruism, arousing selfishness and uncertainties.

Regarding the aforementioned negative factors on donation, it is important to emphasize the importance of two of them: fear of death and respect for the integrity of the body that are not essentially linked to ignorance and/or bad information. Surveys on the behavior of university students regarding the implication of fear of death as an inhibition factor in the acceptance of organ donation and transplants were investigated in different studies. These surveys showed that negative attitudes toward organ donation were associated with higher fears of death and dying of the self and less strongly with higher fears of the death and dying of others. A study showed that students without donor card and with reservations about donation scored significantly higher fear of physical destruction. Possible implications of these findings for medical education and future research are suggested. It was mentioned that given the urgency, attitude toward organ donation should be considered a civic responsibility transforming an unfortunate yet inevitable event into something that positively affects someone else [20–22].

Body integrity, it also remains a central issue for negative behavior toward organ donation. Fear of mutilation is the fear of losing any part of our body structure, the idea of having limits in the mobility of our body or of losing the integrity of any organ, part of the body or natural function. These ideas can generate ethical and moral inhibitory behaviors regarding the treatment that our bodies or those of loved ones receive at the time of death. These reflections regarding the conservation of the body's image play a significant role in the decision of families toward donation [23].

Understanding that those factors can limit the potential supply of available organs for transplantation, the suggestion that our body after death as a unique and irreplaceable source of health should be considered an educational challenge in the search to modify socio-psychological behaviors deeply structured in people's mind. Educational procedures searching the best way to spread this notion should be deeply analyzed by experts in social, psychological and religious questions.

Public education, mainly through the media, non-governmental organizations and lectures by experts, has been the main strategy to change social attitudes toward organ donation. It is important to highlight that the results of these educational endeavors have not been completely satisfactory, as the crisis remains almost unchanged. Although the public is more aware about transplantation issues, there remains a shortage of donated organs.

The increasing number of patients on waiting lists and their daily mortality is a clear expression of the insufficient impact of social education programs to date. The consequence of this inadequate social response is that at least 22 unreasonable deaths occur everyday on organ donation waiting lists [24].

Highlighting the serious situation, Matas and Hays considered that the United States educational policy has had little effect on organ donation [25]. For that reason, the author suggested that making organ donation financially neutral for donors should be supported as one solution to this serious problem. However, it should be considered that this strategy might generate a new type of social injustice and inequality. In addition, it should be noted that there has been several criticisms of the educational social programs on organ donation. Many authors believe that the current methodology is useless and is a needless economic investment [26, 27].

Paradoxically, none of these authors suggested thoughtful modifications to the educational methodologies in order to achieve a more positive social response to organ donation.

2.1. Potential reasons for the present crisis

2.1.1. The message to the public has been inadequate

From the earliest times of the transplantation era, the philosophy used for educational purposes has relied on the concept that organ donation is an expression of altruism and solidarity, a "gift" that will save or improve someone's life. In fact, several surveys have shown that, in general, people are open to donate their organs (or those of a family member) after death. However, when facing the moment of grief, a high percentage of people fail to remember this commitment and consequently the "gift of life" is questioned and does not come to fruition.

The inadequate societal response to the persistent lack of donated organs encourages the following conceptual changes in the philosophy of the organ donation message:

1. Organ shortage is a health emergency.
2. Our body after death is a unique source of health for everyone.
3. Sharing our bodies after death should be acknowledged as a tacit social agreement for a common welfare.

4. Organ donation is not giving life, it is sharing life.
5. Throughout our lives we are all potential organ and tissue recipients.

Successful implementation of these ideas requires acknowledgment by state health and education institutions, scientific societies, organ sharing organizations and representatives of monotheistic religions.

2.1.2. The message has not been effectively transmitted

Undoubtedly, a scientifically programmed and continuously disseminated MEDIA campaign will have an important influence on the improvement of social behavior toward transplantation and donation.

Nevertheless, on the other hand, the MEDIA can transmit prejudicial and negative information and the myths most commonly perpetuated as:

1. Premature declaration of death.
2. Transference of personality traits from donor to recipient.
3. Criminal black market for organs.
4. Corruption in the medical community.
5. Organ allocation systems, which allow celebrities to get transplants first.

A recent study has shown that mass media can generate a conflicting image of organ donation. The inadequate information is responsible for a negative attitude on the part of many potential donors. Investigations on the effects of MEDIA on donation have shown that when people are not in favor, they often mention the negative effect of television programs [28]. The myths transmitted were more believed by the viewers, than by those who did not see these programs. The same phenomenon occurred regarding the donation between spectators and non-spectators.

Although these are not the only myths that the general public believes to be true, the media is a powerful support for them. A well-programmed and persistently disseminated media campaign might have an important influence on improving society's knowledge of organ donation and transplantation.

It has been proposed that the ability of the press to correct negative misinformation might be fundamentally improved with the collaboration between specialists in transplants and journalists in the drafting of news or recommendations on donation and transplantation to society [29].

The decision of an organ donor is one of the most important and significant behavior of a current world citizen.

A public debate regarding organ donation can inform and stimulate many people to be donors.

Proposed solutions:

1. Legal measures
2. Financial incentives
3. Expanding donors
4. Education

1. Legal measures

Laws about organ transplantation have been passing attempts to provide a better system of organ donation and distribution and to encourage individuals to volunteer as organ donors.

In USA, in 1968, The Uniform Anatomical Gift Act was the first effort at providing a national organ and tissue donation policy. The act created a uniform legal procedure for persons who wish to donate organs and for hospitals and medical institutions that want to accept them. A 1986 federal law requires all hospitals participating in Medicare or Medicaid to implement a "required request" policy. Hospitals are required to discuss with potential donors and their families "the option of organ and tissue donation and their option to decline" [30].

Consent and altruism remain core values of organ donation. The term consent is typically defined as a subject adhering to an agreement of principals and regulations.

Two types of legislation concerning organ donations are at present valid worldwide:

1. Informed consent or "opt in" (only those who have given explicit consent are donors or the expressed voluntary of their families in case of death).
2. Presumed consent or "opt out" (who has not refused to express their consent to the donation is a donor).

People have thus to register if they do not want to donate their body.

Presumed consent is one of a number of different varieties of consent. The paradigm of consent in biomedical ethics is to express consent. It appears in the Uniform Anatomical Gift Act's framework for organ donation as well as in rules of voluntary, informed consent in both therapy and research involving human participants.

On the other hand presumed consent has always been perceived as the "best" system for society in terms of organ donations.

However, in both systems, the family has something to say, especially for the deceased who did not sign anything while alive.

Proposals to introduce presumed consent should have full knowledge of their organization and results in the countries in which this legal instrument is in force. In practice, the citizen is informed that his non-registration as a non-donor means that he is a donor. The experience has shown that, in general, the presumed consent has not nullified the will of the families.

In Spain and Italy, it is considered that the increase in donation is the exponent of a better institutional management rather than the result of the presumed consent law.

In France according to the 1976 "Caillavet Law", a person is presumed to have consented to organ donation if he or she has never explicitly said otherwise to close relatives. But even for organs and tissue, where there is no such legal confusion, the "Caillavet Law" has not been applied uniformly in all French hospitals because there was no centralized administration in France to coordinate people's wishes.

France has modified its law on organ donation. All people are donors at death unless they record their refusal in an official registry. The new law provides for the procurement of organs, even against the wishes of the family.

Spain is routinely cited as a successful example of presumed consent. But in Spain, the next-of-kin still has veto power. Most of the growth in donation rates there happened well after the passage of presumed consent legislation.

Some people do not trust the government or the health care system. Many of them are afraid that that signing a donor card may make physicians give up on them too soon, especially if the hospital is likely to lose money on their care.

This legislation, if enacted, must take into account this relatively frequent fear of the people.

Changing the law will not be sufficient. As the experience with presumed consent in Western Europe shows, education of the public and constant training of hospital personnel are essential to achieve the improvement of the structured medical organization for the increase of organ procurement.

Another possibility for increasing donors has been developed with the modification of it acceptance criteria. This means the alternative to consider the use of donors with different medico-surgical conditions that may diminish part of their chances of long-term success.

On the other hand, improvement in the detection, prevention and better therapeutic of the pathologies leading to terminal organ failure, provides alternatives by reducing the number of requiring organs for transplantation.

It is complex to establish whether the presumed consent can justify various social behaviors in countries with or without that type of legal measure.

The medical-social people behaviors are adapted to the degree of education on the subject, the quality and formation of the responsible medical organizations and the economies of each one of the countries.

In particular, the participation of a medical group trained in excellence in the psychosocial methodology of approaching families at the time of the grief of the loss of a loved one, is undoubtedly a factor of principal importance for a positive result regarding the family response [31].

Some critics claim that presumed consent is a "fiction" [32]. However, the conception of presumed consent as tacit and silent overcomes the notion of being a fiction. Sometimes it can be a concretely effective consent, according to the characteristics and organization of the institutional resources, as well as to the competence, understanding and motivation of the people.

With some notable exceptions, previous studies consider that, in practice, the laws of presumed consent have not achieved more important levels in the behavior of people toward donation [33]. In addition, it has been suggested that these results are related to the fact that, despite the law, the consent of the family is usually required [31, 32].

Finally, with respect to the effectiveness of laws concerning the mode of consent, we believed that hardly a law can change the moral and ethical behavior of the people.

2. Financial incentives

Financial incentives are considered any material gain or value obtained by those who consent directly to the process of obtaining organs, whether to the donor, the succession of the donor or the family of the donor.

The arguments in favor of financial incentives for organ donation are based on the hope that such a system will increase the supply of organs safeguarding the basic ethical concern of saving lives.

A set of reimbursement of funeral expenses has also been suggested as a direct "milder" means of incentive for donation.

Finally, a form of "insurance for the donor" has been suggested, for which an individual agrees in advance of the donation, with a payment to their beneficiaries that will only take place after the donation.

The concept that financial incentives can offer a possible solution to the shortage of organ donors in progress has been considered and debated among experts in the field of transplantation, ethics, law and economics [34].

The essential conception of altruistic donation, unchanged in general in the last 50 years, has not been able to overcome the constant lack of organs, with a critical permanent increase in mortality on the waiting list. This constant reality has motivated the justification by different authors to invoke a fundamental change of the current altruistic criterion: financial incentives to facilitate organ donation.

It has been specifically pointed out in this regard that the current system generates financial gains for all concerned: doctors, coordinators, social workers, hospitals, pharmaceutical laboratories, etc. Consequently, it has been described as unjust and insensitive to the families of the donors and a source of basic distrust on the part of the public, that the donor and the family are the only ones that do not directly benefit from the donation process, which therefore, some type of compensation must be defined [35].

Finally, those who promote financial incentives for organ donation conclude that their motives are ethical because they are based on concern for patients and saving lives and not only on abstract theories and issues without concrete answers.

Pilot programs are proposed to evaluate the potential effects of financial incentives for organ donation instead of rejecting this proposal on the basis of theoretical disadvantages not yet tested [36]. This means that it is time to use incentives to reward people who are willing to save the life of a stranger through donation.

Those who support the establishment of economic incentives consider that our current transplant system is inadequate for the task of increasing the volume of organs necessary to save lives. Altruism is not enough, incentive pilot trials are needed [37].

On the other hand, opposed to financial incentives base their objections on the argument that the altruistic system has not been correctly promoted.

It is pointed out that there would be a decrease in respect for life and the sanctity of the human body, and a loss of the personal relationship that currently exists in the donation process [38].

Great concern has also been expressed regarding a potential phenomenon of rich versus poor. Ironically, this type of incentive would be mainly aimed at racial communities of significant poverty [39].

Economic necessity should not be linked in a coercive way to consent to obtain organs. This money would be better spent more on education for medical communities regarding the need for organ donation through the current system to make the society understand the fundamental benefit for its future of donation and organ transplantation.

Beyond that the proposed incentives can be negative for potential donors, it has been argued that the financial gain of the family of the donor has not resolved at all the economic problem motivating the acceptance of economic incentive to donation.

On the other hand, the relative failure of the medical community to participate in the donation process will not be improved by the incentives directed to the potential donor [40].

In the discussion of the problem of acceptance of economic incentives for organ donation, it is convenient to mention the Iranian program of transplants. In this country, a system for payment of organ donation coordinated by the government has been implemented with significant results. Actually, a candidate for transplantation in Iran can get a kidney from a cadaver, living relative, or a living stranger.

However, in contrast to most countries, 76% of kidneys come from strangers; only 12% of kidneys are from deceased donors.

This significant difference makes it necessary to consider the obvious poverty-donation relationship, which notwithstanding any image of responsibility on the part of the state, does not excuse an unavoidable presumption of social injustice, ethically not compatible with the basic principles of ethics in organ transplants.

Those who oppose the financial incentives for organ donation predict the possible loss of control of this process by the government bureaucracy and the "organ traffickers" with a tremendous increase in the cost of administrative requirements [39].

Until it is available through universally accepted surveys as accurate and representative, the feasibility and effect of financial incentives for organ donation remain questionable.

3. Expanding donors

One important factor in the number of transplantations, currently performed, is the growing acceptance of marginal grafts, which are defined as organs at increased risk for poor function or failure that may subject the recipient to greater risks of morbidity or mortality [41].

The persistent "organ shortage" remains with an increase of 8% organ transplants per year. The annual growth of patients on the waiting list is 22% and its mortality is 18%.

This reality has conditioned a modification of the classic acceptance criteria for an organ donor. Currently, donors regarded as "expanded criteria donors" with potentially suboptimal organs have been included.

Simultaneously, the number of cadaveric organ donors has remained relatively static, with only a 4% increase per year. Most of this incrementally small increase has been through the use of "expanded" donors, reflected by the fact that the uses of donors older than 50 years old increased by 24% per year while those younger than 50 years increased by only 1.5% per year [42].

As it was mentioned, to increase the potential donor supply, the implementation of presumed consent and financial incentives for donation have been proposed, nevertheless public attitude toward presumed consent would probably not be acceptable. On the other hand, there has been resistance to financial incentives to the donor family because of the perceived danger of this escalating to the selling of organs as currently taking place in Southeast Asia and India [42].

Efforts to expand the donor pool are therefore limited to expand the criteria for the use of "suboptimal" organs.

Mainly, suboptimal donors are considered when donors are less than 5 years old or older than 65, donors with moderate decrease in renal function, donors with antibodies positive against hepatitis C, donors with type 2 diabetes or with moderate arterial hypertension and particularly the use of donors with cardio-circulatory death [42].

Essential characteristics of these suboptimal donors:

Older donors: the general refusal to use kidneys from older donors is due to the normal structural changes in the aging kidney.

However, these changes may not occur in all donors. For this reason, it has been considered that the older donor should be evaluated individually for its renal function at the time of death. Renal biopsy can be used in donors older than 50 years or with a history of significant hypertension. An organ that presents a glomerular sclerosis less than 20% and with mild interstitial fibrosis is acceptable to be implanted.

It is important in these cases to implement the system called Old to Old, it does means, old donors kidneys for old donor receptors.

It is very important in these kidneys the evaluation of the cold ischemia time (CIT). Kidneys with CIT of more than 48 h have a graft survival of 38% compared to kidneys with CIT less than 48 h, which had a very acceptable graft survival of 76% at 1 year.

Nefrotoxic injury with medication or rejection may also limit the long-term final result of these organs [43].

The hypertensive and diabetic donor: patients who received cadaveric kidneys from donors with a history of either diabetes or hypertension ("non-ideal") were compared with recipients of "ideal" organs. Although the overall graft survival of the non-ideal organs was somewhat less (69% versus 74%), these differences were not significant. Again, these kidneys should be evaluated on an individual basis by biopsy and donor history [42].

The donor with hepatitis C: the use of the hepatitis C (HCV) + donor organ has been controversial and was a subject of debate. Nevertheless, today advances in the treatment of hepatitis C have change acceptance criteria for these donors.

Prevalence of HCV positivity in organ donors has been reported to be between 2 and 6% with contradictory data with respect to the risk of transmission of HCV from positive organ donors [44].

Non-heart beating donors (NHBD): the use of NHBD has been increasing all over in recent years. In controlled and uncontrolled trials, delayed graft function is 60–80% of cases. Nevertheless, no matter this consequence of longer periods of warm ischemia, long-term results and graft survival rates are excellent [45].

Until other options such as xenotransplantation or tissue engineering become realistic, the challenge for the millennium will be to identify which donor organs previously considered suboptimal can be safely used to expand the organ donor pool.

Paired kidney donation: increased living donation (LD) rates are determined by less invasive approaches to donor nephrectomy and by the excellent long-term results.

In recent years, a number of strategies have been introduced to expand living donation programs beyond the classical direct donation, to overcome immunological barriers of blood group or HLA sensitization of recipients.

New strategies in LD include paired kidney exchange. In order to overcome the sometimes difficult barriers of incompatibility in blood groups or the hyper immunized receptor, the pair kidney donation technique has been a significant advance.

The procedure consists of combining the pair of incompatible donor recipients with each compatible member of different pair. Other alternative programs are: altruistic donation, altruistic donor chains and list exchange programs, and desensitization of hyper immunized patients and transplantation across the blood-type barrier [46].

The transplant community is challenged to address the ongoing crisis in organ transplant access. A discarded organ may be a missed opportunity to save a life. While careful judgment and prospective monitoring is crucial, a blanket "no" to these organs will help neither you nor your patients [47].

4. Education

The teaching of basic concepts regarding transplanting and organ donation has been insufficient.

An efficient education on the need to modify the current reluctant negative behavior toward organ donation by society constitutes a potential possibility to improve this urgent medical-social crisis. Education and information will increase the value of altruism by protecting the population from exploitation, increasing the meaning and value of organ donation [48, 49].

Organ donation and transplantation education at all levels of society have been a matter of interest for decades. Nevertheless, the results observed to date must be considered inadequate because organ donation and procurement have not improved worldwide. With regard to medical education on transplantation, multiple polls show a severe lack of knowledge [3–7].

When searching for new alternatives to modify ancestral prejudices and barriers inhibiting the use of the body after life, priority should be given to youth education starting with children in schools.

The rationale of this proposal is that young people, particularly children, are free of prejudices, and are able to easily learn new ideas, sometimes much more easily than adults. Modern psychology suggests that childhood is the best developmental stage to start prevention programs against harmful prejudices. In addition, new notions learned by children at schools can be a way to offer clear and unprejudiced knowledge to their families [50, 51].

The central task of education is to implement facilities to learn; it should produce learning people. The truly human society is a learning society, where grandparents, parents and children are students together.

At present, young people have not been sufficiently informed of their future organ transplant needs and their potential role in the development of educational programs.

No one has yet realized the wealth of sympathy, the kindness and generosity hidden in the soul of a child. The effort of every true education should be to unlock that treasure [52].

Organ and tissue donation can also involve children. Because of its sensitivity, this topic requires careful decision-making. Children have the ability to carefully reflect on this subject and enjoy participating in family discussions about it [53].

Shoenberg consider that teaching young people about organ transplantation is not particularly difficult. He considered that helping young people understand the problem of transplant increases the possibility that they clearly understand its importance. Probably young people in response to this teaching will discuss this issue with their families or with their peers, thus multiplying the educational effect. Intense and persistent educational efforts focused specifically on young people are relatively rare. Consequently, this leading educator not related to medicine, suggested that "the transplant community has to offer strong stimuli that induce professors in various places to assume such a task" [54].

Undoubtedly, the insufficient results of people's education, without significant changes over the decades, indicate the need to review the current methodology of teaching society about this severe crisis, consequently of their current behavior toward organ donation.

The introduction to the permanent curricula of study, in the different levels of education; structured by a commission of experts, that will analyze the insufficient achievements obtained with the current education methodology.

Introducing a new conceptual line of teaching that will provides new approaches and even new slogans to be transmitted to society, could be a necessary test in a search for a progress in the results so far obtained.

Clarify fundamental concepts previously mentioned and up-to-date information on organ donation and transplantation will help to understand fears and prejudices generated by ignorance.

Previous information to the teachers by experts in social communication and specialists in transplants will be fundamental as an initial step for the realization of a new program of education of the youth with transmission to the whole society.

Recent experiences in Argentina and Canada, inspired by the previously described conceptual suggestions, have produced positive results. In their responses to a questionnaire completed after the class, students (aged 10–16 years, from households of different socio-economic levels) showed a clear understanding of the concepts taught, and a coherent and logical interpretation of the problem.

The pilot trial consisted in a 45 min course followed by discussion and questions, with the following purposes:

1. Evaluate the possibility of application of the project.
2. Assess in countries with socio-economic differences, the understanding and acceptance of basic concepts concerning organ donation.

Materials and methods

- Mixed school in Argentina.
- Average age 12.9 years [11–14].
- Girls school in Canada.
- Secondary school: 45 students.
- Average age 14 years [13–16].

The following where the main topics included in the lecture:

1. History of transplantation.
2. Brain death.
3. Cadaveric and living donor.
4. Mortality on the waiting list.
5. Religious attitudes toward transplantation and organ donation.

This pilot test highlights the usefulness of a stable and universal introduction transplantation subjects in the curriculum of youth education [50].

2.2. The role of international organizations responsible for health and education

Considering the stagnant rates of organ donation, it is important to mention that in the search for possible solutions the potential role of a different educational strategy has not yet been significantly promoted by the World Health Organization (WHO) and international transplantation societies.

In contrast, it is interesting to note that the WHO and The Transplantation Society have developed an intense and positive legal and ethical interest into the serious problem of organ commerce and transplant tourism. It would be of great utility to promote joint activity by the WHO, UNESCO and Transplantation Societies, and religious authorities, in order to generate international consensus meetings, looking for efficient educational policies and search for other possible solutions to this global social emergency.

3. Conclusions

Organ and tissue transplants provide the possibility of new life and improved health and well being. However, the number of patients who died due to lack of donated organs increases daily. The main cause of this paradox is inadequate social behavior regarding organ donation, both in life and after death. Education at all levels of society may offer the possibility of improving this critical situation. In this chapter, we suggest a change of methodology based primarily on a modification of the message. We emphasize the need to focus education at an early age, starting with primary school and intensifying it at the university level, especially in medical sciences.

In the USA from 1988 to 2010, donation-related policies on organ donation and transplantation increased in number from 7 to 50. That is great progress with intentions to improve a crisis. Nevertheless as remarked by Chatterjee et al. strategies to encourage organ donation have had no observable effect [55]. Millions of dollars have been unsuccessfully spent on the education of society seeking to change feelings toward organ donation [27]. Consequently, international figures have suggested the controversial need to institute legal and economic incentives to living and deceased donors [37].

The current contradiction is that the global success of organ transplantation is growing as fast as the waiting list and the mortality of its members.

Fundamental measures looking to improve the shortage of donated organs have been scientific and technical; however, there has not been a significant increase in the number of organs and tissues obtained for transplantation. Almost inexplicably, society's communication and education methodology has remained practically unchanged over time. It is clear that human behavior regarding organ donation should be critically analyzed to identify the most effective solutions for the shortage of donated organs. The virtual absence of positive attempts to modify human behavior concerning organ donation suggests a scientific stalemate for crisis resolution by the main protagonists. A change in the current philosophy of social education policies regarding organ donation and transplants is clearly necessary, as recognition and support by international health and education organizations will undoubtedly confirm this need.

As we have previously discussed, should be of critical importance to consider. In the development of new educational plans, the complex barriers to donation, deeply established in social behavior: fear of death and respect for the integrity of the body.

These psychological inhibitions have not been primarily considered in the educational programs. In particular, should be of interest that people can realize some crucial concepts such as that today the dead body represents a unique irreplaceable source of health.

An educational program developed by experts in sociology, psychology and theologians should be essential to carefully planned potential solutions of these real barriers to donation A change in transplant and organ donation education programs, efficiently reviewed, may be a challenge to change the inadequate people's behavior and the tragic consequences of organ failure. The persistence of current reality becomes an unanswered uncertainty.

We consider it of interest at the end of this article to hypothesize why the positive results obtained at an educational level in schools at Argentina and Canada, which have been internationally reported in specialized journals, have not been repeated, particularly in the analysis of the structural changes that have been suggested to carry out concerning education and the message to Society.

Models of social education whose qualities can generate important changes in individual behaviors can be resisted. All potential interested that has experienced long time traditional establishment educational programs usually develop resistance to a change.

Certainly, this resistance to educational changes, especially increases when it modifies ideas set up in the consciousness of people through the time.

The introduction of these educational changes with the aforementioned characteristics also seeks the learner's autonomy and the maximum development of their ability to change concepts firmly established in their knowledge.

In fact, these innovations cannot be taken in isolation or generated at individual levels. Undoubtedly they require the support of official or private institutions responsible for international education policies.

Dealing with ideas that will modify long-held concepts typically produces anxiety and worry.

Obviously, we can think, following concepts mentioned by Schoenberg in 1991 expressed "the transplant community has to offer strong stimuli that induces professors in various places to assume such a task" [54], that even for the main protagonists of the dilemma of organ shortage, the professionals responsible for the practice of transplantation, the influence of traditional educational establishment have not been totally overcome.

In practice, every action to modify this crucial problem should be supported by International Transplant Societies through discussions and forums, which must include, in particular, leading international organizations in education and preventive health policies such as WHO and UNESCO.

Alternatives to improve people's knowledge should be carefully planned so as to avoid the possibility that organ donation becomes equivalent to Shakespeare's disturbing reality of the dramatic symbol of "to be or not to be".

Conflict of interest

The author certifies that they have NO affiliations with or involvement in any organization or entity with any financial interest or non-financial interest in the subject matter or materials discussed in this manuscript.

Author details

Félix Cantarovich

Address all correspondence to: felix.cantarovich@orange.fr

Faculty of Medical Sciences, Catholic University Argentine, Buenos Aires, Argentina

References

[1] World Centric. Social and Economic Injustice (Online). 2003. Available from: http://worldcentric.org/conscious-living/social-and-economic-injustice

[2] Cantarovich F, Heguilen R, Abbud Filho M, et al. An international opinion poll of well-educated people regarding awareness and feelings about organ donation for transplantation. Transplant International. 2007;**20**(6):512-551

[3] Bardell T, Hunter DJ, Kent WD, Jain MK. Do medical students have the knowledge needed to maximize organ donation rates? Canadian Journal of Surgery. 2003;**46**(6):453-457

[4] Liu H, Peng X, Zhang S, Qiao X, Hao Y. Posthumous organ donation beliefs of college students: A qualitative study. International Journal of Nursing Sciences. 2015;**2**(2): 173-177. DOI: 10.1016/j.ijnss.2015.04.012

[5] Chung CK, Ng CW, Li JY, et al. Attitudes, knowledge, and actions with regard to organ donation among Hong Kong medical students. Hong Kong Medical Journal. 2008;**14**(4): 278-285

[6] Makara-Studzińska M, Kowalska A, Wdowiak A, Krys-Noszczyk K. Knowledge and opinions of nurses about organ transplantation in a Polish hospital. Journal of Pre-Clinical and Clinical Research. 2013;**7**(1):48-52

[7] Perelman School of Medicine at the University of Pennsylvania. Organ Donation. Science Daily's, Science News (Online). 2017. Available from: https://www.sciencedaily.com/releases/2017/04/170410110849.htm

[8] Universal Declaration on Bioethics and Human Rights, established by United Nations Educational, Scientific and Cultural Organisation (UNESCO). http://www.unesco.org/new/en/social-and-human-sciences/themes/bioethics/bioethics-and-human-rights/

[9] Mahowald MB. Self-preservation: An argument for therapeutic cloning, and a strategy for fostering respect for moral integrity. The American Journal of Bioethics. 2004;**4**(2):56-66

[10] Nicholi II AM. C.S. Lewis and Sigmund Freud: A Comparison of Their Thoughts and Viewpoints on Life, Pain and Death (Online). 1997. Available from: http://www.independent.org/publications/article.asp?id=1668

[11] O'Carroll RE, Foster C, McGeechan G, Sandford K, Ferguson E. The "ick" factor, anticipated regret, and willingness to become an organ donor. Health Psychology. 2011; **30**(2):236-245. DOI: 10.1037/a0022379

[12] Sade RM. Brain death, cardiac death and the dead donor rule. Journal of the South Carolina Medical Association. 2011;**107**(4):146-149

[13] Applbaum AI, Tilburt JC, Collins MT, Wendler D. A family's request for complementary medicine after patient brain death. Journal of the American Medical Association. 2008;**299**(18):2188-2193. DOI: 10.1001/jama.299.18.2188

[14] Scheper-Hughes N. Organ Stealing: Fact, Fantasy, Conspiracy or Urban Legend? (Online). 1996. Available from: http://pascalfroissart.online.fr/3-cache/1996-scheperhughes.pdf

[15] Cantarovich F. Organ commerce. Transplantation Proceedings. 1999;**31**(7):2958-2961. DOI: 10.1016/S0041-1345(99)00626-0

[16] Cantarovich F. Influence of socioeconomic and ethical factors on people's behaviour regarding the use of cadaveric organs. Transplantation Proceedings. 2005;**37**(2):539-542. DOI: 10.1016/j.transproceed.2004.12.039

[17] Machnicki G, Seriai L, Schnitzler M. Economics of transplantation: A review of the literature. Transplantation Reviews. 2006;**20**(2):61-75. DOI: 10.1016/j.trre.2006.05.001

[18] Chugh KS, Jha V, Chugh S. Economics of dialysis and renal transplantation in the developing world. Transplantation Proceedings. 1999;**31**(8):3275-3277

[19] Matesanz R, Miranda B. Organ donation—The role of the media and of public opinion. Nephrology, Dialysis, Transplantation. 1996;**11**(11):2127-2128

[20] Strenge H. Fear of death and willingness to consider organ donation among medical students. Psychotherapie, Psychosomatik, Medizinische Psychologie. 1999;**49**(1):23-28

[21] Lester D. Organ donation and the fear of death. Psychological Reports. 2005;**96**(3): 769-770. DOI: 10.2466/pr0.96.3.769-770

[22] Kodan A. The Irrational Fears of Organ Donation. The University of Maryland Independent Student's Newspaper, 2017. The Diamondback (Online). Available from: http://www.dbknews.com/2017/04/25/organ-donation-myth-transplant-list/

[23] Viens AM. Bodily integrity as a barrier to organ donation. In: Jox RJ, Assadi G, Marckmann G, editors. Organ Transplantation in Times of Donor Shortage, Chapter the Ethics of Organ Donation: Foundations and Challenges, Chapter 3. 2016. pp. 19-26. https://eprints.soton.ac.uk/370030/

[24] Kim WR, Therneau TM, Benson JT, et al. Deaths on the liver transplant waiting list: An analysis of competing risks. Hepatology. 2006;**43**(2):345-351

[25] Matas AJ, Hays RE. Transplantation: Little effect of state policies on organ donation in the USA. Nature Reviews. Nephrology. 2015;**11**(10):570-572. DOI: 10.1038/nrneph.2015.113

[26] Lawlor M, Kerridge I, Ankeny R, Billson F. Public education and organ donation: Untested assumptions and unexpected consequences. Journal of Law and Medicine. 2007;**14**(3):360-366

[27] Tabarrok A. Life-saving Incentives: Consequences, Costs and Solutions to the Organ Shortage (Online). Library of Economics and Liberty; 2009 Available from: http://www.econlib.org/library/Columns/y2009/Tabarroklifesaving.htm

[28] Morgan SE, Harrison TR, Long SD, et al. Family discussions about organ donation: How the media influences opinions about donation decisions. Clinical Transplantation. 2005;**19**:674-682. DOI: 10.1111/j.1399-0012.2005.00407

[29] Matesanz R. Organ donation, transplantation, and mass media. Transplantation Proceedings. 2002;**35**:987-989. DOI: 10.1016/S0041-1345(03)00266-5

[30] Crowe S, Cohen E. Organ Transplantation Policies and Policy Reforms. (Staff Discussion Paper) (Online). 2006. Available from: https://bioethicsarchive.georgetown.edu/pcbe/background/crowepaper.html

[31] Rithalia A, McDaid C, Suekarran S, et al. A systematic review of presumed consent systems for deceased organ donation. Health Technology Assessment. 2009;**13**(26):iii, ix-xi, 1-95. DOI: 10.3310/hta13260

[32] Erin CA, Harris J. Presumed consent or contracting out. Journal of Medical Ethics. 1999; **25**(5):365-366

[33] Johnson EJ, Goldstein DG. Defaults and donation decisions. Transplantation. 2004; **78**:1713-1716

[34] Dala AR. Philosophy of organ donation: Review of ethical facets. World Journal of Transplantation. 2015;**5**(2):44-51. DOI: 10.5500/wjt.v5.i2.44

[35] Clark P. Financial incentives for cadaveric organ donation: An ethical analysis. The Internet Journal of Law, Healthcare and Ethics. 2005;**4**(1):1-11

[36] Ubel PA, Bryce CL, Siminoff LA, Capla AL, Arnold RM. Pennsylvania's voluntary benefits program: Evaluating an innovative proposal for increasing organ donation. The Greenwall Foundation is funding an evaluation of this controversial pilot program. Health Affairs. 2000;**19**(5):206-211. DOI: https://www.healthaffairs.org/doi/abs/10.1377/hlthaff.19.5.206

[37] Working Group on Incentives for Living Donation. Incentives for organ donation: Proposed standards for an internationally acceptable system. American Journal of Transplantation. 2012;**12**(2):306-312. DOI: 10.1111/j.1600-6143.2011.03881.x

[38] Brown RCH. Social values and the corruption argument against financial incentives for healthy behaviour. Journal of Medical Ethics. 2017;**43**(3):140-144. DOI: 10.1136/medethics-2016-103372

[39] Graham WK, Livingston JP. Perspectives on financial incentives to induce live donor kidney donation scholarships in exchange for the gift of life. Saint Louis University Journal of Health Law and Policy. 2009;**2**(2):347-358

[40] Arnold R, Bartlett AR, Bernat S, et al. Financial incentives for cadaver organ donation: An ethical reappraisal. Transplantation. 2002;**73**(8):1361-1367

[41] Foster R, Zimmerman M, Trotter JF. Expanding donor options: Marginal, living, and split donors. Clinics in Liver Disease. 2007;**11**(2):417-429. DOI: 10.1016/j.cld.2007.04.00

[42] Jordan ML, Shapiro R, Vivas CA, et al. High-risk donors: Expanding donor criteria. Transplantation Proceedings. 1999;**31**(1-2):1401-1403

[43] Kayler L, Yu X, Cortes C, et al. Impact of cold ischemia time in kidney transplants from donation after circulatory death donors. Transplant Direct. 2017;**3**(7):e177. DOI: 10.1097/TXD.0000000000000680

[44] Trotter PB, Summers DM, Ushiro-Lumb I, et al. Use of organs from hepatitis C virus positive donors for uninfected recipients: A potential cost-effective approach to save lives? Transplantation. 2017 Nov 22. DOI: 10.1097/TP.0000000000002033 [Epub ahead of print]

[45] Perico N, Ruggenenti P, Scalamogna M, et al. Tackling the shortage of donor kidneys: How to use the best that we have. American Journal of Nephrology. 2003;**23**:245-259. DOI: 10.1159/000072055

[46] Ferrari P, de Klerk M. Paired kidney donations to expand the living donor pool. Journal of Nephrology. 2009;**22**(6):699-707

[47] Axelrod D. Expanding the Donor Pool. XYN Management (Online). Available from http://xynmanagement.com/expanding-donor-pool/

[48] Sotiropoulos GC, Brokolaki EI. Living organ donation: Is there still place for altruism? Hepatogastroenterology. 2004 Jan;**51**(55):516-518

[49] Childress JF. How can we ethically increase the supply of transplantable organs? Annals of Internal Medicine. 2006;**145**(3):224-225

[50] Cantarovich F, Cantarovich M, Falco E, et al. Education on organ donation and transplantation in elementary and high schools: Formulation of a new proposal. Transplantation. 2010;**89**(9):1167-1168. DOI: 10.1097/TP.0b013e3181d2fe98

[51] Gonzalez-Mena J, Pulido-Tobiassen D. Teaching diversity: A place to begin early [Online]. Early Childhood Today. 1999 Available from: https://www.scholastic.com/teachers/articles/teaching-content/teaching-diversity-place-begin-0/

[52] Lloyd Yero J. The Meaning of Education Teacher's Mind Resources 2001-2002 [Online]. Available from: https://fr.scribd.com/document/20635703/Teacher-s-Mind-Resources-Http-Www-teachersMind-com

[53] Siebelink MJ, Verhagen AAE, Roodbol PF, et al. Education on organ donation and transplantation in primary school; teachers' support and the first results of a teaching module. PLoS One. 2017;**12**(5):e0178128. DOI: 10.1371/journal.pone.0178128

[54] Shoenberg RS. The Reports of the Surgeon General. The Surgeon General's Workshop on Increasing Organ Donation: Background Papers: 'Planting the Seed: Organ Transplantation Education for Children, Youth and Young Adults'; 1991. pp. 181-198. https://profiles.nlm.nih.gov/ps/access/nnbczk.pdf

[55] Chatterjee P, Venkataramani AS, Vijayan A, et al. The effect of state policies on organ donation and transplantation in the United States. JAMA Internal Medicine. 2015;**175**(8):1323-1329. DOI: 10.1001/jamainternmed.2015.2194

2

Current Situation of Organ Donation in China

Yingzi Ming, Baoren Tu and Quan Zhuang

Abstract

The shortage of organs is a worldwide challenge for transplantation. To alleviate such organ shortage and keep pace with the world's development and experience on organ transplantation, the pilot program of organ donation after citizen death (DCD) has been carried out in China, with support and attention from the Chinese government. From 2010, with the joint efforts of the government and medical workers for these years, a series of laws, regulations and related process management have been formulated, and great achievements have been made in DCD work. Currently, the main source of organs in China has come from DCD. However, some difficulties still restrict organ donation rates. Firstly, resistance to organ donation in China is often due to the conventional view among citizens. Secondly, some medical workers do not fully understand the definition and diagnosis criteria of brain death and therefore do not uphold and promote DCD work. Thirdly, the existing laws and institutions for organ transplantation fail to implement and remain defective. Nevertheless, China has made a firm and strong stride in DCD work. In order to carry out DCD work better, Chinese government, people and medical workers have to do much more.

Keywords: organ donation, transplantation, China, DCD, OPO

1. Introduction

Organ transplantation in China began in the 1960s and has gone through semicentennial of hard work and development [1]. With the continuous development of the technology in transplantation, we have made great progress in organ transplantation and have gradually improved and completed in aspects of operation technology, long-term patient maintenance, transplantation-related scientific research and transplant-related management. At the same time, more and more patients with end-stage organ failure get prompt treatment and long-term survival. The curative effect has been recognized by the public. At present, it has become a routine treatment in our country.

However, from the 1960s to 2006, organ transplantation in China lacks supporting and supervision of specialized regulatory and law [2]. Due to the specificity of organ transplantation, which involves various of parts and links, it requires strict and orderly management of the identification, assessment, procurement, preservation, function maintenance, registration, distribution of organ resources and selection, evaluation, postoperative maintenance of recipient and other aspects. All these need to establish a scientific donation system at the national level to ensure the legal operation of organ transplantation, to guarantee the legal rights and benefits of the donor and the recipient, to ensure the quality of transplanted organs and the fair distribution and rational use of organs. The selection of recipient should also be based on the severity of illness rather than the other requirements. Meanwhile, strict control indications to ensure the quality of medical care and safety of recipients.

In 2007, our country promulgated "the Regulations on Human Organ Transplantation" (hereinafter referred to as "the Regulations") [3], which marks that our organ transplantation has embarked on a legal track [4]. After the relevant departments took a series of positive measures, initial results were obtained. The objective of implementing the "the Regulations" is to establish an ethical and sustainable organ transplant system. In the past, there were some serious problems in organ transplantation in our country, such as organ trading, tourism transplanting, opaque distribution, and so on. In the meantime, due to the lack of voluntary organ donation, there had been a history of reliance on organs of deceased prisoners [5]. These are all serious mismatches with the development of our country's modernization and seriously restrict the sustainable development of organ transplantation [6]. It is not only difficult to guarantee the quality and safety of transplantation but also undermine the image of our civilized power. With the rapid and steady development of all walks of life in our country, the firm establishment of legal system, the increasing emphasis on health of people and the increasing demands on the quality of life, the medical industry in our country has become the industry which needs more improvement. The development of organ transplantation in our country has entered a crucial stage.

Since the 1980s, China began to try organ donation-related work in the light of international advanced experience. In June 1986, experts from various disciplines in China drafted the first draft "Brain death criteria," and in 1995 and 2003, they repeatedly modified and improved the draft. In July 1997, the first brain-dead organ was donated in Shanghai, and two cases of kidney transplantation were successfully performed. In February 2001, the second case of brain-dead organ donation and the first DBD liver transplantation were performed in Nanjing, China. In July 2005, the first case of donation after cardiac death (DCD) was successfully performed in Guangzhou, China. The first case of DBD heart transplantation in China was successfully performed in July 2006. The first DBD lung transplantation in China was obtained in March 2007. The successes of these attempts have also inspired our continued search [7].

In view of the declining source of cadaver donation in our country, living donors are in violation of the international principle of "no injury" to healthy people. In order to avoid the trade of organs, our country strictly investigates and limits the donor's status and relatives' scope [8]. Living donors cannot be the major source of organ transplantation. China urgently needs to establish a sustainable organ donation and transplantation system in line with social ethics and China's national conditions. In August 2009, the Red Cross of China and the former Ministry of Health held a conference for human organ donation work in Shanghai to jointly announce the establishment of a human organ donation system and promote DCD across the country [9].

2. The gradual processing of DCD work in China

After a long period of deliberation and discussion by health authorities and scholars of transplantation and law, China started pilot work of organ donation and procurement in 2010, that is, donation of cardiac death (DCD). Chinese Red Cross, entrusted by the ministry of health, hosted the pilot work. Since then, China's organ transplantation has entered a new stage [10].

In March 2010, the Ministry of Health (now the China Health and Family Planning Commission) and the Red Cross Society issued a document to carry out organ donation pilot work in 10 provinces and cities in China. The 10 provinces and cities are Tianjin, Liaoning, Shanghai, Jiangsu, Zhejiang, Fujian, Jiangxi, Shandong, Hubei and Guangdong [11]. Since Hunan Province had begun organ donation work and made some achievements before that, in June 2010, the Ministry of Health and the Red Cross General Union jointly approved Hunan Province to join the pilot provinces for organ donation [12]. At the same time, a document was issued on the "Organ Donation Pilot Work Program." Several requirements were put forward in the work of the 11 provinces and cities: (1) to establish the organization structure and team of organ donation work; (2) do a good job of personnel training; (3) to ensure the start of this work and ensure the work funding; (4) attach great importance to propaganda work; (5) explore the establishment of compensation and relief mechanism and incentive mechanism to ensure the sustainable and healthy development of donations; and (6) on the basis of common goals and principles, explore the formulation of implementation rules in line with the actual conditions in the region. In July 2010, the "Guidance to Chinese Organ Donation after Cardiac Death pilot work," which was written by the former Ministry of Health and the Red Cross of China together with related experts, was published in "Chinese Journal of Organ Transplantation" and initiated the DCD pilot work in China [13]. At the same time, the "Organ Donation Pilot Work Program" has also been formulated, which specified the duties and institutional framework of organ donation system and preliminary scheme of donation work process (**Figures 1** and **2**).

2.1. The determination and classification of DCD

International classification of cardiac death organ donation is mainly based on the Maastricht standard established in 1995. In view of the immature conditions of legislation on brain death in our country, our country has formulated the DCD classification standard of China according to China's national conditions so that the combination of "brain death" and "cardiac death" is well applied, in which way can also avoid the misunderstanding in our country's cultural identity and make the donation procedure comply with the law. In 2011, the Ministry of Health issued

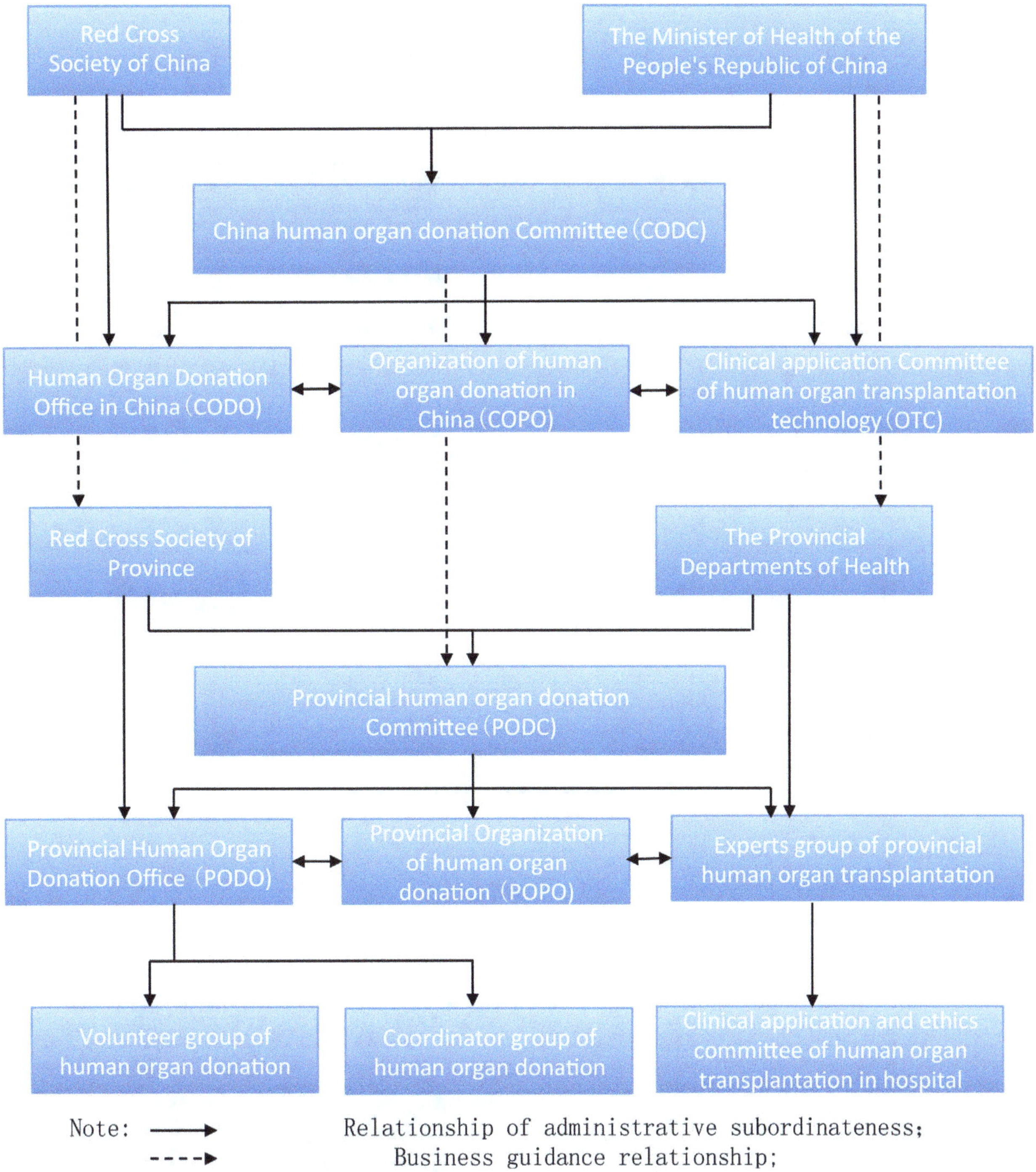

Figure 1. The structural chart of Chinese human organ donation system [11].

"Notice of the General Office of the Ministry of Health on Initiating Cardiac Death Donor Organ Transplantation" and proposed "China Classification Criteria" and related definitions:

1. Definition of DCD: DCD refers to the organ donation after the citizen's death. In the past, it was also called non-heart beating donation (NHBD)
2. DCD classification: Currently, the DCD classification standard as defined by the 1995 Maastricht International Conference in Holland is adopted internationally. According to China's national conditions combined with internationally accepted standards, in February 2011, the

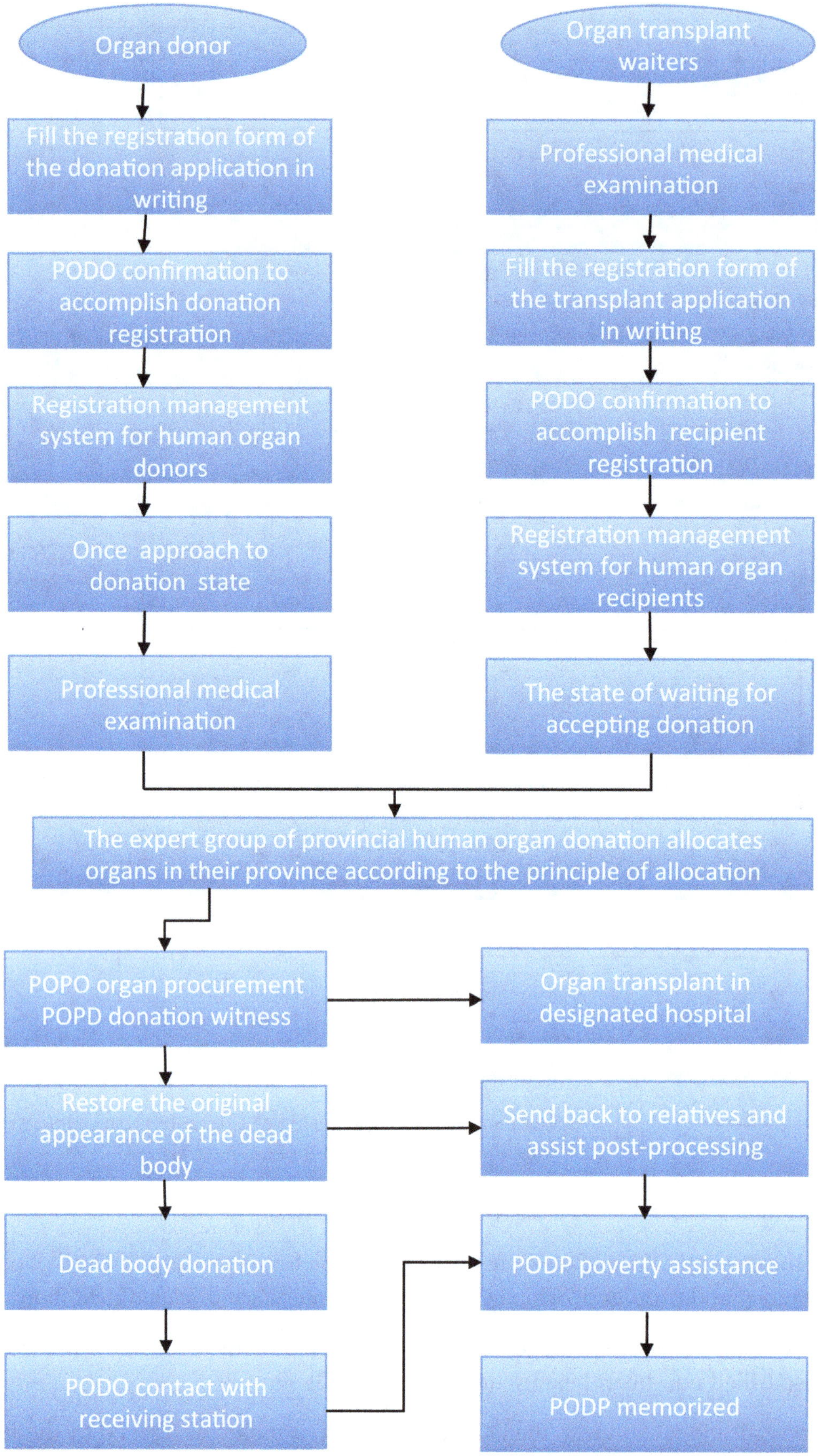

Figure 2. The process chart of Chinese human organ donation work [11].

China Human Organ Transplantation Technology Clinical Application Committee passed and announced the Chinese human organ donation classification standers, that is, the following three categories:

China Category I (C-I): This includes internationally standardized donation after brain death (DBD), that is, brain death cases. After rigorous medical examination, the indicators of potential donors are in line with the latest international and current domestic brain death standards (China Journal of Cerebrovascular Diseases, 2009 Volume 6, Issue 4), by the Ministry of Health commissioned by the agency-certified brain death experts who clearly identified it as brain death. Family members also come under this category, who fully understand the situation and choose to stop the treatment and donate organs, at the same time, having obtained the approval and support from the hospital and relevant leading departments.

China Category II (C-II): Internationally standardized cardiac death organ donation (DCD) includes the I–III case of the Maastricht standard classification.

China Category III (C-III): This includes donation after brain death awaiting cardiac death (DBCD). Similar to Maastricht's standard class IV, it is a controlled type and meets the diagnostic criteria for brain death. Since the brain death law has not yet been established, and family members cannot accept donations of organs under cardiac beating, donations should be made according to the DCD procedure, that is, life support should be removed, and donations should be made after cardiac arrest. The C-III is in line with China National conditions [14].

2.2. The pilot project of DCD has been carried out smoothly

In March 2012, the National Health and Family Planning Commission (formerly the Ministry of Health) and the Red Cross Society jointly held a wrap-up meeting on the organ donation pilot work throughout the country in Hangzhou, Zhejiang Province, and summarized their experience in organ donation work [15]. After 2 years of pilot work, under the joint promotion of the Red Cross and the National Health and Family Planning Commission, the Pilot Regions had to do a lot of work and achieved initial success in setting up sound organizations, applying for specialized agencies, revising of laws, exploring relief mechanisms, standardizing work processes and coordinating training, guiding the public in a scientific way and carrying out scientific assessments. As of March 15, 2012, the pilot completed a total of 207 donations, contributing 546 organs and saving more than 500 lives [16]. In August 2012, the National Health and Family Planning Commission and the Red Cross jointly issued the "Opinions on Further Promoting human organ donation work" (Zhonghong Zi, No. 39) in order to continue this steady progress. It specified the guiding ideology, basic principles, work objectives and specific measures for human organ donation. It also announced the organizational structure and responsibilities of the organ donation system and the organ donation process after the death of Chinese citizens, including eight important aspects, which are registration, donation evaluation, donation confirmation, organ acquisition, organ distribution, body processing, memory and humanitarian aid [17]. On March 25, 2013, the National Health and Family Planning Commission and the Red Cross jointly held a video conference on organ donation work throughout the country, demanding to carry our organ donation work in the whole country this year [18]. As of August 14, 2014, 169 units completed 2107 human donations and 5787 organs were donated, saving the lives of more than 5000 patients by transplants [19].

3. Organ donation work procedure after Chinese citizens' death

On August 1, 2012, the Red Cross Society of China and the Ministry of Health published the "Opinion on Further Promoting human organ donation work (Zhonghong Zi, No. 39)," officially announcing the organ donation process after the death of Chinese citizens. The main contents include enrollment registration, donation evaluation, donation confirmation, organ acquisition, organ distribution, body processing, memory, humanitarian assistance, and so on (**Figure 3**).

DCD organ procurement process (**Figures 4–7**).

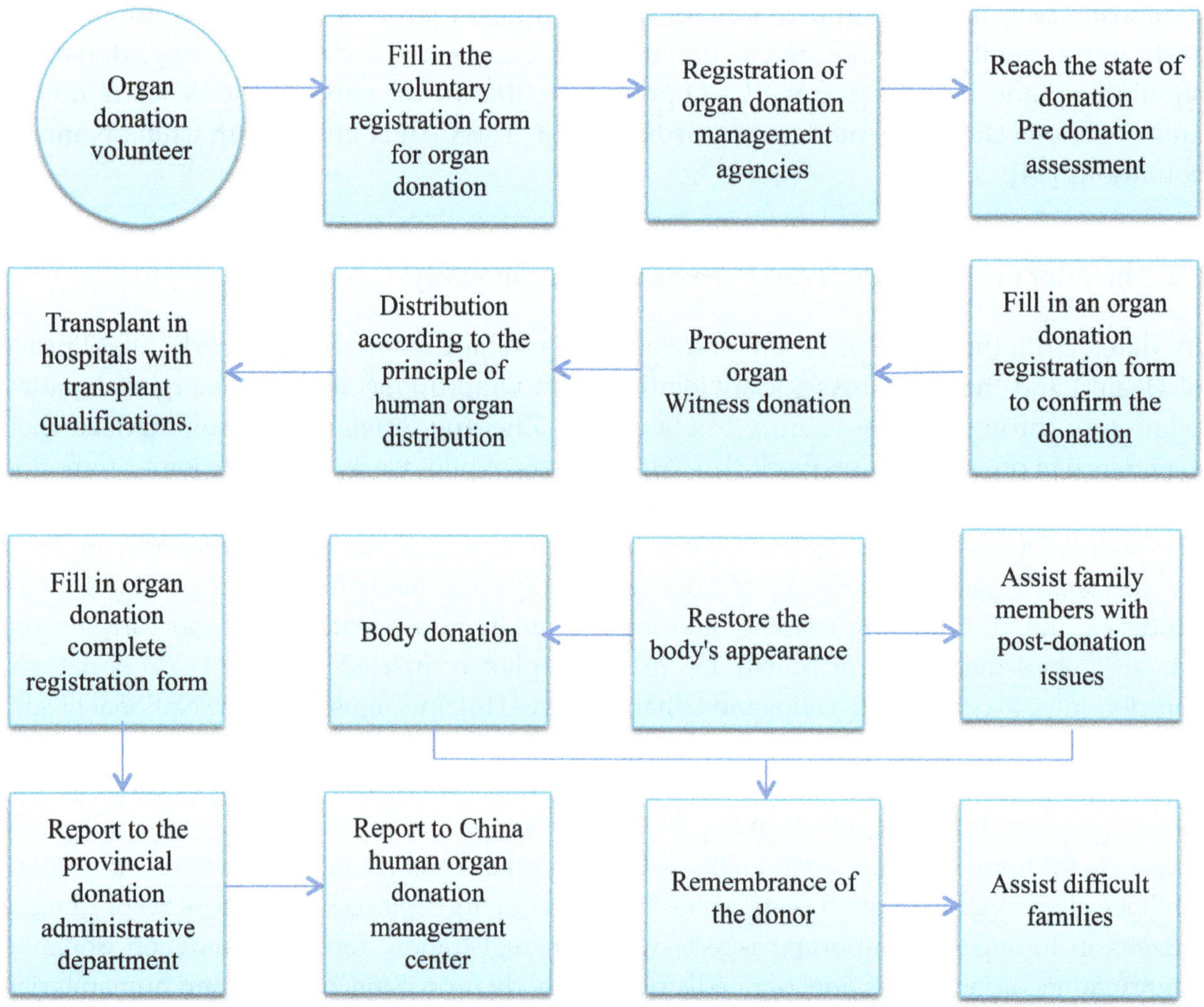

Figure 3. The process chart of Chinese DCD work [11].

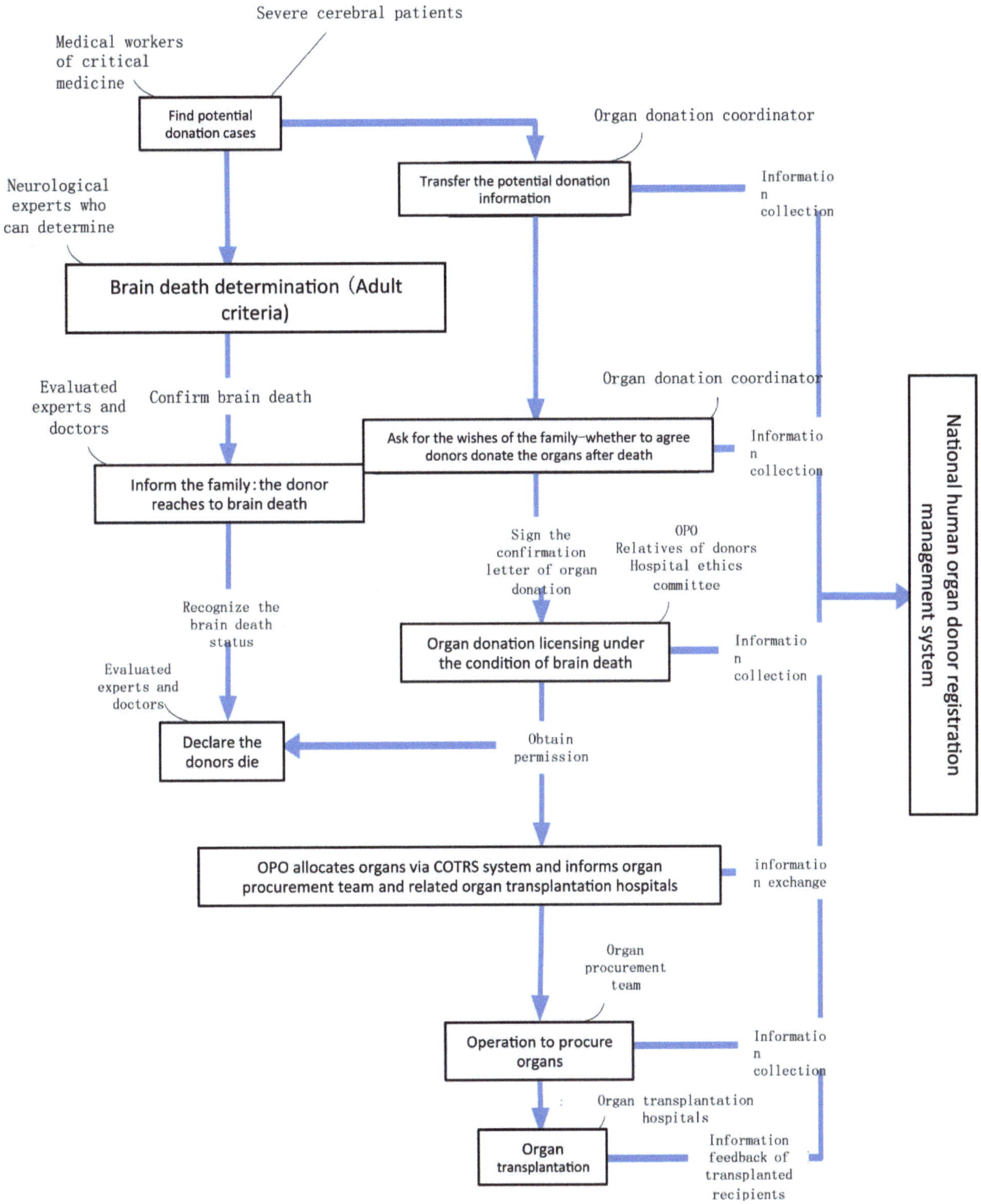

Figure 4. Flow chart of organ donation and procurement (C-I) [20].

The distribution of organs is based on the following seven basic principles of "Basic Principles for the Allocation and Sharing of Human Organs in China (2010 edition)" [21]:

1. The distribution and sharing of human organs should meet the medical needs.

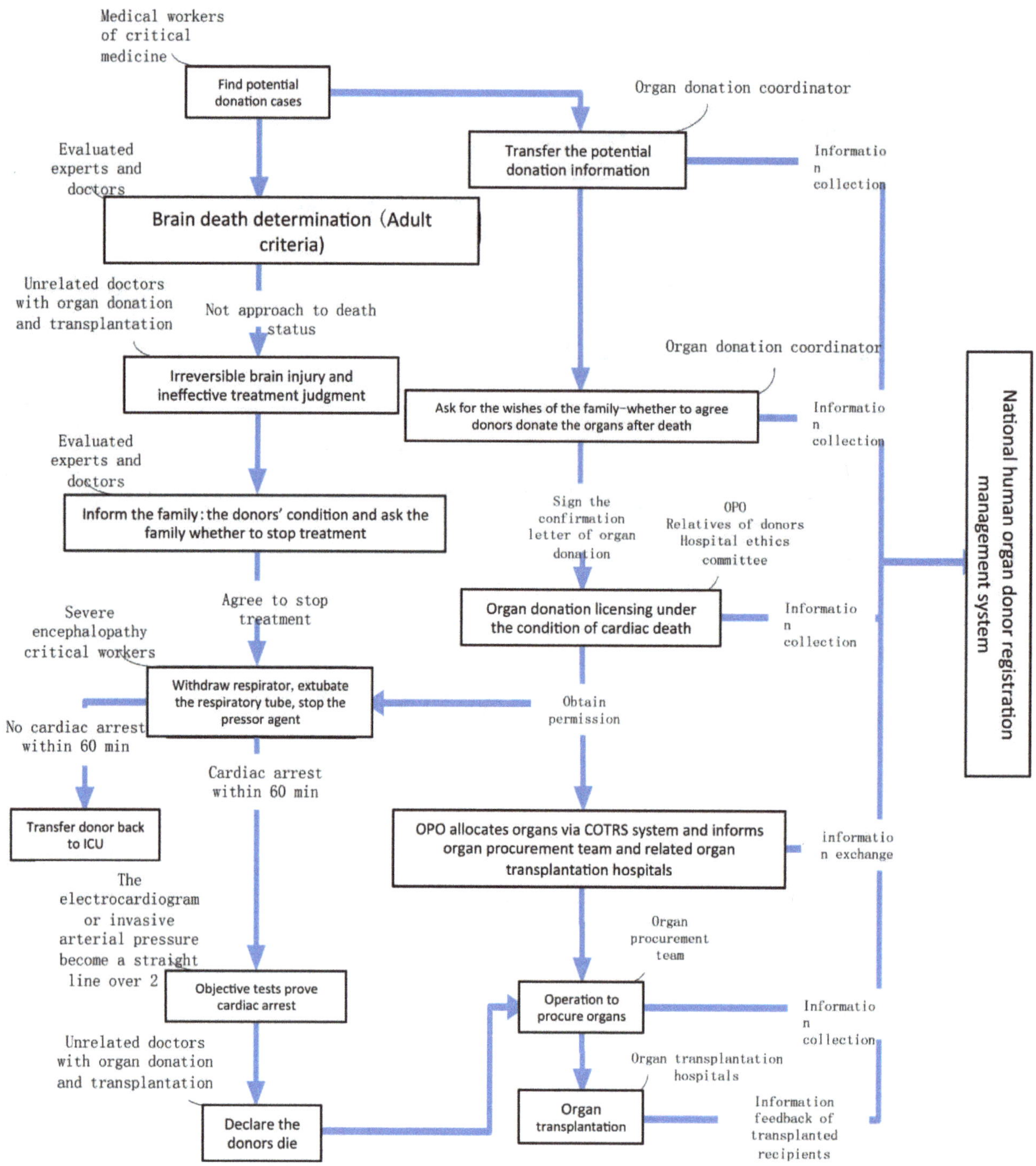

Figure 5. Flow chart of organ donation and procurement (C-II) [20].

2. The transplant hospital has the right, based on sound medical judgment, to refuse to accept unsuitable organs for transplant wait-ins.

3. Human organ distribution and sharing must take place according to the transplantation of hospitals, provinces (municipalities and autonomous regions), three levels of organ distribution and sharing level by level:

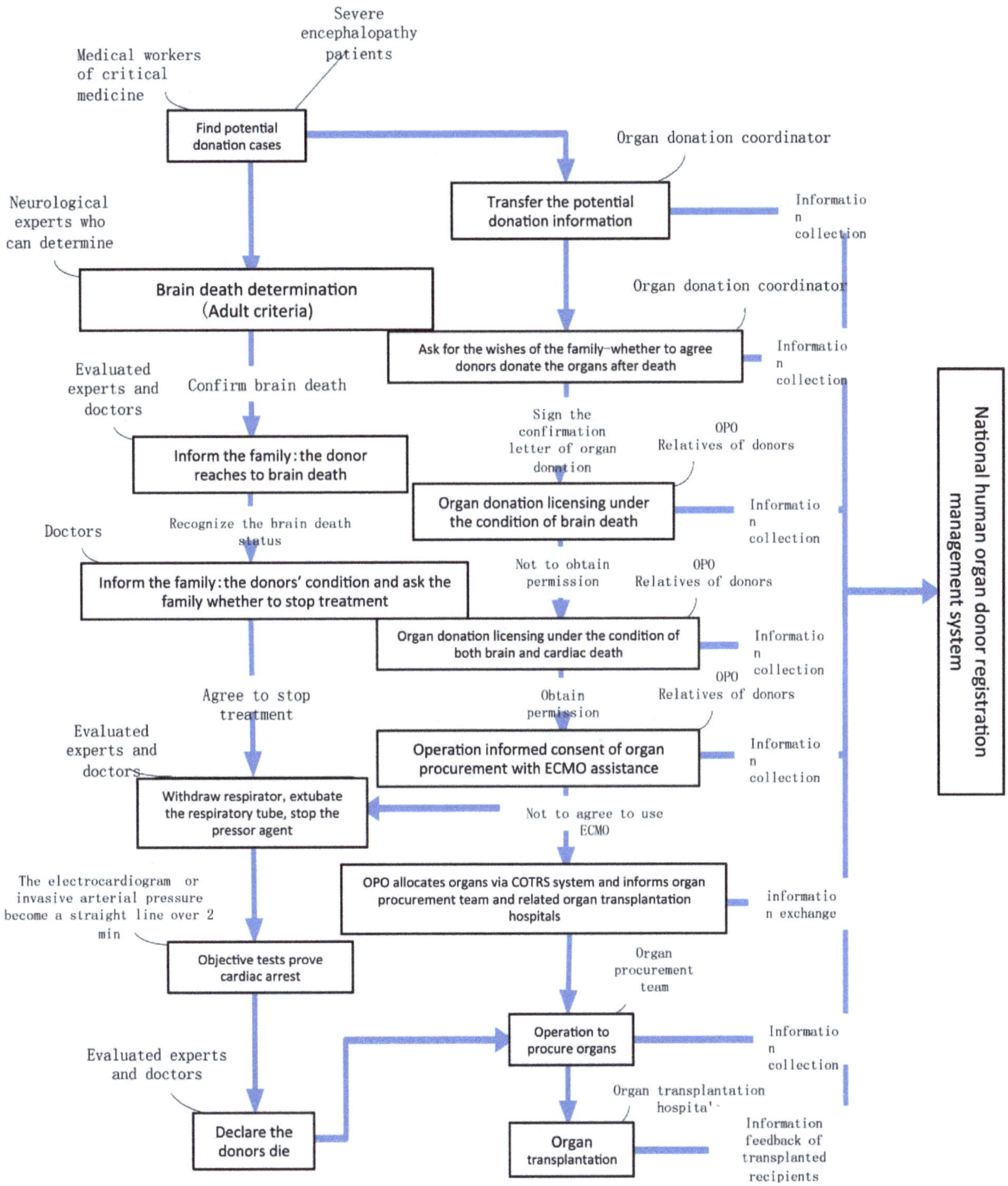

Figure 6. Flow chart of organ donation and procurement (C-III) without ECMO assistance [20].

4. Human organ distribution and sharing process should avoid the waste of organs to maximize the patient's chance of receiving a transplant and improve the efficiency of organ distribution.

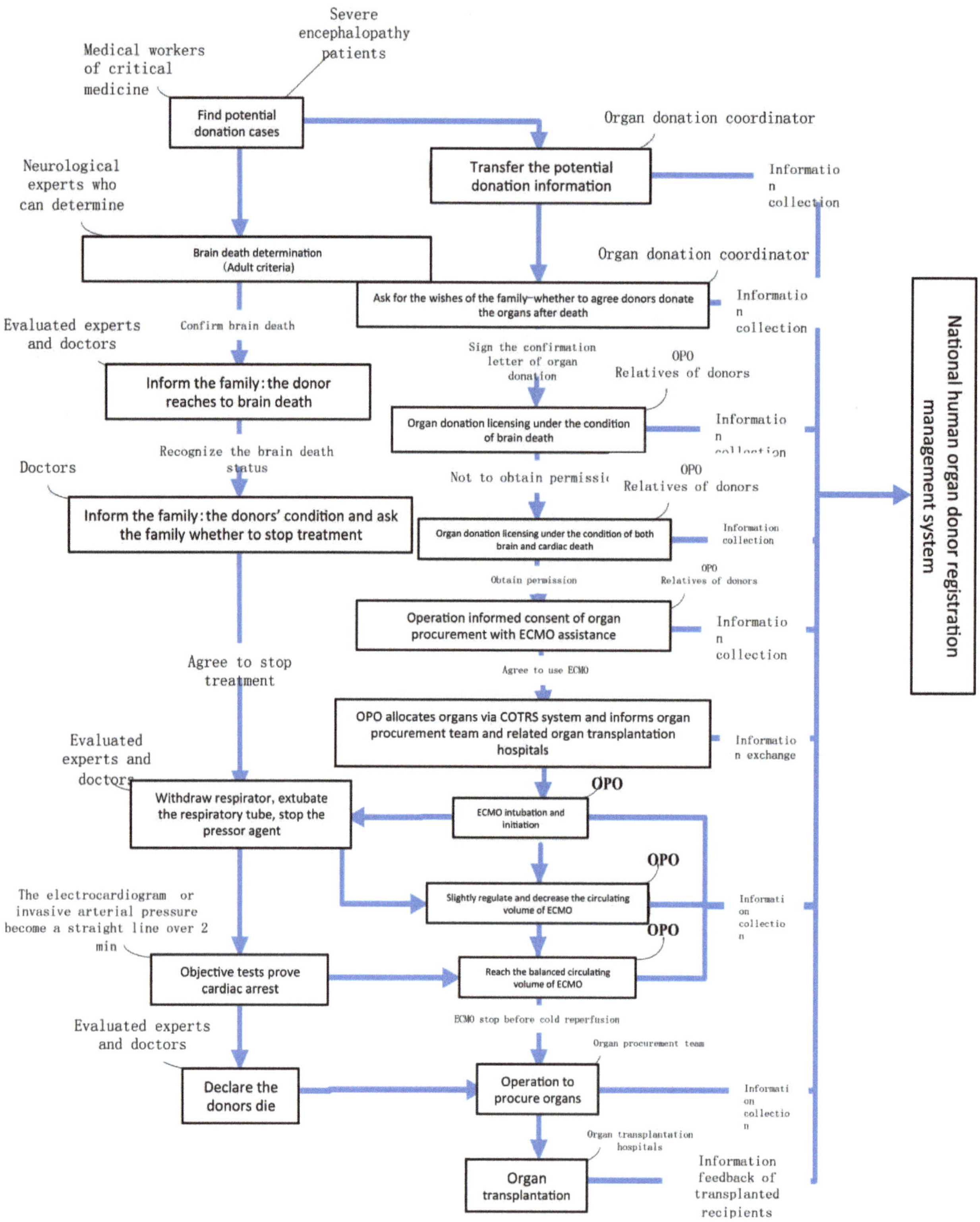

Figure 7. Flow chart of organ donation and procurement (C-III) with ECMO assistance [20].

5. To optimize the matching quality of organs and recipients and improve the postoperative survival rate and quality of life of transplant recipients, on the premise of ensuring the lowest possible death rate in the transplant waiting list.

6. To ensure the fairness of organ distribution and reduce the physical, pathological and geographical differences caused by uneven distribution of organs.
7. Regularly review and amend human organ distribution and sharing policies.

With the progress of the human organ donation pilot work in our country, in order to further standardize organ procurement, distribution and transplantation, the National Health and Family Planning Commission issued the "Regulation on the Administration and Accession of Human Donated Organs (Trial Implementation)" in 2013. The regulation further develops the organizational structure and normative process of organ procurement and distribution system. It also has consolidated the legal basis for the establishment of the organ procurement and distribution system in our country. Not only does it promote the birth of organ procurement organization (OPO) but it also empowers the China Organ Transplant Response Systems (CORS) (www.cot.org.cn) to exercise the power of organ distribution. The regulation compulsively demands that donated organ must be distributed through the organ distribution system, and organizations or individuals cannot allocate donated organs outside the organ distribution system to ensure the origin and fairness of organ donation. At the same time, it requires OPOs to obtain the organ according to the china organ donation after cardiac death classification standard [22].

In order to guarantee the implementation of laws, regulations and policies, the medical database associated with it has also been gradually improved in recent years. Following the establishment of the four major scientific systems of kidney, liver, heart and lung transplantation, the China Organ Transplant Response Systems (CORS), China Organ Transplant Surgeon Registration System and Human Organ Donation Coordinator Registration System have also been constructed and put into use one after another. Since the "Regulations" were implemented through April 30, 2015, the organ distribution system has performed a total of 6170 organ matches, including 1738 liver and 4432 kidneys. Among them, 83.2% (5136 cases) were assigned to wait in hospital and 16.8% (1034 cases) were shared with other transplant hospitals in and outside the province. According to the statistics, the organ distribution system calculates the matching list for no more than 8 s and takes an average of 1.2 h for organ sharing [23]. The organ distribution system operates efficiently without human intervention. Through the assistance and data exchange between the various systems, invisible monitoring network of Chinese organ procurement and transplant is formed, which means that China's organ transplant, based on the legal management, further deepens scientific information management.

4. The composition and responsibilities of the DCD working group

The DCD team includes the donor's responsible doctor, organ donation coordinator, member of human organ procurement organization (OPO), surgical group, anesthesiologist, organ donation management committee, organ transplantation ethics committee, and so on. The above members constitute the DCD working group to participate in the DCD implementation process, each of which does its job, divides the labor and cooperate and jointly decides the key procedures.

4.1. DCD working group

1. The donor's responsible doctor: the doctor participates in the entire donation process except for the removal of the organ. Major responsibilities: find potential donors, have a preliminary assessment of potential donors with donation conditions; responsible to inform the families of patients, after the family members express the intention to terminate treatment; contact the Provincial organ Donation Committee (PODC); submit the basic information of potential donors; assist in organ donation coordination and discuss organ donation matters with family members; consult with family members to decide to remove cardiopulmonary support treatment; responsible for the implementation of the removal; confirm and announce the death of the donor; carry out necessary medical intervention of donors before donation; fill DCD records; review the case and report to the hospital organ donation committee and hospital organ transplant ethics committee.
2. Organ donation coordinator: the main responsibility is to discuss the organ donation with the family members and obtain the legal documents such as the donation of informed consent and so on. The organ donation coordinator is trained and qualified by the Red Cross.
3. Organ donation evaluation expert: the team is composed of high-quantified chief physicians or above-ICU physicians, neurologists and surgeons and is mainly responsible for confirming whether the patient meets organ donation conditions.
4. OPO group: the team is mainly responsible for organ removal and not participating in the removal of cardiopulmonary support.
5. The Hospital Organ Donation Committee/The Hospital Organ Transplant Ethics Committee: the team checks whether the relevant legal documents for supervision and donation are perfect, whether the donation process accords with the informed consent principle and supervises the DCD reporting medical records and record management.
6. Other related members, including the anesthesiologist, operation staff, and so on, mainly assist the OPO team to complete the organ procurement [24].

4.2. Organ procurement organization

1. Constituent conditions: The Organ Organization (OPO) is established by provincial health administration department and comprises one or several human organs' organ transplant surgeons, neurologists, critical care physicians and nurses under the unified leadership of the Health and Family Planning Commission. The OPO must establish a team of human organ donation coordinators with specialized skills and qualifications. OPO also needs to formulate medical standards of identifying and screening potential donors, to establish standard human donation organs' procurement, technical specifications and provide specialized personnel and equipment to ensure the quality of organ procurement.

2. Responsibilities: (1) appropriate medical assessment of potential donors in their service area; (2) in accordance with the "Regulations," sign the human organ donation informed consent or other human organ donation legitimacy document with the donors or their spouse, adult children, parents (or other legal guardians), and so on. (3) maintenance of organ donation; (4) entry of clinical data and legal documents of potential donors and donated organs into CORT; (5) use of organ distribution system to start donation of organs; (6) acquire, save and deliver donated organs and confirm the transfer of donated organs according to the distribution result of the organ distribution system and the hospital with human organ transplantation qualification where the organ transplant recipients who obtained the organ are located; (7) carry out medical treatment on the remains of donors according to ethical principles and participate in the memory and condolences work; (8) protect the personal information of donors, recipients and waiters and protect their legal rights and interests; (9) organize relevant medical staff in medical institutions within the scope of their services to participate in professional training and assist the executive on the regular OPO coordinator training and assessment, conduct scientific research and academic exchanges; and (10) publicity and education on knowledge of human organ donation to the general public [25].

4.3. Division principle of OPO service areas

In order to encourage and promote effective DCD work in all the provinces and avoid unnecessary competition and looting, under the coordination of the health administrative departments, various provinces and cities established a number of independent OPO organizations and divided the service scope of OPO organizations at the same time. The OPO group must comply with the following principles [26]:

1. Provincial OPOs cannot procure organs across provinces.
2. Each OPO cannot procure organs across their own service area.
3. All organs must be assigned to the China Organ Transplant Response System for uniform distribution.
4. Each OPO has a priority in the allocation of its organs but should ensure that organs will be used effectively.

The number of OPOs varies from province to province. Most provinces adhere to the principle of free combination among transplant hospitals. For example, hospitals that are more advanced in DCD work and have a higher transplantation professional level and can carry out multiple organ transplants can form independent OPOs. A strong transplant center can lead a weaker transplant center to form an OPO. An experienced transplant center can lead an inexperienced transplant center to form an OPO. To avoid organ waste, centers that only can carry out one kind of transplantation can form an OPO with centers that can carry out multiple kinds of transplantation.

Taking Hunan as an example: With a population of 67.83 million (in 2015), Hunan Province has a total area of 211,800 km^2 and a total of 14 cities and 122 counties. There are eight hospitals in the province that can carry out organ transplants, of which three hospitals can carry out a variety of organ transplants and the remaining five can only carry out kidney transplantation; there are a total of four existing OPOs in Hunan Province and under the joint consultation divided into four OPO service areas [27].

In order to carry out the work of DCD better, each transplantation hospital has set up some working groups: the OPO leadership group, the DCD ethics committee, the DCD work hospital coordination group, the full-time coordinator team, the OPO procurement group, the DCD work post-processing group, and so on. The composition and responsibilities of each group are as follows [28]:

1. OPO leadership group

   Composition: includes the hospital main party and government leaders, functional departments and potential DCD clinical department leaders and transplant center responsible person.

   Responsibilities:

   1. to protect the development of DCD work and provide a good platform for collaboration;
   2. to carry out publicity work inside and outside the DCD and regularly report to the higher authorities;
   3. regular inspection, to grasp the legality of the DCD process;
   4. to give DCD work in financial support and financial supervision; and
   5. to protect, such as ambulances, equipment, care, medical, legal and other aspects of support to ensure the smooth flow of DCD work.

2. DCD Working Coordination Group: Composed of the Medical Services Department, the Department of Health, Propaganda Department, the vehicle team, the hospital legal adviser, potential DCD medical department director, nurse and coordinators.

3. DCD Ethics Committee

   Composition: Includes the management, medical, psychological, nursing, pharmacy, law, ethics, community representatives and other aspects of the composition of the residents.

   Responsibilities:

   1. confirming and identifying that medical institutions have the relevant qualifications and conditions;
   2. discuss and approve DCD organ transplantation and confirm that the donor source is legitimate and matching type is reasonable;
   3. to confirm that the donor and the recipient of the documents meet the requirements of legal documents, that there is no sale of human organs;

4. to confirm whether necessary inspections have been given to the donors and recipients to ensure clinical efficacy.

4. DCD determination group

   Composition: Includes the brain death or DCD identification of neurological and surgical experts. Requirements:

   1. experts in determination group at least are associated experts and
   2. experts must undergo a specific brain death and DCD training.

5. OPO procurement group

   Composition: Includes professional transplantation medical staff and related staff.

   Responsibilities:

   1. receive DCD-related information and DCD authentication written information;
   2. evaluation of donor quality;
   3. assess the recipient indications, contraindications, general condition and timing of surgery; and
   4. being responsible for the acquisition, preservation and transshipment of organs.

6. DCD post-processing group

   Composition: Formed by the Medical Department, the vehicle team, the Propaganda Department, logistics department, coordinators and Red Cross staff, and so on.

   Responsibilities:

   1. body maintenance;
   2. coordinate with the relevant departments and arrange the cremation;
   3. communicate and coordinate with relevant departments and arrange the implementation of the cemetery and the memory activities;
   4. cooperate with the Red Cross in publicity; and
   5. deal with other left-over issues after DCD work.

DCD work in Hunan Province has always been in a leading position in the country. The success of DCD work in Hunan Province is mainly attributed to the strong support and cooperation of the Provincial Health and Family Planning Commission, the Red Cross Society and the transplant hospitals. **Figure 1** shows DCD in eight hospitals in Hunan Province for 2010–2016 and **Figure 2** shows implementation of DCD in China. The work of organ transplantation in China is also known as the "Hospital president project" and all the transplant centers that have better development are fully supported by their presidents [29].

5. Chinese organ donation coordinator

5.1. Basic requirements of coordinator

"There is no organ transplant without organ donation, no organ donation without coordinator" [30]. This fully demonstrates the importance of coordinators in organ donation and transplantation. At present, there are two main types of coordinators in China: Red Cross Coordinator and OPO Coordinator.

Based on relevant regulations "Management of human organ donation coordinator" promulgated on June 1, 2013, the coordinator shall meet the following conditions [31]:

1. has good conduct and loves organ donation career
2. has medical and other related disciplines' specialist qualifications
3. has at least 2 years of work experience
4. are formal or hired personnel of local regulatory agencies or persons recommended by medical institutions

According to the "Regulation on Procurement and Distribution of Human Donated Organs (Provisional)" issued by the National Health and Family Planning Commission, the OPO coordinator should meet one of the following conditions:

1. bachelor's degree or above in medical college, holds a valid "People's Republic of China physician practicing certificate", with more than 2 years of clinical work experience and is a licensed doctor engaged in medical work in medical institutions.
2. has a college degree on nursing or above and has "People's Republic of China nurse practicing certificate." The person must have more than 2 years of clinical nursing experience and is a registered nurse engaged in clinical nursing activities in a medical institution.

In addition, the coordinator should also have a serious working attitude, a certain degree of communication skills and language skills as well as good psychological quality and psychological endurance. Only in this way can we properly handle the relationship with donors and their families, do a good job in organ donation coordination and push forward the donation of human organs [32].

5.2. Coordinator training in China at the current stage

From 2010 to 2012, the Chinese Red Cross is mainly responsible for the training of coordinators. After the establishment of China Organs Donation Administration Center after 2013, it specially undertook the training of coordinators and organized 4–5 training courses each year. It invited experts in medicine, law, ethics and psychology from all over the country to give lectures and organized domestic relevant experts who compiled the "Training Materials on Human Organ Donation Coordinator in China" (the first and second volumes) [33]. The coordinators were required to attend relevant studies and pass the qualification examination.

At present, a management system of coordinators with rigorous management, impartial examination and scientific training has been formed, which has delivered a large number of high-quality coordinators for the DCD work in China and, at this stage, and has made great contributions to the successful development and promotion of DCD work in China.

5.3. Organ donation coordinator working procedures in current China

1. discover potential DCD donors [31]
2. report the information and wait for evaluation
3. after the assessment team finds that it meets the conditions of donation, communicate with potential DCD family members
4. after donors' family members agree to donate, witness the completion of China organ donation registration form and family's informed consent
5. witness the work of the OPO team to ensure that all work is conducted in a reasonable and lawful manner
6. assist in the burial, memory and other post-processing work
7. assist the aftermath of the donors' family members
8. assist in completing legal instruments related to organ donation

6. China's current DCD work archives establishment and management

The organ donation archive is a strong evidence of DCD's legal compliance but also important information for late summing up experience and conducting scientific research. With the increasing number of DCDs, the management of donors' archives is becoming increasingly important. Establishing a set of scientific and standardized donor archive management standards is of great significance to promote the sustainable development of DCD [34].

Since the launch of the pilot DCD program in China in 2010, great attention has been paid to the collection of archives and data. All provinces and transplant hospitals have done a great deal of work and summed up some experience. For each case of donation, corresponding archives were set up and collected the important information. In the early stage, it is mainly the collection and preservation of paper materials; the project basically includes the following [35]:

1. China organ donation completion form
2. China organ donation registration form
3. donor and their relatives' ID cards
4. donor's basic information table

5. donor comprehensive evaluation table
6. potential organ donor's family informed consent
7. brain death determination family member's application form
8. brain death determination family's informed consent
9. brain death determination form
10. the donor electroencephalogram inspection report
11. DCD organ transplant ethics form
12. donor management form
13. organ procurement record form
14. the donor discharge diagnosis/patient history information
15. the HLA matching report
16. the recipient information
17. recording video or photo material throughout the process of organ donation
18. donor medical death certificate
19. cremation certificate
20. organ donation process record form

However, there are also some problems. For example, the standard norms are not uniform, and the paper materials are not conducive to long-term preservation; inspection and data statistics are inefficient. Through continuous discussion and exploration and the cooperation of various field experts, we have made use of information technology and Internet technology to develop an organ transplant file management system that is suitable for China. The

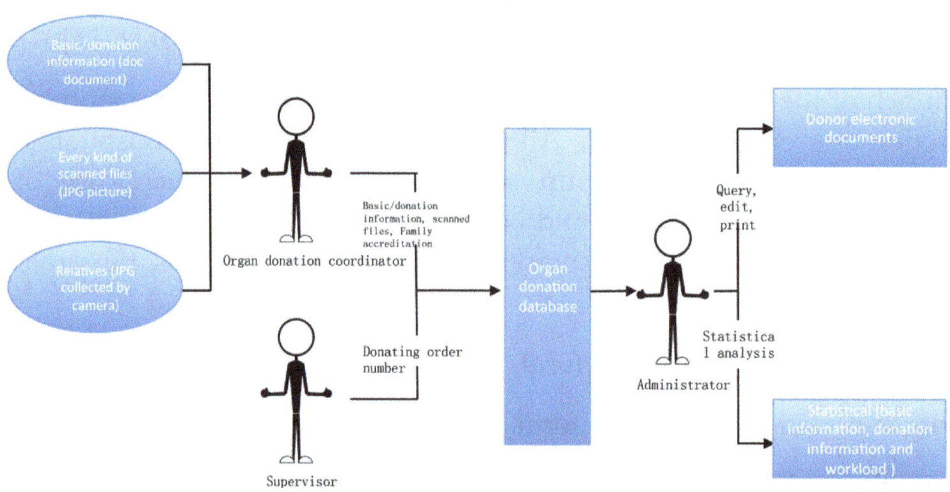

Figure 8. Flow chart of organ transplant file management system [33].

registration of this system basically covers all the information and data above. The process is as follows (**Figure 8**):

Real-time reporting, monitoring of implementation, data analysis and follow-up were conducted in every case of this organ donation database to ensure the regulation of DCD work and also accumulated a large amount of data and laid the foundation for the long-term development of DCD.

7. China's DCD organ donation problems

7.1. Organ donation and transplantation supply and demand situation is still grim

At present, great progress has been made in organ donation and transplantation in our country. With the continued development of our society and economy, especially the improvement of the levels of medical service, it is still a huge challenge to solve the contradiction between the rapid growth of people's health needs and the overall shortage of service provision. About 300,000 end-stage organ failure patients in our country need organ transplantation each year, yet the number of organ transplants is less than 20,000 each year. From a global perspective, the number of organ donations in our country is at the forefront, but the donation rate per million population needs to be improved. How to improve the organ donation rate so that more patients receive prompt treatment is still the long-term goal of our work.

7.2. Citizens lack the correct understanding of organ donation

First of all, under the influence of "maintaining the integrity of the body" and the wrong "death concept," Chinese citizens' willingness to organ donation is not strong, and due to the fact that the law relating to brain death is still lacking in our country, it also hinders the practice of "brain death" standard to a certain extent in our country. Secondly, the lack of social propaganda makes citizens lack the recognition of the donation process and give up donation. Coupled with the wrong public opinion, such as some exaggerated organ buying and selling speech, etc., also make citizens concern whether the use of donated organ is properly or not, which mislead citizens' cognition of organ donation, affecting their willingness to donate. At the same time, most medical workers have not been involved in organ donation and are not familiar with the criteria for determining brain death, the classification and conditions of organ donation and their reluctance to ask their patients' families' attitudes and wishes toward organ donation, which also hinder the discovery of potential organ donors.

7.3. Organ donation and transplantation-related systems still need to be sound

China's organ donation worked from scratch, achieved by leaps and bounds. At present, we have initially established a donation and transplantation system for human organs in line with China's national conditions, culture and social ethics. However, all aspects of system design and legal norms still need to be explored and developed in practice. To establish a sound organ donation and transplantation system that is compatible with the level of social-economic development level, improve a more equitable and efficient organ distribution system and to scientifically plan the regional distribution of transplanted hospitals so as to ensure the equalization of organ transplant services for all citizens, we also need to keep it up.

For example, various provinces in China have formed an independent organ procurement organization (OPO) and delineated their corresponding service scope. Unlike other countries, most of the OPOs in China are composed of transplant medical teams in organ transplant hospitals. This form is advantageous in the initial stage of DCD work, but with the development of this work, some disadvantages are also exposed, such as the limitation of organ distribution and the irrational division of service areas, and so on, which all need to be constantly adjusted and improved in following-up work.

At present, there are two organ donation registration websites in China: organ donation administration center website by the Chinese Red Cross and "Shi and Suo" organ donation registration website administered by the National Health and Family Planning Commission. Current organ donation and transplantation network systems include the donor system, China organ transplant response system (CORTS). The use of websites is yet to be promoted, just as CORTS, a site that plays a major role in organ allocation, the number of patients who have registered on CORTS for transplantation has a large discrepancy from the actual number of 300,000 patients who are waiting for transplant. Compared with the UNOS website in the United States, the COTRS website in our country did not give full play to its functions, and lacked the legal effect and administrative system. Its authority and compulsion needed to be improved [36, 37].

8. The achievements and prospective of China's DCD work

After several years of hard work, China has made gratifying achievements in the work of DCD. Some of the figures are shown in **Figures 9–19**:

China has successfully resumed the transition from relying on the judicial channels to procuring organs through the voluntary donation of citizens. The reform is the result of the concerted efforts of the top leadership of the country, relevant departments, social organizations, the vast majority of transplant medical personnel and Red Cross workers, who obtained the understanding of society and the recognition of the international community. Based on the guiding principles set by the relevant international organizations and based on the actual social and economic development and cultural traditions in China, we adopted methods suited to China's national conditions and promoted the continuous progress of organ donation and transplantation in China. After several years of pilot research, the influence of organ donation after citizen death to our society has surpassed that of the transplant medical service itself. Such love charity is gradually becoming a common practice in China. With the joint efforts of the health administrative departments, the Red Cross Society and the transplant medical institutions, organ donation after citizen death has taken a solid first step. However, China has a large population, huge demand for organ transplants and some traditional concepts are still affecting us. In particular, we are still in the process of improving laws and regulations, strengthening government supervision and departmental coordination, clarifying responsibilities of all parties, refining work processes and strengthening international exchanges and cooperation. There is still a lot of work to do [38].

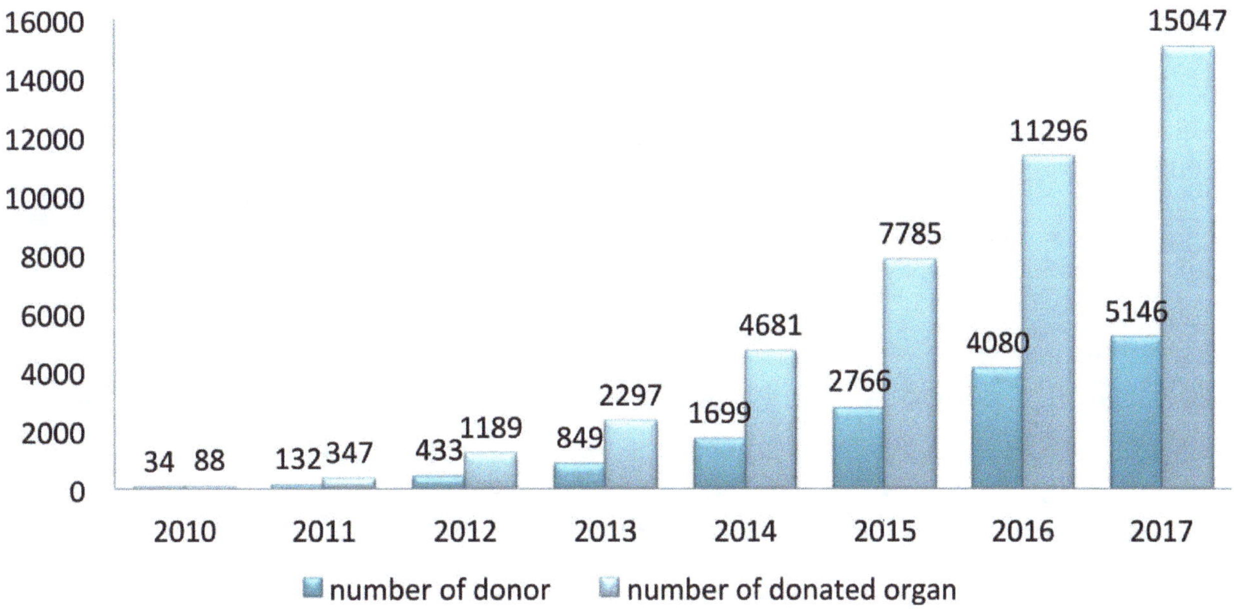

Figure 9. Overview of organ donation according to the data of China organ donation administrate center, by the end of 2017 [data from China organ donation administrate center].

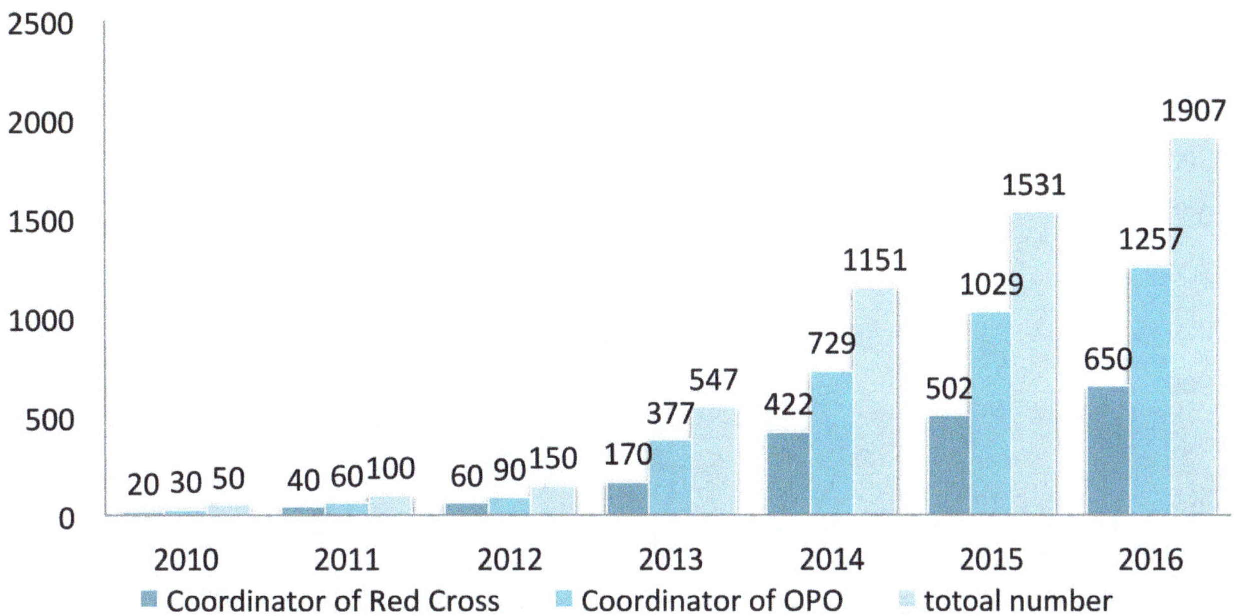

Figure 10. The change of the number of coordinators according to China organ donation administrative center [data from China organ donation administrate center].

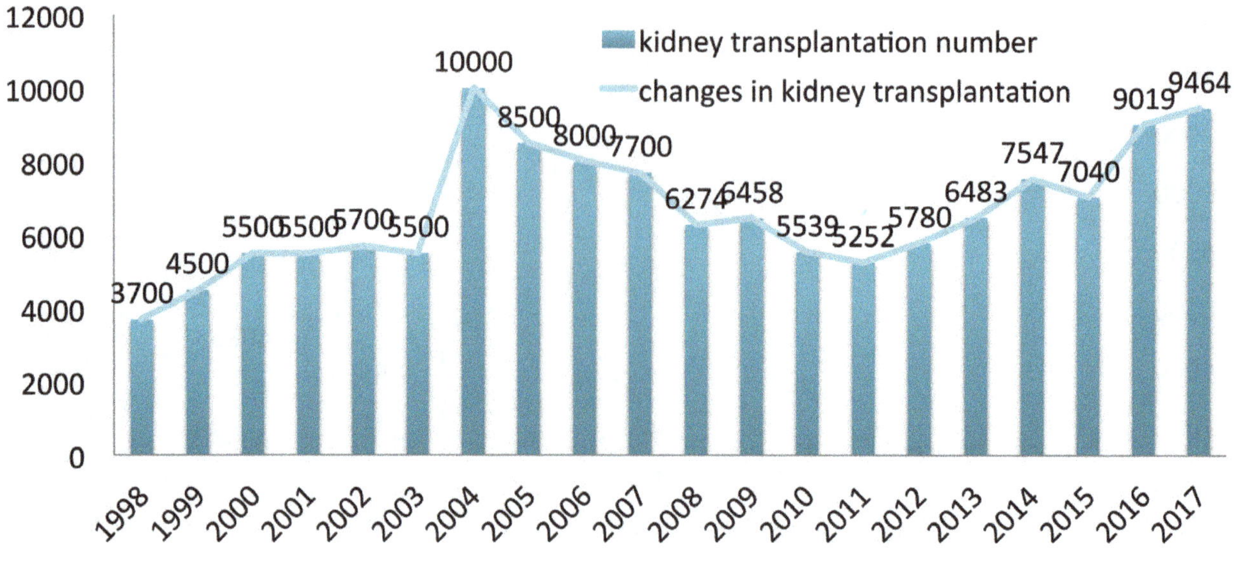

Figure 11. Annual data on kidney transplantation (20 years) [data from Chinese scientific registration of kidney transplantation (CSRKT)].

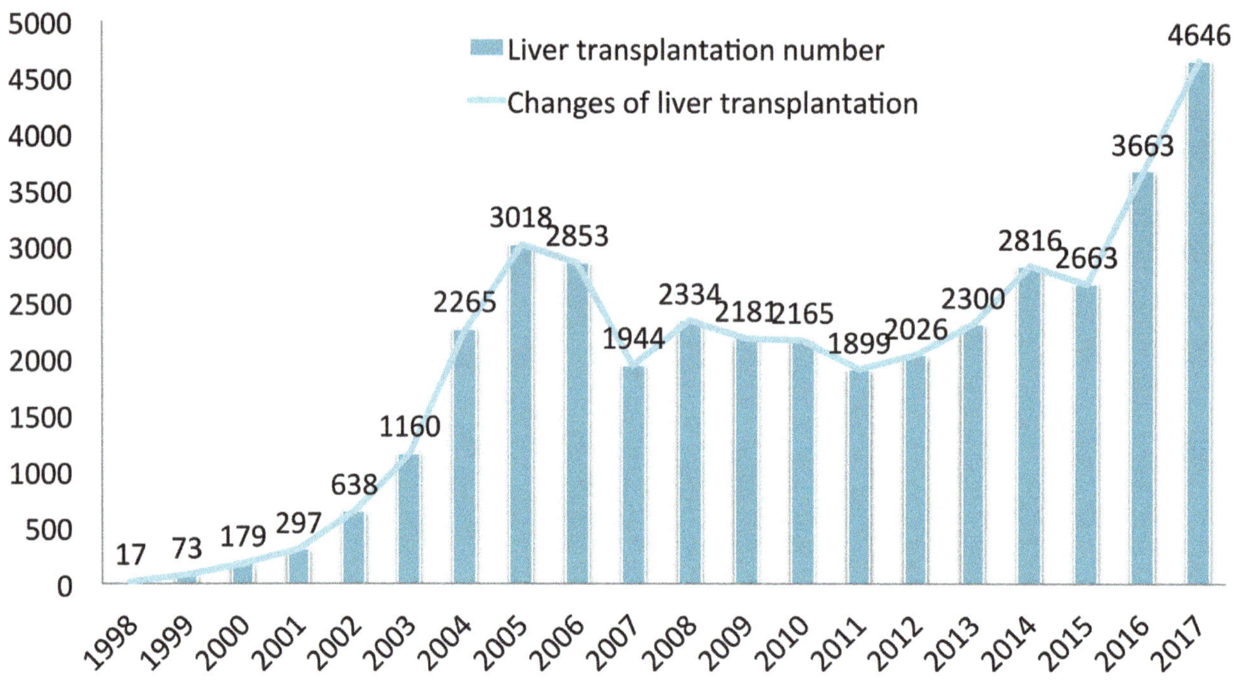

Figure 12. Annual data on liver transplantation (20 years) [data from Chinese liver transplantation registration].

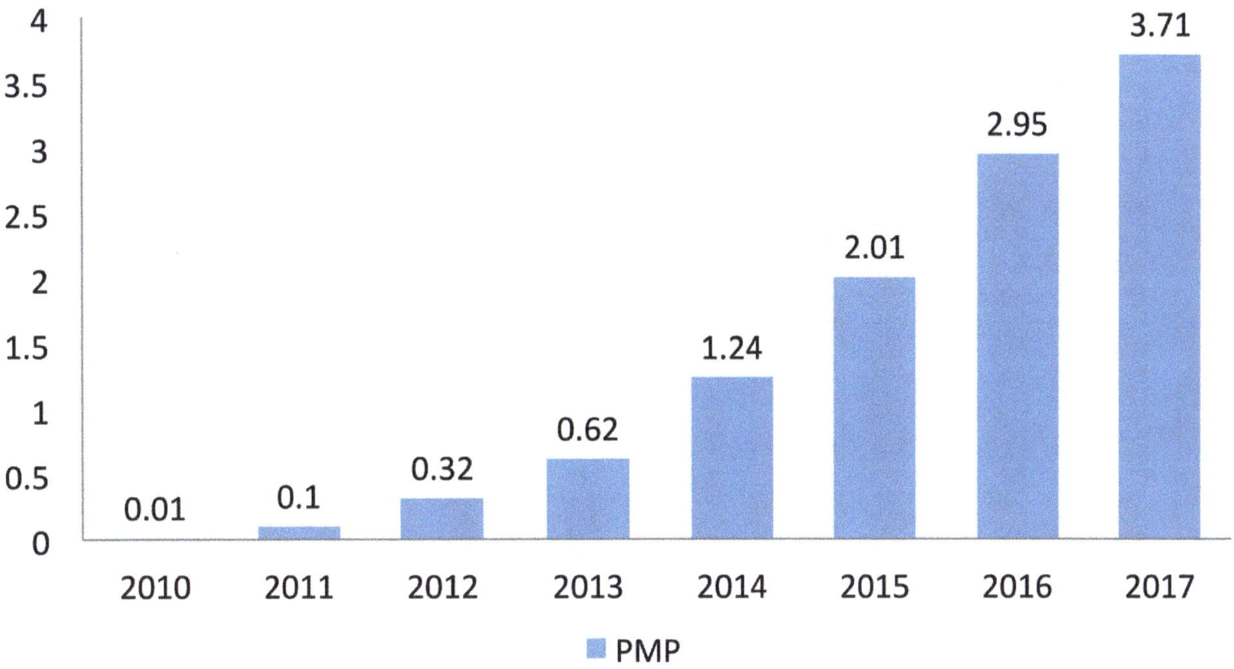

Figure 13. Annual data on organ donation PMP [data from China organ donation administrate center].

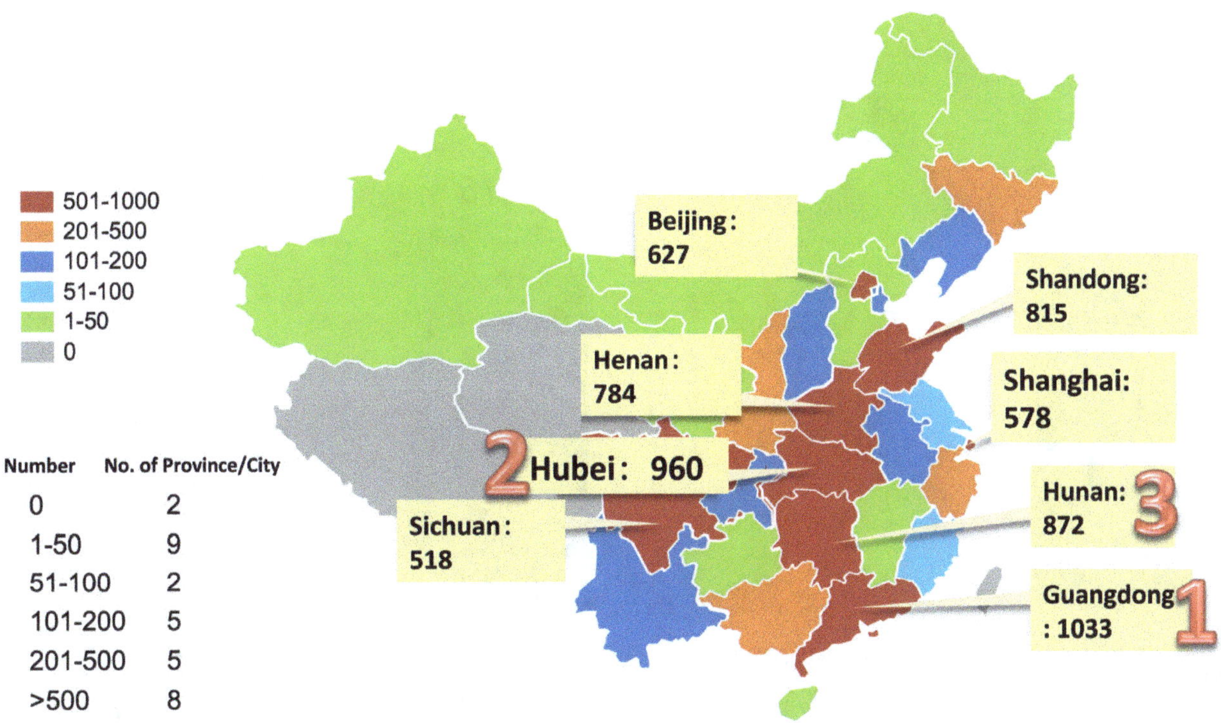

Figure 14. The overview of kidney transplant in 2016 [data from Chinese scientific registration of kidney transplantation (CSRKT)].

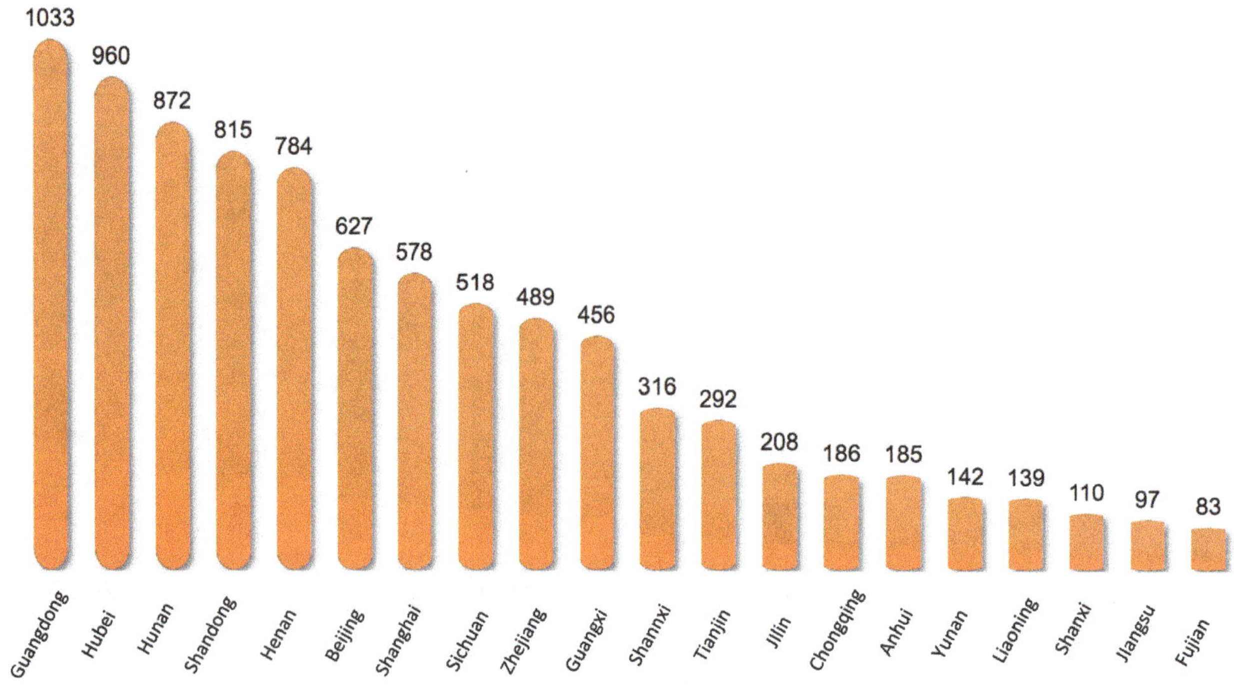

Figure 15. Number of kidney transplantations in each province in 2016 top 20 [data from Chinese scientific registration of kidney transplantation (CSRKT)].

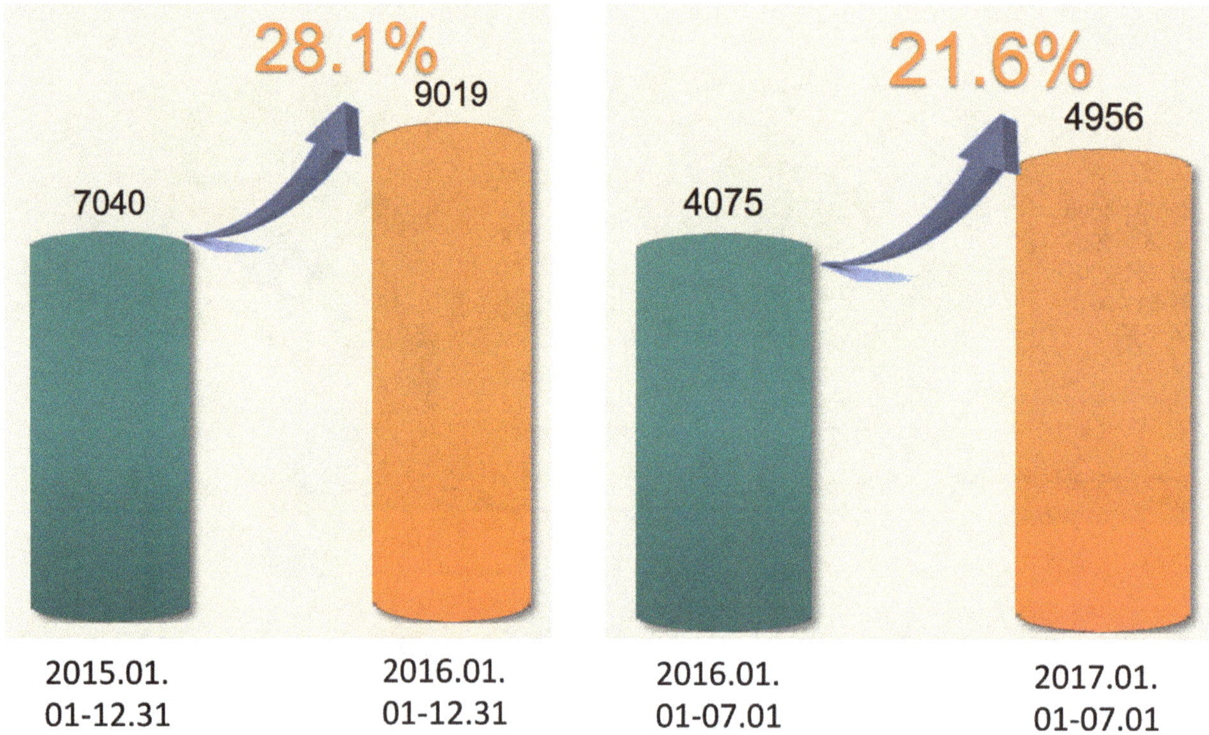

Figure 16. During the same time period, the number of kidney transplantations has been continously increasing, that is, more than 20% [data from Chinese scientific registration of kidney transplantation (CSRKT)].

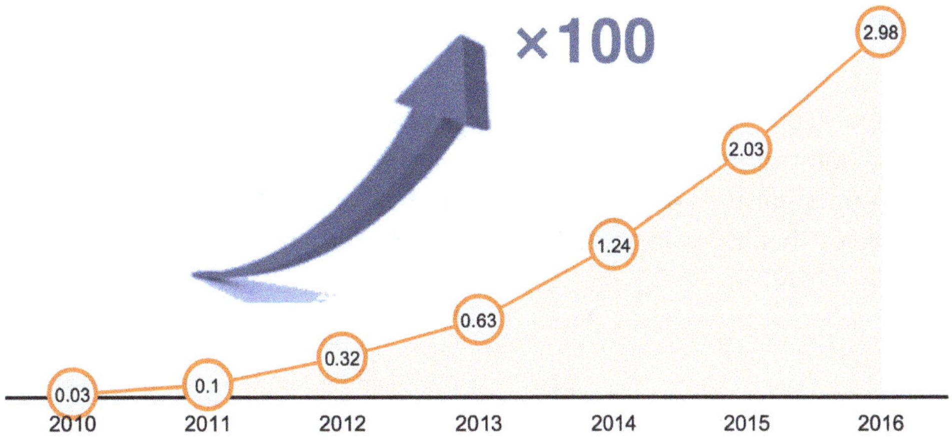

Figure 17. The increasing of donation rate [data from Chinese scientific registration of kidney transplantation (CSRKT)].

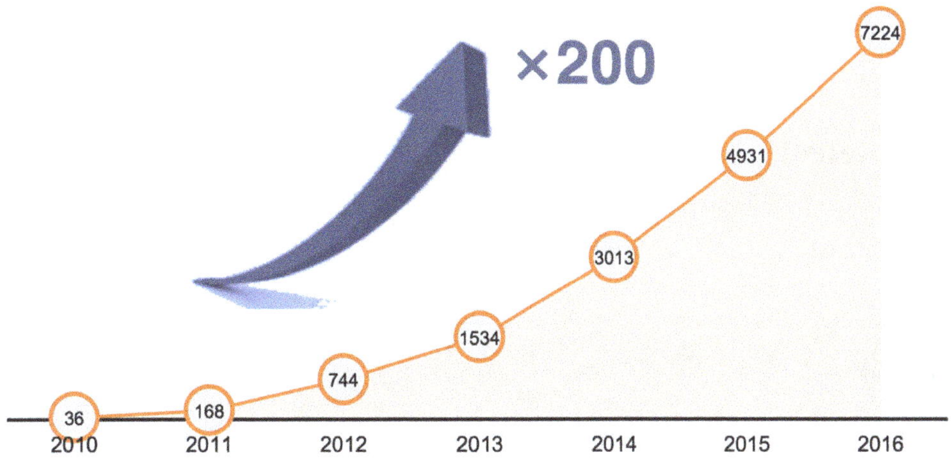

Figure 18. The increasing of DCD cases [data from Chinese scientific registration of kidney transplantation (CSRKT)].

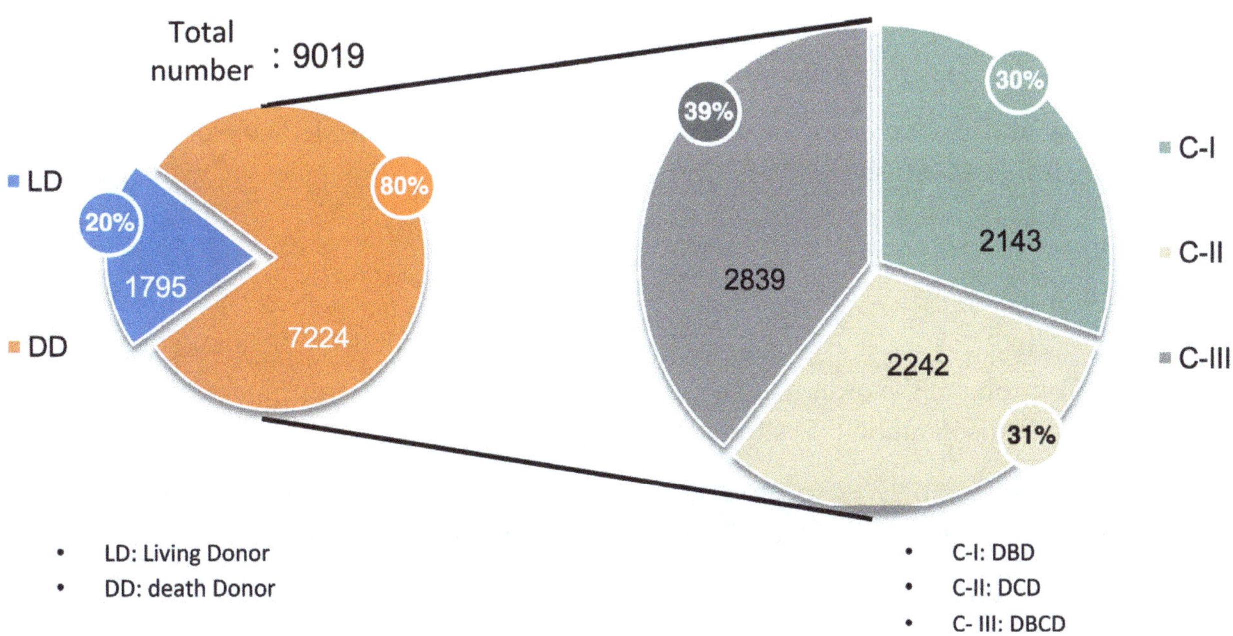

Figure 19. Organ donation in our country is based on death donors at current stage.

9. Conclusion

The shortage of organs was the bottleneck of transplantation. According to Chinese own features and the international development situation, China has carried out DCD work, which is fruitful, innovative and achievable. This has guaranteed the organ donation issue of China to develop healthily and sustainably. Although there is still some imperfection, Chinese DCD work will be better and better with our continuous promotion and international help.

Acknowledgements

This work was supported by grants from the National Natural Science Foundation of China (No. 81771722 and 81700658) to YZ.M and Q.Z.

Conflict of interest

No conflict of interest.

Author details

Yingzi Ming[1,2]*, Baoren Tu[1,2] and Quan Zhuang[1,2]

*Address all correspondence to: myz_china@aliyun.com

1 Transplantation Center of the third Xiangya Hospital, Central South University, Changsha, Hunan, China

2 Engineering and Technology Research Center for Transplantation Medicine of National Ministry of Health, Changsha, Hunan, China

References

[1] He X. To promote the orderly development of organ donation in China. Chinese Journal of Organ Transplantation (Electronic Edition). 2010;**4**(2):7-9

[2] Huang J. Key initiatives to promote the healthy development of organ transplant in China. Chinese Journal of Organ Transplantation. January 2011;**32**(1)

[3] Regulations on Organ Transplantation. State Council Order No. 491

[4] Huang J. The development process of organ donation in China. Chinese Critical Care Medicine Intensive Case Med. May 2017;**3**(2)

[5] Huang J. Speech at the national human organ donation pilot conference. 2010.3.2

[6] Huang J. To create organ donation and transplantation system that is in line with China's national conditions. Chinese Journal of Surgery. January 2013;**51**(1)

[7] Chen Z. Twenty five years wear a sword—Global organ shortage and transplant crisis and China's new road. Chinese Journal of Organ Transplantation (Electronic Edition). November 2010;**4**(4)

[8] Regulations on Regulating Living Organ Transplantation by The Ministry of Health. The Ministry of Health Order [2009] No. 126

[9] Huang J. Speech at National Organ Donation Conference. 26 August 2009

[10] Letter of the Ministry of Health on Entrusting the Red Cross Society of China to carry out Organ Donation Work. The Ministry of Health Order [2010] No. 25

[11] Notice on Printing Organ Donation Pilot Work Program. The Red Cross of China Order [2010] No. 13

[12] Approval on Including Hunan Province into Organ Donation Pilot Work. The Red Cross of China Order [2010] No.68

[13] Chinese Medical Association Organ Transplantation Group. China organ donation after cardiac death work guidance. Chinese Journal of Organ Transplantation. July 2010;**31**(7)

[14] Chinese Medical Association Transplantation Branch. China organ donation after cardiac death work guidance (the second version). Chinese Journal of Organ Transplantation. December 2011;**32**(12)

[15] Declaration of China's human organ donation pilot work summary meeting. 23 March, 2012

[16] Linna Hao. The Speech of Chinese Red Cross President on National Human Organ Donation Pilot Work Summary Meeting [Internet]. 2012. Available from: http://www.chinanews.com/jk/2012/03-22/3764262.shtm [Accessed: 2018-01-20l]

[17] Chinese Red Cross the Ministry of health Opinion on Continuing Promoting Organ Donation Work. The Red Cross of China Order [2012] No. 39

[18] Huang J. Speech at a National Video Conference on Human Organ Donation. 25 February, 2013

[19] Huang J, He X, editors. Theory and Practice of Organ Donation after Citizens' Death. ISBN: 978-7-117-20121-1

[20] China Organ Donation Work Guidance (the fourth version)

[21] Notice of the Ministry of Health on printing Fundamentals of Human Organ Distribution and Sharing in China and Core Policies of Liver and Kidney Transplantation. The Ministry of Health Order [2010] No. 113

[22] Provisions on the Administration of the Procurement and Distribution of Donated Organs (trial). The Ministry of Health Order [2013] No. 11

[23] China Organ Transplant Response System (COTRS). Available from: https://www.cot.org.cn/

[24] China Organ Donation Work Guidance. August 2013;**1**:P55-P56

[25] China Organ Donation Work Guidance (the fourth version). August 2015:P21-P22

[26] New Regulations on the Administration of Organ Procurement Organization. China Hospital CEO. Sept 2013;17. ISSN 1674-3989

[27] Ming Y. Speech on China-Beijing International Organ Donation Conference. Oct 2016

[28] Ye Q. Speech on Chinese Medical Doctor Association Organ Transplant Annual Meeting. Dec 2015

[29] Ming Y. Speech on 14th Congress of International Society for Organ Donation and Procurement (ISODP). Sept 2017

[30] Gao X. Standardized training, strict management, law-based promoting human organ donation coordinator team building. Prac International Journal of Organ Transplantation (Electronic Version). Mar 2015;**3**(2)

[31] Notice on Printing The Management Method of Organ Donation Coordinator (trial). The Red Cross of China Order [2011] No.65

[32] Ming Y. Discussion on the building of organ donation coordinator teams. Organ Transplantation. Sep 2014;**5**(5)

[33] China Organ Donation Coordinator Training Material (two volumes)

[34] Chen Yao, Bingyi Shi etc. Construction of organ donation files management system. Hospital Administration Journal of PLA. 30 Oct 2016;**23**(10)

[35] Ye Q. The organizational construction of organ procurement organization. Speech on China Organ Donation Coordinator Training Session. 2015

[36] Yu H. Rational thinking on increasing the donation rate of citizens' organ in our country. Medicine and Philosophy. Jun 2012;**33**(454)

[37] Yu H. Countermeasures for the transplantation dilemma in China. Medicine and Society. Sept 2012;**25**(10)

[38] Chen Z. Efforts to create a new situation of organ transplantation with Chinese characteristics. 21 Aug 2015

3

Diagnosis, Treatment, and Outcomes of Antibody-Mediated Rejection in Kidney Transplantation

Vasishta S. Tatapudi and Bonnie E. Lonze

Abstract

Antibody mediated rejection remains an important barrier to optimal long-term outcomes after kidney transplantation. Donor specific antibody, while not the formidable barrier to transplantation it once was, remains a major risk factor for antibody mediated rejection and its consequences of premature graft failure. Recent advances in understanding of the cellular and molecular mechanisms of antibody production and antibody-mediated injury have led to refinements in diagnostic techniques, and have paved the way for the development of novel therapies to treat rejection and prolong allograft function. The purpose of this chapter is to review the current level at which we understand the pathophysiology of antibody mediated rejection, describe the current diagnostic criteria for antibody mediated rejection, and discuss available and emerging treatments as well as their outcomes.

Keywords: kidney transplantation, donor specific antibody, antibody mediated rejection

1. Introduction

The first successful kidney transplant was performed between identical twins by Joseph E. Murray and his colleagues at the Peter Bent Brigham Hospital in 1954 [1]. Since then, the field of kidney transplantation has progressed immensely owing to greater understanding of the immune mechanisms underlying allograft rejection at a cellular and molecular level and development of increasingly potent immunosuppressive drug therapies [2]. Today, kidney transplantation is considered the treatment of choice for patients with end stage renal disease (ESRD) since it is associated with lower mortality and cardiovascular morbidity while offering

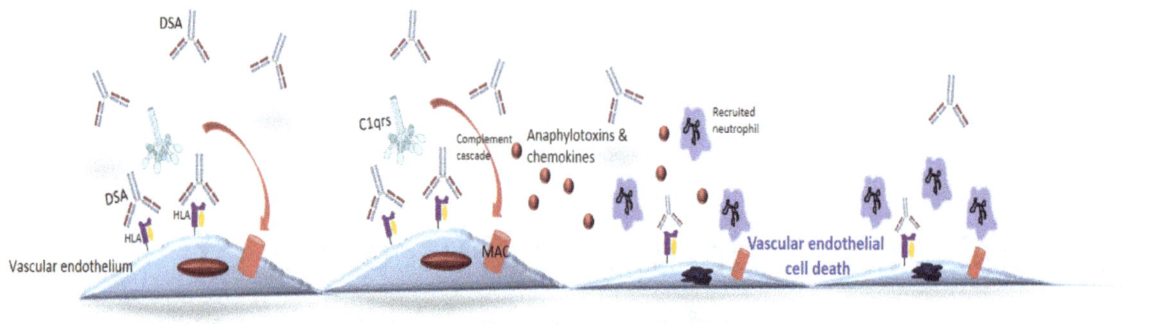

Figure 1. In AMR, DSAs bind to human leukocyte antigens on graft vascular endothelium. This is followed by activation of complement, membrane attack complex-mediated cellular injury and infiltration of mononuclear cells. Reproduced with permission from Montgomery et al. [4].

improved quality of life [3]. However, allograft rejection remains a major impediment to the longevity of renal allografts. Recognition of donor antigens as "non-self" by the host immune system elicits humoral and cell mediated immune responses that if left unchecked result in the destruction of the allograft (**Figure 1**).

2. Human leukocyte antigen (HLA) system and allograft rejection

Human leukocyte antigens (HLA) play a vital role in host defense against foreign pathogens and in immune surveillance of tumors. These antigens are encoded by the major histocompatibility complex (MHC) which is a family of genes that encompasses a 3.6 million base pair genomic region, 6p21, on the short arm of chromosome 6 [5]. The MHC complex is divided into three regions representing three classes of genes—classes I, II, and III. The HLA genes that are involved in the immune response belong to classes, I and II [6]. Class I antigens are expressed on all nucleated cells whereas class II antigens are expressed only on professional antigen presenting cells (APCs)—dendritic cells, B-cells, and macrophages [7]. In the setting of infection, pathogen derived foreign antigens are presented to T-cells as peptides on the surface of major histocompatibility complex (MHC) molecules expressed on the surface of APCs. The ensuing signaling cascade results in the activation, proliferation, and differentiation of naïve T lymphocytes into subtypes with distinct cytokine profiles. Type 1 helper T (Th1) cells drive the cellular immune response mediated by CD8+ cytotoxic T lymphocytes, and type 2 helper T (Th2) cells drive B-cell mediated humoral immune response [2].

The heterogeneity of human MHC molecules enables the immune system to protect us from a variety of foreign pathogens. However, in the context of transplantation between genetically distinct individuals, these MHC polymorphisms elicit immune responses that can result in rejection of the allograft [7]. Two pathophysiologically distinct flavors of renal allograft rejection are recognized—cell mediated, and antibody mediated rejection. Both these types of rejection can manifest as acute or chronic clinicopathologic variants. Acute cell mediated rejection is characterized by infiltration of the allograft by effector T cells resulting in the typical features such as tubulitis, interstitial inflammation and in more advanced cases, endothelial arteritis [2, 8].

3. Clinical relevance of antibody mediated rejection

AMR is estimated to occur in 3–10% of transplant recipients and it represents 20–30% of episodes of acute rejection [7]. Although less common than cell mediated rejection, AMR is generally recognized to have a worse prognosis and requires different forms of therapy [9]. In the 1960s anti-HLA antibodies were recognized as a cause for allograft rejection following reports of hyperacute antibody mediated rejection in patients with antibodies reactive to donor lymphocytes [10, 11]. Patel and Terasaki's landmark study documented immediate graft failure in 24 of 30 (80%) of the patients with circulating donor reactive antibodies identified by a positive cytotoxicity crossmatch [12]. This led to the universal practice of antibody screening by complement dependent cytotoxicity (CDC) crossmatch prior to renal transplantation and the avoidance of transplantation in patients with a positive crossmatch. Therefore, until the mid-1980s, acute cellular rejection, as opposed to antibody mediated rejection (AMR), was considered the major barrier to successful [13]. The advent of calcineurin inhibitors (CNIs) in the 1980s led to a significant decline in incidence of acute rejection and a consequent improvement in short term graft survival rates [14]. Today, cellular rejection seldom causes graft loss [15]. However, contemporary data suggests that these gains have not led to sustained improvement in long-term graft survival [16]. Reasons for the lack of improvement in long-term graft survival have been a topic of much debate and most late graft losses were attributed to either chronic allograft nephropathy (CAN) or death with a functioning graft [17]. Although, the multifactorial nature of late renal allograft loss makes therapeutic intervention challenging [18] prevention and treatment of AMR holds the key to optimizing long term graft survival.

Exposure to non-self HLA by way of pregnancy, blood transfusion or transplantation may lead to the development of circulating anti-HLA antibodies. ESRD patients who are sensitized to HLA by prior exposure have a prolonged wait-time for transplantation and reduced transplant rates. Removal of pre-formed circulating donor specific antibodies (DSA) by various desensitization techniques allows transplantation of many of these biologically disadvantaged patients [19–21] However, such HLA incompatible kidney transplants recipients are at increased risk for developing AMR. A high percentage of episodes of AMR are difficult to treat and may cause immediate graft loss or delayed transplant glomerulopathy [22]. Therefore, AMR remains a significant impediment to the success of transplantation in this subset of patients.

4. Diagnosis of antibody mediated rejection

The Banff classification schema has been used internationally for scoring and classifying kidney transplant pathology findings since its first iteration was published in 1993. However, earlier versions dealt with AMR in an imprecise manner. The development of more sophisticated methods of detection of DSAs by means of solid-phase assays together with the sensitivity and specificity of C4d staining in peritubular capillaries in identifying AMR paved the way for rigorous morphological classification of AMR [23]. The cornerstones for the diagnosis for AMR are (1) Histologic evidence of acute tissue injury; (2) Evidence of current/recent antibody interaction with vascular endothelium; (3) Serologic evidence of DSAs. The updated 2015 Banff classification system recognizes acute active AMR and chronic active AMR and outlines detailed criteria for the diagnosis of each (**Table 1**) [24].

Acute/active AbMR	All three features must be present for diagnosis. Biopsies showing histological features plus evidence of current/recent antibody interaction with vascular endothelium or DSA, but not both, may be designated as suspicious for acute/active ABMR. Lesions may be clinically acute or smoldering or may be subclinical; it should be noted if the lesion is C4d-positive or C4d-negative, based on the following criteria: 1. Histologic evidence of acute tissue injury, including one or more of the following: • Microvascular inflammation ($g^a > 0$ in the absence of recurrent or *de novo* glomerulonephritis, and/or $ptc^b > 0$) • Intimal or transmural arteritis ($v^c > 0$) • Acute thrombotic microangiopathy in the absence of any other cause • Acute tubular injury in the absence of any other apparent cause 2. Evidence of current/recent antibody interaction with vascular endothelium, including at least one of the following: • Linear C4d staining in peritubular capillaries (C4d2 or C4d3 by IF on frozen sections or C4d >0 by IHC on paraffin sections) • At least moderate microvascular inflammation ([g + ptc] ≥2), although in the presence of acute T-cell mediated rejection (TCMR), borderline infiltrate, or infection; ptc ≥2 alone is not sufficient, and g must be ≥1 • Increased expression of gene transcripts in the biopsy tissue indicative of endothelial injury, if thoroughly validated 3. Serologic evidence of DSAs (HLA or other antigens) Biopsies suspicious for AMR on the basis of meeting criteria 1 and 2 should prompt expedited DSA testing
Chronic active ABMR	All three features must be present for diagnosis. As with acute/active ABMR, biopsies showing histological features plus evidence of current/recent antibody interaction with vascular endothelium or DSA, but not both, may be designated as suspicious, and it should be noted if the lesion is C4d-positive or C4d-negative, based on the criteria listed: 1. Histologic evidence of chronic tissue injury, including one or more of the following: • TG ($cg^d > 0$), if no evidence of chronic thrombotic microangiopathy; includes changes evident by EM only • Severe peritubular capillary basement membrane multilayering (requires EM)c • Arterial intimal fibrosis of new onset, excluding other causes; leukocytes within the sclerotic intima favor chronic ABMR if there is no prior history of biopsy-proven TCMR with arterial involvement but are not required 2. Evidence of current/recent antibody interaction with vascular endothelium, including at least one of the following: • Linear C4d staining in peritubular capillaries (C4d2 or C4d3 by IF on frozen sections, or C4d >0 by IHC on paraffin sections) • At least moderate microvascular inflammation ([g + ptc] ≥2), although in the presence of acute TCMR, borderline infiltrate, or infection, ptc ≥2 alone is not sufficient and g must be ≥1 3. Serologic evidence of DSAs (HLA or other antigens): • Biopsies suspicious for AMR on the basis of meeting criteria 1 and 2 should prompt expedited DSA testing

C4d staining without evidence of rejection	All three features must be present for diagnosis: 1. Linear C4d staining in peritubular capillaries (C4d2 or C4d3 by IF on frozen sections, or C4d >0 by IHC on paraffin sections 2. g = 0, ptc = 0, cg = 0 (by light microscopy and by EM if available), v = 0; no TMA, no peritubular capillary basement membrane multilayering, no acute tubular injury (in the absence of another apparent cause for this) 3. No acute cell-mediated rejection (Banff 1997 type 1A or greater) or borderline changes

g-glomerulitis, ptc-peritubular capillaritis, v-vasculitis, cg-chronic glomerulopathy (transplant glomerulopathy)

Table 1. Criteria for antibody mediated rejection as outlined by the Banff 2015 Meeting Work Group [24].

Glomerular and/or peritubular capillary infiltration with polymorphonuclear leukocytes and/or macrophages represents microvascular inflammation and is the classic histologic feature of acute tissue injury in acute AMR (**Figure 2**). However, intimal or transmural arteritis, acute TMA and ATN can also denote acute AMR (**Figure 3**). Splitting or double contouring of the GBM (transplant glomerulopathy) as well as severe multi-lamination of peritubular capillary basement membrane are histologic features of chronic AMR. Detection of inert complement split product, C4d in peritubular capillaries by IF or IHC indicates antibody interaction with vascular endothelium (**Figure 4**). However, recognizing that complement independent pathways may be involved in the etiopathogenesis of AMR, the Banff classification also sets forth certain criteria (listed in **Table 1**) that allow for the diagnosis of acute or chronic AMR in patients without detectable C4d staining. Demonstration of circulating DSAs is a pre-requisite for diagnosis of AMR. Noting that non-HLA DSAs may result in clinical and histopathologic findings indistinguishable from AMR, Banff criteria for serologic evidence of DSAs require detection of either DSAs directed against donor HLA or "other" antigens [24].

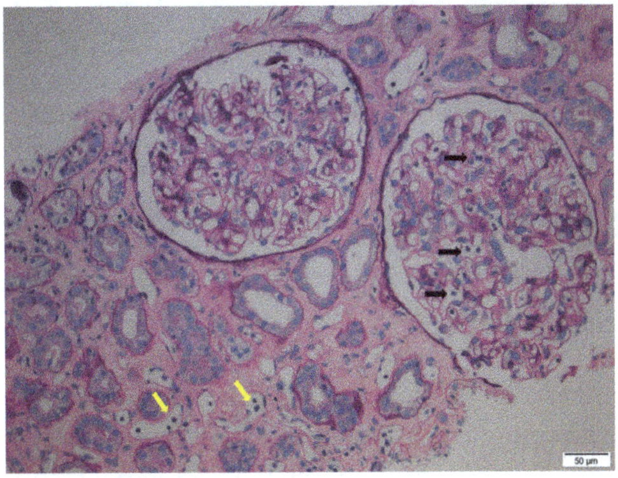

Figure 2. Black arrows show infiltrating polymorphonuclear leukocytes in glomerular capillary loops (glomerulitis) in a patient undergoing acute oliguric antibody mediated rejection. Yellow arrows point to demarginated polymorphonuclear leukocytes in peritubular capillaries (peritubular capillaritis). Pathology slides courtesy: Dr. Ming Wu, Department of Pathology, NYU Langone Medical Center.

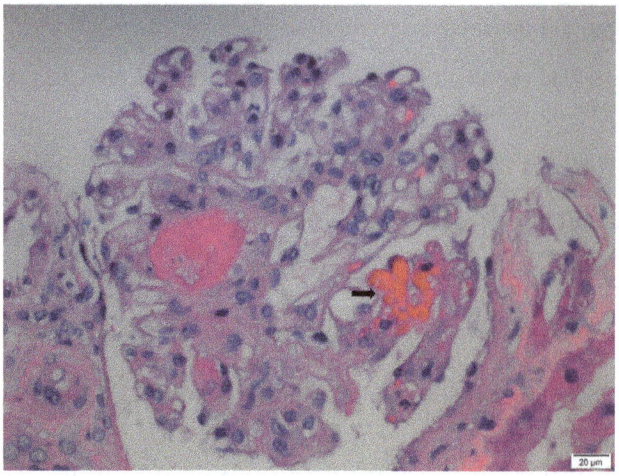

Figure 3. Platelet fibrin thrombi in glomerular capillary loops (black arrow) due to acute thrombotic microangiopathy in a patient with acute antibody mediated rejection. Pathology slides courtesy: Dr. Ming Wu, Department of Pathology, NYU Langone Medical Center.

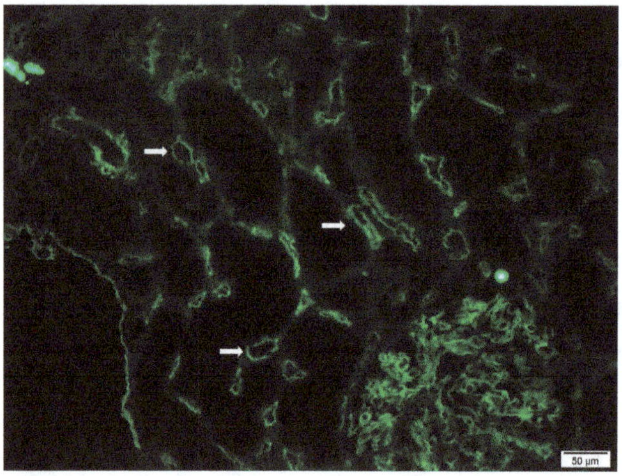

Figure 4. Immunofluorescence staining showing diffuse linear C4d positivity in peritubular capillaries (white arrows). Pathology slides courtesy: Dr. Ming Wu, Department of Pathology, NYU Langone Medical Center.

5. HLA antibody detection assays

5.1. Calculated panel reactive antibody (cPRA)

In the complement-dependent cytotoxicity (CDC) assay, recipient serum is mixed with donor lymphocytes and complement is supplemented. Presence of DSAs is indicated by the appearance of cytotoxicity. The CDC crossmatch was principal technique for detecting DSAs in kidney transplant candidates till the mid-1980s [12, 15]. The panel reactive antibody (PRA) assay, a simple test that predicts the likelihood of a transplant candidate finding a HLA compatible donor (with a negative CDC crossmatch). This test involves treating a panel of cells derived from a pool of individuals representative of the local donor population with recipient serum and noting the percentage of cells that develop cytotoxicity. Therefore, a patient with a high PRA percentage can be predicted to be HLA incompatible with a majority of the potential donors. Consequently, such patients have prolonged wait times for transplantation and may die waiting for a compatible organ [25]. The emergence of more sensitive solid phase assays that employ HLA antigen-coated beads have revealed a greater prevalence of pre-sensitization to HLA in potential transplant recipients than was previously appreciated. Using these sensitive techniques of HLA antibody detection (in recipient serum) in conjunction with modern HLA typing methods (to determine donor HLA typing), we can now estimate a transplant candidate's calculated panel reactive antibody (cPRA). This is an alternative to standard PRA testing. Transplant centers can designate HLA antigens to which the patient has been sensitized as "unacceptable." The cPRA is computed from HLA antigen frequencies among kidney donors in the United States and represents the percentage of actual organ donors that express any "unacceptable" HLA antigens [25]. One of the key elements of the Organ Procurement and Transplantation Network's (OPTN) new Kidney Allocation System (KAS) introduced in December 2014 is to allocate additional points to waitlisted kidney transplant candidates based on a CPRA sliding scale [26]. The aim of this policy is to increase access to transplantation for sensitized candidates [27]. Soon after the new KAS came into effect, the proportion of transplants being performed in patients with CPRA >98% rose from 2.4 to 13.4% [28]. Therefore, the new KAS appears to be accomplishing the goal of equitable allocation of scarce deceased donor organs to highly sensitized patients who are biologically disadvantaged.

5.2. HLA antibody detection assays

Techniques for detection of HLA antibodies in transplant candidates have evolved considerably since the 1960s when the traditional cell-based complement dependent cytotoxicity (CDC) assay was first developed. Modern flow-cytometry and solid phase assays are far more sensitive than the CDC crossmatch. In the CDC crossmatch, recipient serum is incubated with donor lymphocytes, along with complement. A positive crossmatch is said to occur when DSAs present in the recipient serum bind the corresponding antigens expressed on the surface of donor T or B lymphocytes and activate complement leading to cell lysis [29]. The flow cytometry crossmatch (FCXM) developed in the 1980s was shown to be more sensitive than the CDC crossmatch and can detect lower strength, but clinically significant antibodies that are imperceptible to the CDC crossmatch [30]. In the FCXM, like the CDC crossmatch, donor-specific anti-HLA antibodies, if present in the recipient serum, bind HLA molecules on the surface of donor T or B lymphocytes. The flow cytometry technique detects these HLA bound anti-HLA antibodies by means of secondary fluorescein-labelled antihuman IgG [29]. The advent of solid phase assays for HLA antibody screening in the 1990s has redefined what it means to be sensitized to HLA. There are two varieties of solid phase assays – enzyme linked immunosorbent assay (ELISA) based methods and single antigen bead based methods. Single antigen bead based assays may employ either a flow cytometry platform or a Luminex platform to detect HLA [31]. The Luminex platform employs fluorochrome impregnated microbeads that are coated with specific HLA molecules. Donor-specific anti-HLA antibodies, if present in the recipient serum, bind HLA molecules coated on the surface of the beads. The microbeads are then incubated with phycoerythrin (PE)-labeled anti-human IgG antibodies. The Luminex dual laser system identifies the specificity of the bound anti-HLA antibodies[Ref]. The Luminex based assay has now become the most popular method of HLA antibody detection, both due to its superior sensitivity, as well as its ability to identify the antigenic specificity of the detected HLA antibody [29].

6. Treatments for antibody mediated rejection

The success of desensitization techniques, which enabled transplantation in the setting of pre-existing DSA, represented a breakthrough in the ability to offer transplantation to highly-sensitized patients, who previously had little hope of receiving a transplant [32–34]. But early success was tempered by observations of antibody rebound, early AMR, and suboptimal long-term graft survival [35, 36]. Thus the ability to successfully perform incompatible transplants and optimize long-term outcomes is contingent upon the ability to successfully treat AMR. The first reported efforts at allograft rescue in the setting AMR employed similar techniques as were used for desensitization, namely, techniques that remove or reduce circulating antibody [37]. While removal of antibody remains the cornerstone of AMR therapy, improved understanding of the pathophysiological mechanisms of antibody production and antibody mediated injury have yielded several adjunctive treatment options which are now in various stages of application or new development. For treatment of AMR, no standard protocols exist. Published reports are generally small patient series, and reported techniques vary based on center-specific experience and expertise, as well as center-specific access to emerging therapies [38–40]. Thus, randomized-controlled trial data do not exist for most of these treatments. Meta-analyses are limited by patient heterogeneity, treatment regimen heterogeneity and sample size [39, 41]. Below are brief descriptions of currently existing treatment modalities, though it is important to understand that these are rarely, if ever, used as monotherapies. Most AMR treatment strategies employ a technique for antibody removal in combination with adjunctive agents to minimize antibody production and/or act at the level of the graft to minimize antibody-mediated injury.

6.1. Therapeutic plasma exchange

Though often referred to simply as "plasmapheresis," the procedure utilized in the treatment of AMR is more accurately described as therapeutic plasma exchange (TPE). While plasmapheresis [42] technically describes plasma removal without replacement, TPE entails plasma removal with replacement of a substitute colloid component. A 1–1.5 L plasma volume exchange generally removes approximately 70% of plasma components, including anti-HLA antibodies [43]. For immunoglobulins, the durability this treatment differs dependent upon the tissue compartments in which each immunoglobulin subclass resides. IgM, which resides solely in the intravascular space, and does not significantly repopulate by re-equilibration following TPE, much unlike IgG and IgA. Re-equilibration into the intravascular space generally means that for IgG present in high concentration initially in the serum, multiple TPE treatments are required to make measurable impact on the circulating concentration [44–46]. Rates of antibody removal with TPE, as well as characteristics of rebound following treatment vary with antibody subclass and specificity, and mechanistically this remains poorly understood [47]. TPE was one of the first reported successful strategies for treatment AMR and remains a cornerstone of most current treatment protocols [37, 38, 48, 49].

6.2. Immunoadsorption

Immunoadsorption (IA) is a therapy not available worldwide, but where applied has been used successfully in both desensitization and treatment of AMR. IA has the benefit of specifically removing circulating IgG, while sparing desired plasma protein components such as clotting factors [50]. IA can rapidly and efficiently deplete IgG after a small number of treatments [51–53]. A single randomized controlled trial reporting IA plus pulse steroid compared to pulse steroid alone as treatment for AMR was stopped early after an excessive number of graft failures in the control group [54].

6.3. Intravenous immune globulin (IVIG)

The precise mechanisms of IVIG action both in desensitization and in treatment of AMR remain unclear, but there is evidence to support that it is multimodal [55, 56]. IVIG has been shown to have inhibitory effects on B-cells [57–59], antigen presenting cells [60], and on complement [61, 62]. IVIG in the treatment of AMR has been reported as high-dose therapy (1–2 gm/kg) used without plasma exchange treatments [63–65], and more commonly, as low-dose therapy (100 mg/kg/dose) used in combination with TPE [39, 40, 66].

6.4. Splenectomy

Removal of the spleen, the largest lymphoid organ in the body, is postulated to deplete the plasma cell reservoir, and thereby yield a rapid decrease in circulating HLA antibody in patients with severe acute rejection [67, 68]. Due to its associated morbidity, splenectomy is generally reserved as a rescue therapy [67, 69–71] when all other less invasive interventions are failing and a graft is at risk for imminent loss. Potentially less morbid alternatives to operative splenectomy, including angioembolization or splenic irradiation, may prove to be beneficial in select patient situations [72].

6.5. B-cell and plasma cell targeted medical therapies

Rituximab (Rituxan®, Genentech) is a monoclonal antibody directed against the B-cell CD20 antigen [73]. This recombinant antibody is constructed as a chimeric protein with human IgG_1 constant regions linked to murine anti-human CD20 variable regions [74]. Binding of rituximab to CD20 leads to antibody-dependent complement-mediated cytotoxicity and apoptosis of the bound cell. Rituximab thereby depletes the memory B-cell population and this is hypothesized to, in turn, reduce the plasma cell population and decrease HLA-antibody production [75–77]. Rituximab has been used as an adjunctive therapy in combination with various treatment modalities including: IVIG [78], TPE plus steroid pulse [79, 80], and TPE plus IVIG [66, 81]. While rituximab was perhaps the earliest used adjunctive agent in the treatment of AMR, to date only a single randomized controlled trial of its use has been performed, in which it was compared to placebo in addition to standard therapy (TPE with low dose IVIG). No difference was observed in this underpowered study though there was a trend toward improved outcomes with the addition of rituximab [82].

Whereas the postulated effect of rituximab on antibody-production is indirect, bortezomib (Velcade®, Takeda Oncology) acts directly at the level of the antibody-producing plasma cell. Bortezomib is a proteasomal inhibitor that depletes circulating plasma cells by inducing apoptosis [83–85]. The first reported use bortezomib in transplant recipients was in a small series where graft salvage was attempted in the cases of AMR refractory to therapies including TPE, IVIG, and rituximab [86]. Following bortezomib therapy, circulating DSA strength has been reported to decrease substantially [87], though interestingly, class I and class II DSAs may be not be reduced with equal efficacy [88]. Bortezomib, like rituximab, has been used in combination with TPE, with and without steroids and rituximab [89–92] and is thoroughly reviewed elsewhere [85].

6.6. Complement inhibition

The realization that the tissue injury associated with AMR was, at least in part, mediated by the complement cascade led to the hypothesis that complement inhibition may afford tissue-level protection while TPE or other antibody removing techniques were implemented. The first reported use of the terminal complement inhibitor eculizumab (Soliris®, Alexion Pharmaceuticals) was in a patient with severe accelerated oliguric AMR who was deemed an inappropriate candidate for a rescue splenectomy [93]. With TPE, IVIG, rituximab, and eculizumab, recovery of renal function was achieved. Several reports describe the use of eculizumab as a salvage therapy, either in lieu of or in combination with splenectomy [94–96], but reports of successful salvage are not universal [97]. Eculizumab's mechanism of action of action led to studies of its pre-emptive use in incompatible kidney recipients at high risk for AMR, and while eculizumab may decrease the incidence of AMR [98], it does not prevent it [99].

Additional complement inhibitors have since become available and are being evaluated for their relative efficacy in AMR. C1-esterase inhibitor (C1-INH) is an endogenous protein that is a more proximal inhibitor of the complement cascade and is commercially available as a purified plasma preparation (Berinert®, CSL Behring, and Cinryze®, Shire). A recently reported double-blinded randomized controlled trial of C1-INH as an add-on to standard TPE therapy for AMR suggested a benefit in terms of improved long term renal allograft function in those who received C1-INH [100]. Like eculizumab, C1-INH may have promise in the prevention of AMR in high-risk patients [101], or as a graft protective agent in the setting of severe or treatment refractory AMR [102].

6.7. IL-6 inhibition

IL-6 is a pro-inflammatory cytokine with properties that activate numerous cell lines including B-T- and plasma cells. Tocilizumab (Actemra®, Genentech)is a humanized monoclonal antibody which blocks IL-6 signal transduction by binding and inhibiting the IL-6 receptor [103]. In animal models, IL-6/IL-6R signaling has been found to promote renal injury [104] and may be associated with the injury of acute rejection [105]. In human studies, it may affect a decrease in HLA antibody production [106]. A recent trial of tocilizumab in patients with refractory chronic AMR reported improved long-term graft survival rates in those who received tocilizumab [107].

7. Outcomes and unanswered questions

Generally reported estimates of the incidence of AMR are around 7% for all recipients [108], and may be as high as 50% among recipients of HLA-incompatible grafts [109, 110]. Despite improved abilities to diagnose and treat AMR, it remains an important cause of premature graft loss [111, 112]. Clinically silent AMR identified on biopsy in the setting of normal renal function, if left untreated, is associated with a two-fold increased risk of graft loss [109, 113]. If the AMR is clinically apparent and associated with graft dysfunction, the risk of graft loss can increase to six-fold [109]. Even when recognized and treated promptly, AMR portends recurrent AMR, and ultimately, chronic AMR and transplant glomerulopathy [114, 115].

The pathophysiology of AMR and the molecular mechanisms of antibody-mediated injury have never been better understood, however the fact that such heterogeneity is observed clinically from case to case suggests that much remains yet to be clarified. The spectrum of AMR severity, acuity, and treatability is broad and not easily predictable even when clinical parameters appear relatively constant. While some lines of evidence suggest that any DSA [116, 117] even historical DSA not present at transplant [111], has the potential to be harmful, others have reported clinically silent DSA that, although detectable, has no apparent impact the incidence of rejection or on long-term outcomes [118]. Whether sensitization alone, not just DSA, is an independent risk factor for AMR, is unclear [115]. Whether this variability lies in the DSA specificity, in differential expression of the target HLA molecules on the allograft, or on other factors, remains to be determined. Multiple lines of evidence suggest that complement activating, C1q-binding DSA are associated with greater risks for rejection and for worse outcomes [119–122], compared to non-C1q binding DSAs. The ability to identify and test for the more virulent DSAs may prove to be of benefit in terms of surveillance and directing treatment. There is evidence that class II DSA is associated with worse long-term outcomes [123–125], and poorer responses to treatments [126] compared to class I DSAs. What underlies this difference, remains uncertain. Whether, and how, antigens vary in terms of their immunogenicity and risks for inciting AMR, remains to be determined. Whether any of the available therapies is optimally suited for different DSA patterns or specificities, or AMR phenotypes, also remains to be determined.

Perhaps the most effective means of minimizing the risks of AMR may be in maximizing efforts to prevent it. Experience with HLA-incompatible transplant recipients have demonstrated, both in single-center and multi-center series, that long-term outcomes are inversely correlated with the starting crossmatch strength [19, 20]. Thus careful attention paid to donor selection, and making any effort possible to minimize incompatibility, can pay great dividends in the long-term post-transplant [115]. And while prevention will not always be feasible, the ability to more readily and accurately detect AMR will enable more rapid treatments and improve the chances of their success. Just as new agents are being developed to remove antibody [127], and interrupt the pathways that impart antibody-mediated injury, so too are innovative, increasingly specific, and less invasive procedures for the diagnosis of AMR. The ability to identify AMR, and perhaps even characterize AMR phenotypes based on gene expression profiles in biopsy tissue [128, 129] should allow a clearer determination of AMR severity and ultimately help guide therapy. The identification of serum and/or urinary biomarkers [130–133] should enable better surveillance, earlier diagnosis of AMR, and prompt treatment to prevent irreversible tissue injury. Ultimately, optimizing the diagnosis and treatment of AMR will lead to greater graft longevity and thus, better utilization of this vastly limited resource.

Author details

Vasishta S. Tatapudi and Bonnie E. Lonze*

*Address all correspondence to: bonnie.lonze@nyumc.org

NYU Langone Health, Transplant Institute, New York, NY, USA

References

[1] Harrison JH, Merrill JP, Murray JE. Renal homotransplantation in identical twins. Surgical Forum. 1956;**6**:432-436

[2] Nankivell BJ, Alexander SI. Rejection of the kidney allograft. The New England Journal of Medicine. 2010;**363**(15):1451-1462

[3] Tonelli M et al. Systematic review: Kidney transplantation compared with dialysis in clinically relevant outcomes. American Journal of Transplantation. 2011;**11**(10):2093-2109

[4] Montgomery RA, Lonze BE, Tatapudi VS. IgG degrading enzyme of Streptococcus Pyogenes: An exciting new development in desensitization therapy. Transplantation. 2018;**102**(1):2-4

[5] Shiina T, Inoko H, Kulski JK. An update of the HLA genomic region, locus information and disease associations: 2004. Tissue Antigens. 2004;**64**(6):631-649

[6] Klein J, Sato A. The HLA system. First of two parts. The New England Journal of Medicine. 2000;**343**(10):702-709

[7] Womer KL. Immunologic principles in kidney transplantation. In: Feehally J, Floege J, Johnson RJ, editors. Comprehensive Clinical Nephrology. 3rd ed. Philadelphia: Mosby/Elsevier. xviii; 2007. p. 1239

[8] Haas M et al. Banff 2013 meeting report: Inclusion of c4d-negative antibody-mediated rejection and antibody-associated arterial lesions. American Journal of Transplantation. 2014;**14**(2):272-283

[9] Colvin RB. Antibody-mediated renal allograft rejection: Diagnosis and pathogenesis. Journal of the American Society of Nephrology. 2007;**18**(4):1046-1056

[10] Kissmeyer-Nielsen F et al. Hyperacute rejection of kidney allografts, associated with pre-existing humoral antibodies against donor cells. Lancet. 1966;**2**(7465):662-665

[11] Williams GM et al. "Hyperacute" renal-homograft rejection in man. The New England Journal of Medicine. 1968;**279**(12):611-618

[12] Patel R, Terasaki PI. Significance of the positive crossmatch test in kidney transplantation. The New England Journal of Medicine. 1969;**280**(14):735-739

[13] Tatapudi VS, Montgomery RA. Pharmacologic complement inhibition in clinical transplantation. Current Transplantation Reports. 2017;**4**(2):91-100

[14] Hariharan S et al. Improved graft survival after renal transplantation in the United States, 1988 to 1996. The New England Journal of Medicine. 2000;**342**(9):605-612

[15] Stegall MD, Chedid MF, Cornell LD. The role of complement in antibody-mediated rejection in kidney transplantation. Nature Reviews Nephrology. 2012;**8**(11):670-678

[16] Meier-Kriesche HU et al. Lack of improvement in renal allograft survival despite a marked decrease in acute rejection rates over the most recent era. American Journal of Transplantation. 2004;**4**(3):378-383

[17] Gaston RS et al. Evidence for antibody-mediated injury as a major determinant of late kidney allograft failure. Transplantation. 2010;**90**(1):68-74

[18] Lamb KE, Lodhi S, Meier-Kriesche HU. Long-term renal allograft survival in the United States: A critical reappraisal. American Journal of Transplantation. 2011;**11**(3):450-462

[19] Montgomery RA et al. Desensitization in HLA-incompatible kidney recipients and survival. The New England Journal of Medicine. 2011;**365**(4):318-326

[20] Orandi BJ et al. Survival benefit with kidney transplants from HLA-incompatible live donors. The New England Journal of Medicine. 2016;**374**(10):940-950

[21] Vo AA et al. Rituximab and intravenous immune globulin for desensitization during renal transplantation. The New England Journal of Medicine. 2008;**359**(3):242-251

[22] Burns JM et al. Alloantibody levels and acute humoral rejection early after positive crossmatch kidney transplantation. American Journal of Transplantation. 2008;**8**(12):2684-2694

[23] Racusen LC et al. Antibody-mediated rejection criteria – an addition to the Banff 97 classification of renal allograft rejection. American Journal of Transplantation. 2003;**3**(6):708-714

[24] Loupy A et al. The Banff 2015 kidney meeting report: Current challenges in rejection classification and prospects for adopting molecular pathology. American Journal of Transplantation. 2017;**17**(1):28-41

[25] Cecka JM. Calculated PRA (CPRA): The new measure of sensitization for transplant candidates. American Journal of Transplantation. 2010;**10**(1):26-29

[26] Paramesh AS et al. OPO strategies to prevent unintended use of kidneys exported for high PRA (>98% cPRA) recipients. American Journal of Transplantation. 2017;**17**(8):2139-2143

[27] The New Kidney Allocation System: Resources for Protocols and Processes Webinar. https://www.transplantpro.org/wp-content/uploads/sites/3/KAS_Protocols_Processes_Slides_Script.pdf. Last accessed February 1st, 2018

[28] Stewart DE et al. Changes in deceased donor kidney transplantation one year after KAS implementation. American Journal of Transplantation. 2016;**16**(6):1834-1847

[29] Mulley WR, Kanellis J. Understanding crossmatch testing in organ transplantation: A case-based guide for the general nephrologist. Nephrology (Carlton). 2011;**16**(2):125-133

[30] Cook DJ et al. The flow cytometry crossmatch in kidney transplantation. Clinical Transplants. 1987:409-414

[31] Tait BD et al. Review article: Luminex technology for HLA antibody detection in organ transplantation. Nephrology (Carlton). 2009;**14**(2):247-254

[32] Taube DH et al. Renal transplantation after removal and prevention of resynthesis of HLA antibodies. Lancet. 1984;**1**(8381):824-828

[33] Palmer A et al. Removal of anti-HLA antibodies by extracorporeal immunoadsorption to enable renal transplantation. Lancet. 1989;**1**(8628):10-12

[34] Fauchald P et al. Plasma exchange and immunoadsorption prior to renal transplantation in allosensitized patients. Transplantation Proceedings. 1990;**22**(1):149-150

[35] Higgins RM et al. 5-year follow-up of patients successfully transplanted after immunoadsorption to remove anti-HLA antibodies. Nephron. 1996;**74**(1):53-57

[36] Halloran PF et al. The significance of the anti-class I antibody response. I. Clinical and pathologic features of anti-class I-mediated rejection. Transplantation. 1990;**49**(1):85-91

[37] Montgomery RA et al. Plasmapheresis and intravenous immune globulin provides effective rescue therapy for refractory humoral rejection and allows kidneys to be successfully transplanted into cross-match-positive recipients. Transplantation. 2000;**70**(6):887-895

[38] Archdeacon P et al. Summary of FDA antibody-mediated rejection workshop. American Journal of Transplantation. 2011;**11**(5):896-906

[39] Roberts DM, Jiang SH, Chadban SJ. The treatment of acute antibody-mediated rejection in kidney transplant recipients-a systematic review. Transplantation. 2012;**94**(8):775-783

[40] Burton SA et al. Treatment of antibody-mediated rejection in renal transplant patients: A clinical practice survey. Clinical Transplantation. 2015;**29**(2):118-123

[41] Wan SS et al. The treatment of antibody-mediated rejection in kidney transplantation: An updated systematic review and meta-analysis. Transplantation. 2018;**102**:557-568

[42] Reeves HM, Winters JL. The mechanisms of action of plasma exchange. British Journal of Haematology. 2014;**164**(3):342-351

[43] Winters JL. Plasma exchange: Concepts, mechanisms, and an overview of the American Society for Apheresis guidelines. Hematology American Society of Hematology Education Program. 2012;**2012**:7-12

[44] Okafor C et al. Introduction and overview of therapeutic apheresis. Journal of Clinical Apheresis. 2010;**25**(5):240-249

[45] Williams ME, Balogun RA. Principles of separation: Indications and therapeutic targets for plasma exchange. Clinical Journal of the American Society of Nephrology. 2014;**9**(1):181-190

[46] Ward DM. Conventional apheresis therapies: A review. Journal of Clinical Apheresis. 2011;**26**(5):230-238

[47] Yamada C et al. Efficacy of plasmapheresis on donor-specific antibody reduction by HLA specificity in post-kidney transplant recipients. Transfusion. 2015;**55**(4):727-735 quiz 726

[48] Cardella CJ et al. Effect of intensive plasma exchange on renal transplant rejection and serum cytotoxic antibody. Transplantation Proceedings. 1978;**10**(3):617-619

[49] Pascual M et al. Plasma exchange and tacrolimus-mycophenolate rescue for acute humoral rejection in kidney transplantation. Transplantation. 1998;**66**(11):1460-1464

[50] Schwenger V, Morath C. Immunoadsorption in nephrology and kidney transplantation. Nephrology, Dialysis, Transplantation. 2010;**25**(8):2407-2413

[51] Belak M et al. Technical and clinical experience with protein a immunoadsorption columns. Transfusion Science. 1994;**15**(4):419-422

[52] Pretagostini R et al. Immunoadsorption with protein a in humoral rejection of kidney transplants. ASAIO Journal. 1996;**42**(5):M645-M648

[53] Bohmig GA et al. C4d-positive acute humoral renal allograft rejection: Effective treatment by immunoadsorption. Journal of the American Society of Nephrology. 2001;**12**(11):2482-2489

[54] Bohmig GA et al. Immunoadsorption in severe C4d-positive acute kidney allograft rejection: A randomized controlled trial. American Journal of Transplantation. 2007;**7**(1):117-121

[55] Nimmerjahn F, Ravetch JV. Anti-inflammatory actions of intravenous immunoglobulin. Annual Review of Immunology. 2008;**26**:513-533

[56] Jordan SC, Toyoda M, Vo AA. Intravenous immunoglobulin a natural regulator of immunity and inflammation. Transplantation. 2009;**88**(1):1-6

[57] Muta T et al. A 13-amino-acid motif in the cytoplasmic domain of Fc gamma RIIB modulates B-cell receptor signalling. Nature. 1994;**369**(6478):340

[58] Kaneko Y, Nimmerjahn F, Ravetch JV. Anti-inflammatory activity of immunoglobulin G resulting from Fc sialylation. Science. 2006;**313**(5787):670-673

[59] Jordan SC. Intravenous gamma-globulin therapy in systemic lupus erythematosus and immune complex disease. Clinical Immunology and Immunopathology. 1989;**53**(2 Pt 2): S164-S169

[60] Anthony RM et al. Intravenous gammaglobulin suppresses inflammation through a novel T(H)2 pathway. Nature. 2011;**475**(7354):110-113

[61] Spycher M et al. In vitro comparison of the complement-scavenging capacity of different intravenous immunoglobulin preparations. Vox Sanguinis. 2009;**97**(4):348-354

[62] Watanabe J, Scornik JC. IVIG and HLA antibodies. Evidence for inhibition of complement activation but not for anti-idiotypic activity. American Journal of Transplantation. 2005;**5**(11):2786-2790

[63] Jordan SC et al. Posttransplant therapy using high-dose human immunoglobulin (intravenous gammaglobulin) to control acute humoral rejection in renal and cardiac allograft recipients and potential mechanism of action. Transplantation. 1998;**66**(6):800-805

[64] Casadei DH et al. A randomized and prospective study comparing treatment with high-dose intravenous immunoglobulin with monoclonal antibodies for rescue of kidney grafts with steroid-resistant rejection. Transplantation. 2001;**71**(1):53-58

[65] Jordan SC et al. Advances in diagnosing and managing antibody-mediated rejection. Pediatric Nephrology. 2010;**25**(10):2035-2045 quiz 2045-8

[66] Lefaucheur C et al. Comparison of combination plasmapheresis/IVIg/anti-CD20 versus high-dose IVIg in the treatment of antibody-mediated rejection. American Journal of Transplantation. 2009;**9**(5):1099-1107

[67] Locke JE et al. The utility of splenectomy as rescue treatment for severe acute antibody mediated rejection. American Journal of Transplantation. 2007;**7**(4):842-846

[68] Tzvetanov I et al. The role of splenectomy in the setting of refractory humoral rejection after kidney transplantation. Transplantation Proceedings. 2012;**44**(5):1254-1258

[69] Kaplan B et al. Successful rescue of refractory, severe antibody mediated rejection with splenectomy. Transplantation. 2007;**83**(1):99-100

[70] Locke JE et al. Rescue splenectomy for severe acute antibody-mediated rejection. Clinical Transplants. 2006:518-520

[71] Roberti I, Geffner S, Vyas S. Successful rescue of refractory acute antibody-mediated renal allograft rejection with splenectomy--a case report. Pediatric Transplantation. 2012;**16**(2):E49-E52

[72] Orandi BJ et al. Splenic irradiation for the treatment of severe antibody-mediated rejection. American Journal of Transplantation. 2016;**16**(10):3041-3045

[73] Maloney DG et al. IDEC-C2B8 (Rituximab) anti-CD20 monoclonal antibody therapy in patients with relapsed low-grade non-Hodgkin's lymphoma. Blood. 1997;**90**(6):2188-2195

[74] Reff ME et al. Depletion of B cells in vivo by a chimeric mouse human monoclonal antibody to CD20. Blood. 1994;**83**(2):435-445

[75] Becker YT et al. Rituximab as treatment for refractory kidney transplant rejection. American Journal of Transplantation. 2004;**4**(6):996-1001

[76] Genberg H et al. Pharmacodynamics of rituximab in kidney allotransplantation. American Journal of Transplantation. 2006;**6**(10):2418-2428

[77] Lehnhardt A et al. Nodular B-cell aggregates associated with treatment refractory renal transplant rejection resolved by rituximab. American Journal of Transplantation. 2006;**6**(4):847-851

[78] Billing H et al. Successful treatment of chronic antibody-mediated rejection with IVIG and rituximab in pediatric renal transplant recipients. Transplantation. 2008;**86**(9):1214-1221

[79] Faguer S et al. Rituximab therapy for acute humoral rejection after kidney transplantation. Transplantation. 2007;**83**(9):1277-1280

[80] Rostaing L, Guilbeau-Frugier C, Kamar N. Rituximab for humoral rejection after kidney transplantation: An update. Transplantation. 2009;**87**(8):1261

[81] Mulley WR et al. A single low-fixed dose of rituximab to salvage renal transplants from refractory antibody-mediated rejection. Transplantation. 2009;**87**(2):286-289

[82] Sautenet B et al. One-year results of the effects of rituximab on acute antibody-mediated rejection in renal transplantation: RITUX ERAH, a multicenter double-blind randomized placebo-controlled trial. Transplantation. 2016;**100**(2):391-399

[83] Perry DK et al. Proteasome inhibition causes apoptosis of normal human plasma cells preventing alloantibody production. American Journal of Transplantation. 2009;**9**(1):201-209

[84] Everly JJ et al. Proteasome inhibition for antibody-mediated rejection. Current Opinion in Organ Transplantation. 2009;**14**(6):662-666

[85] Ejaz NS et al. Review of bortezomib treatment of antibody-mediated rejection in renal transplantation. Antioxidants & Redox Signaling. 2014;**21**(17):2401-2418

[86] Everly MJ et al. Bortezomib provides effective therapy for antibody- and cell-mediated acute rejection. Transplantation. 2008;**86**(12):1754-1761

[87] Idica A et al. Elimination of post-transplant donor-specific HLA antibodies with bortezomib. Clinical Transplants. 2008:229-239

[88] Philogene MC et al. Differential effect of bortezomib on HLA class I and class II antibody. Transplantation. 2014;**98**(6):660-665

[89] Walsh RC et al. Proteasome inhibitor-based primary therapy for antibody-mediated renal allograft rejection. Transplantation. 2010;**89**(3):277-284

[90] Sureshkumar KK et al. Proteasome inhibition with bortezomib: An effective therapy for severe antibody mediated rejection after renal transplantation. Clinical Nephrology. 2012;**77**(3):246-253

[91] Sadaka B et al. Proteasome inhibition for antibody-mediated allograft rejection. Seminars in Hematology. 2012;**49**(3):263-269

[92] Flechner SM et al. The role of proteasome inhibition with bortezomib in the treatment of antibody-mediated rejection after kidney-only or kidney-combined organ transplantation. Transplantation. 2010;**90**(12):1486-1492

[93] Locke JE et al. The use of antibody to complement protein C5 for salvage treatment of severe antibody-mediated rejection. American Journal of Transplantation. 2009;**9**(1):231-235

[94] Orandi BJ et al. Eculizumab and splenectomy as salvage therapy for severe antibody-mediated rejection after HLA-incompatible kidney transplantation. Transplantation. 2014;**98**(8):857-863

[95] Yelken B et al. Eculizumab for treatment of refractory antibody-mediated rejection in kidney transplant patients: A single-center experience. Transplantation Proceedings. 2015;**47**(6):1754-1759

[96] Kocak B et al. Eculizumab for salvage treatment of refractory antibody-mediated rejection in kidney transplant patients: Case reports. Transplantation Proceedings. 2013;**45**(3):1022-1025

[97] Burbach M et al. Report of the inefficacy of eculizumab in two cases of severe antibody-mediated rejection of renal grafts. Transplantation. 2014;**98**(10):1056-1059

[98] Stegall MD et al. Terminal complement inhibition decreases antibody-mediated rejection in sensitized renal transplant recipients. American Journal of Transplantation. 2011;**11**(11):2405-2413

[99] Bentall A et al. Antibody-mediated rejection despite inhibition of terminal complement. Transplant International. 2014;**27**(12):1235-1243

[100] Montgomery RA et al. Plasma-derived C1 esterase inhibitor for acute antibody-mediated rejection following kidney transplantation: Results of a randomized double-blind placebo-controlled pilot study. American Journal of Transplantation. 2016;**16**(12):3468-3478

[101] Vo AA et al. A phase I/II placebo-controlled trial of C1-inhibitor for prevention of antibody-mediated rejection in HLA sensitized patients. Transplantation. 2015;**99**(2):299-308

[102] Viglietti D et al. C1 inhibitor in acute antibody-mediated rejection nonresponsive to conventional therapy in kidney transplant recipients: A pilot study. American Journal of Transplantation. 2016;**16**(5):1596-1603

[103] Nishimoto N, Kishimoto T. Humanized antihuman IL-6 receptor antibody, tocilizumab. Handbook of Experimental Pharmacology. 2008;**181**:151-160

[104] Nechemia-Arbely Y et al. IL-6/IL-6R axis plays a critical role in acute kidney injury. Journal of the American Society of Nephrology. 2008;**19**(6):1106-1115

[105] Budde K, Waiser J, Neumayer HH. The diagnostic value of GM-CSF and IL-6 determinations in patients after renal transplantation. Transplant International. 1994;**7**(Suppl 1): S97-S101

[106] Vo AA et al. A phase I/II trial of the Interleukin-6 receptor-specific humanized monoclonal (Tocilizumab) + intravenous immunoglobulin in difficult to desensitize patients. Transplantation. 2015;**99**(11):2356-2363

[107] Choi J et al. Assessment of tocilizumab (anti-Interleukin-6 receptor monoclonal) as a potential treatment for chronic antibody-mediated rejection and transplant glomerulopathy in HLA-sensitized renal allograft recipients. American Journal of Transplantation. 2017;**17**(9):2381-2389

[108] Colvin RB, Smith RN. Antibody-mediated organ-allograft rejection. Nature Reviews Immunology. 2005;**5**(10):807-817

[109] Orandi BJ et al. Quantifying renal allograft loss following early antibody-mediated rejection. American Journal of Transplantation. 2015;**15**(2):489-498

[110] Gloor J, Stegall MD. Sensitized renal transplant recipients: Current protocols and future directions. Nature Reviews Nephrology. 2010;**6**(5):297-306

[111] Lefaucheur C et al. Preexisting donor-specific HLA antibodies predict outcome in kidney transplantation. Journal of the American Society of Nephrology. 2010;**21**(8):1398-1406

[112] Sellares J et al. Understanding the causes of kidney transplant failure: The dominant role of antibody-mediated rejection and nonadherence. American Journal of Transplantation. 2012;**12**(2):388-399

[113] Loupy A et al. Subclinical rejection phenotypes at 1 year post-transplant and outcome of kidney allografts. Journal of the American Society of Nephrology. 2015;**26**(7):1721-1731

[114] Everly MJ et al. Reducing de novo donor-specific antibody levels during acute rejection diminishes renal allograft loss. American Journal of Transplantation. 2009;**9**(5):1063-1071

[115] Dunn TB et al. Revisiting traditional risk factors for rejection and graft loss after kidney transplantation. American Journal of Transplantation. 2011;**11**(10):2132-2143

[116] Otten HG et al. Pretransplant donor-specific HLA class-I and -II antibodies are associated with an increased risk for kidney graft failure. American Journal of Transplantation. 2012;**12**(6):1618-1623

[117] Willicombe M et al. Antibody-mediated rejection after alemtuzumab induction: Incidence, risk factors, and predictors of poor outcome. Transplantation. 2011;**92**(2):176-182

[118] van den Berg-Loonen EM et al. Clinical relevance of pretransplant donor-directed antibodies detected by single antigen beads in highly sensitized renal transplant patients. Transplantation. 2008;**85**(8):1086-1090

[119] Lefaucheur C et al. IgG donor-specific anti-human HLA antibody subclasses and kidney allograft antibody-mediated injury. Journal of the American Society of Nephrology. 2016;**27**(1):293-304

[120] Loupy A et al. Complement-binding anti-HLA antibodies and kidney-allograft survival. The New England Journal of Medicine. 2013;**369**(13):1215-1226

[121] Yabu JM et al. C1q-fixing human leukocyte antigen antibodies are specific for predicting transplant glomerulopathy and late graft failure after kidney transplantation. Transplantation. 2011;**91**(3):342-347

[122] Sutherland SM et al. Complement-fixing donor-specific antibodies identified by a novel C1q assay are associated with allograft loss. Pediatric Transplantation. 2012;**16**(1):12-17

[123] Bentall A et al. Five-year outcomes in living donor kidney transplants with a positive crossmatch. American Journal of Transplantation. 2013;**13**(1):76-85

[124] Willicombe M et al. De novo DQ donor-specific antibodies are associated with a significant risk of antibody-mediated rejection and transplant glomerulopathy. Transplantation. 2012;**94**(2):172-177

[125] Freitas MC et al. The role of immunoglobulin-G subclasses and C1q in de novo HLA-DQ donor-specific antibody kidney transplantation outcomes. Transplantation. 2013;**95**(9):1113-1119

[126] Everly MJ et al. Beyond histology: Lowering human leukocyte antigen antibody to improve renal allograft survival in acute rejection. Transplantation. 2010;**89**(8):962-967

[127] Jordan SC, Lorant T, Choi J. IgG endopeptidase in highly sensitized patients undergoing transplantation. The New England Journal of Medicine. 2017;**377**(17):1693-1694

[128] Loupy A et al. Molecular microscope strategy to improve risk stratification in early antibody-mediated kidney allograft rejection. Journal of the American Society of Nephrology. 2014;**25**(10):2267-2277

[129] Safa K, Magee CN, Azzi J. A critical review of biomarkers in kidney transplantation. Current Opinion in Nephrology and Hypertension. 2017;**26**(6):509-515

[130] Blydt-Hansen TD et al. Urinary metabolomics for noninvasive detection of antibody-mediated rejection in children after kidney transplantation. Transplantation. 2017;**101**(10):2553-2561

[131] Nissaisorakarn V et al. Urine biomarkers informative of human kidney allograft rejection and tolerance. Human Immunology. 2018

[132] Erpicum P et al. Non-invasive approaches in the diagnosis of acute rejection in kidney transplant recipients, Part II: Omics analyses of urine and blood samples. Clinical Kidney Journal. 2017;**10**(1):106-115

[133] Dharnidharka VR, Malone A. Biomarkers to detect rejection after kidney transplantation. Pediatric Nephrology. 2017. https://doi.org/10.1007/s00467-017-3712-6

4

Pancreas Retrieval for Whole Organ and Islet Cell Transplantation

Wayne J. Hawthorne, Ahmer Hameed and Henry Pleass

Abstract

For more than five decades, we have been refining advances in pancreas whole organ and islet cell transplantation as clinical therapies to treat the ever-increasing number of patients suffering from type-1-diabetes. Research and clinical practice have contributed to making both whole organ and cellular transplantation viable therapeutic options for a broader range of patients. Furthermore, both forms of clinical transplantation results have progressively improved, due to the ongoing refinement of organ donation and its various technical processes, combined with the evolution of immunosuppression and patient care now offering excellent long-term treatment for both type-1-diabetes and concomitant renal failure. This chapter provides an overview on how this has been undertaken and achieved over decades to ultimately provide outstanding outcomes on par with other organ transplantation results. Briefly, we cover the history of pancreas retrieval procedures, the importance of donor selection, the intricate processes of the organ donor operation, preservation of the pancreas, and the ideal ways to best improve outcomes for transplantation. Improving and providing the optimal donor and preservation conditions underpinning the success of subsequent whole pancreas or islet transplantation as a safe, effective, and feasible therapeutic option for an increasing number of patients suffering from type-1-diabetes.

Keywords: diabetes, insulin, islet, islet cell, islet cell allotransplantation, islet cell transplantation, islet cell isolation, organ perfusion, organ retrieval, renal failure, type 1 diabetes, whole organ transplantation

1. Introduction

Since Kelly and colleagues performed the first whole pancreas transplant in 1966, significant advancements in pancreas transplantation have been made. [1] There was a gap following the first series of whole pancreas transplants due to poor graft outcomes with significant impact from poor organ preservation of the pancreas playing a major role. It took almost 20 years for the development of newer surgical techniques including use of newly developed perfusion solutions, segmental grafts, advances in ductal drainage including bladder drainage, and effective immunosuppression regimens such that whole organ transplantation burgeoned, with great advances made by Sutherland and colleagues at the University of Minnesota [2]. However, it was not until much later following many years of experimental research that pancreata for islet cell isolation and transplantation became a reality. Over the past two decades in particular a great deal of effort has underpinned making islet cell transplantation a viable therapy for a broader range of patients with type 1 diabetes (T1D). Clinical results have progressively improved, now demonstrating outcomes on par with other organ transplants, specifically in terms of insulin independence, and graft and patient survival [3]. We are now at the point where islet cell transplantation, in the form of allotransplantation, like its forebear whole organ transplantation, has become widely accepted as a clinical therapy for patients affected by T1D.

Now more than five decades on and with many organ donor operations having been performed since the advent of organ donor procedures as we know them, we have refined and perfected the organ donor process since the first organ retrieval of a brain dead donor in 1963 [4] and the subsequent adoption of the "Acceptance of Brain Death for Organ Donation" issued by the Ad Hoc Committee of the Harvard Medical School [5]. We have seen an increasing emergence of specialized organ retrieval teams with focus on the overwhelming need to improve organ donor rates for the ever increasing recipient patient population [6]. Always a dedicated surgical pursuit, research into organ donation and the surgical retrieval process for the pancreas and most other organs has often been overlooked in favor of recipient-related research into the prevention of rejection, and improving immunosuppression and tissue matching. This is particularly problematic when it comes to whole pancreas and islet transplantation as the pancreas is a less retrieval tolerant organ than other solid organs, and requires extra attention both during and after retrieval to ensure that the organ's valuable islets, which are especially susceptible to hypoxia and the ischemic insult, are effectively preserved [7, 8].

In this chapter we provide a general overview of Pancreas Retrieval for both Whole Organ and Islet Cell Transplantation, but it should be noted that there are clear overlaps in this process for both whole organ and cellular transplantation. As such the way the processes are performed can be utilized for retrieval for either type of subsequent transplant. Overall, we have seen significant improvements to pancreas transplantation results, in particular in the islet cell arena, due to the significant research undertaken to improve graft outcomes by improving donor selection and organ procurement and preservation [9]. On the recipient side we have also further improved outcomes with changes to the transplant and to the pharmacological treatment of recipients such as newer focused monoclonal immunosuppressive strategies that better control graft rejection [9].

This chapter focuses on the optimal process for deceased donor pancreas retrieval and its role in maximizing graft function and survival. However, with a great number of processes to outline, only the major ones will be covered in this chapter. In particular, we will emphasize major improvements in donor selection, surgical retrieval techniques, pancreas retrieval in the context of multi-organ donors, back-table preparation of the pancreas, perfusion fluid types, and future perspectives including the utilization of technologies such as machine perfusion and persufflation. These factors will be discussed in the context of improved outcomes to the engraftment, function and survival of the transplants. It is also acknowledged that there remains the ongoing need for further improvements to both whole organ and islet cell transplantation, however both techniques clearly offer safe and achievable therapeutic options for the ever-expanding number of patients suffering from T1D [10].

2. Historical timeline

The original retrieval processes of the modern era were initially developed for and used in kidney only retrieval surgery. As per **Figure 1** the procedure first introduced in 1963 utilized cold lactated Ringer's or low-molecular-weight dextran solutions infused directly into the renal artery of the retrieved kidneys, performed only after their removal from the donor [11]. These were the beginnings of modern donor retrieval but they were less than ideal techniques due to the time taken to perfuse the organs, and therefore a number of more active and by far more effective methods of perfusion and cooling of organs were subsequently developed in order to minimize ischemic insult and subsequent damage to organs. These techniques were based upon the concepts from cardiothoracic surgery, involving active patient cooling during procedures to prevent ischemic damage [12, 13]. The transplant fraternity quickly adopted these intravascular perfusion-related cooling techniques, which were standardly utilized as a first step in the preservation of all whole-organ grafts. The currently accepted modern cadaveric donor procedure is performed using some basal form of the *ex situ* techniques developed and performed in the mid to late 60's by Starzl and colleagues [14] for not only kidneys but also incorporating the pancreas and liver. Further refinements saw the perfusion and addition of heparin to the perfusate solutions and also the donor. Ensuring removal of blood by *ex situ* perfusion as described by Belzer et al. [15] resulted in improved but only satisfactory kidney preservation of several days. However, this technique was eventually abandoned in most kidney transplant centers when it was learned that the quality of 2-day preservation was no better than with the simpler *"iced slush"* methods [16].

The underpinning method of *iced slush* for shipping was based around experimental work on kidneys [17]. This research and practice focused on perfusion fluids of differing intracellular and extracellular fluids consisting of electrolytes with varying osmotic and oncotic effects that were infused into the allograft before placing it in a cold storage container. Collins

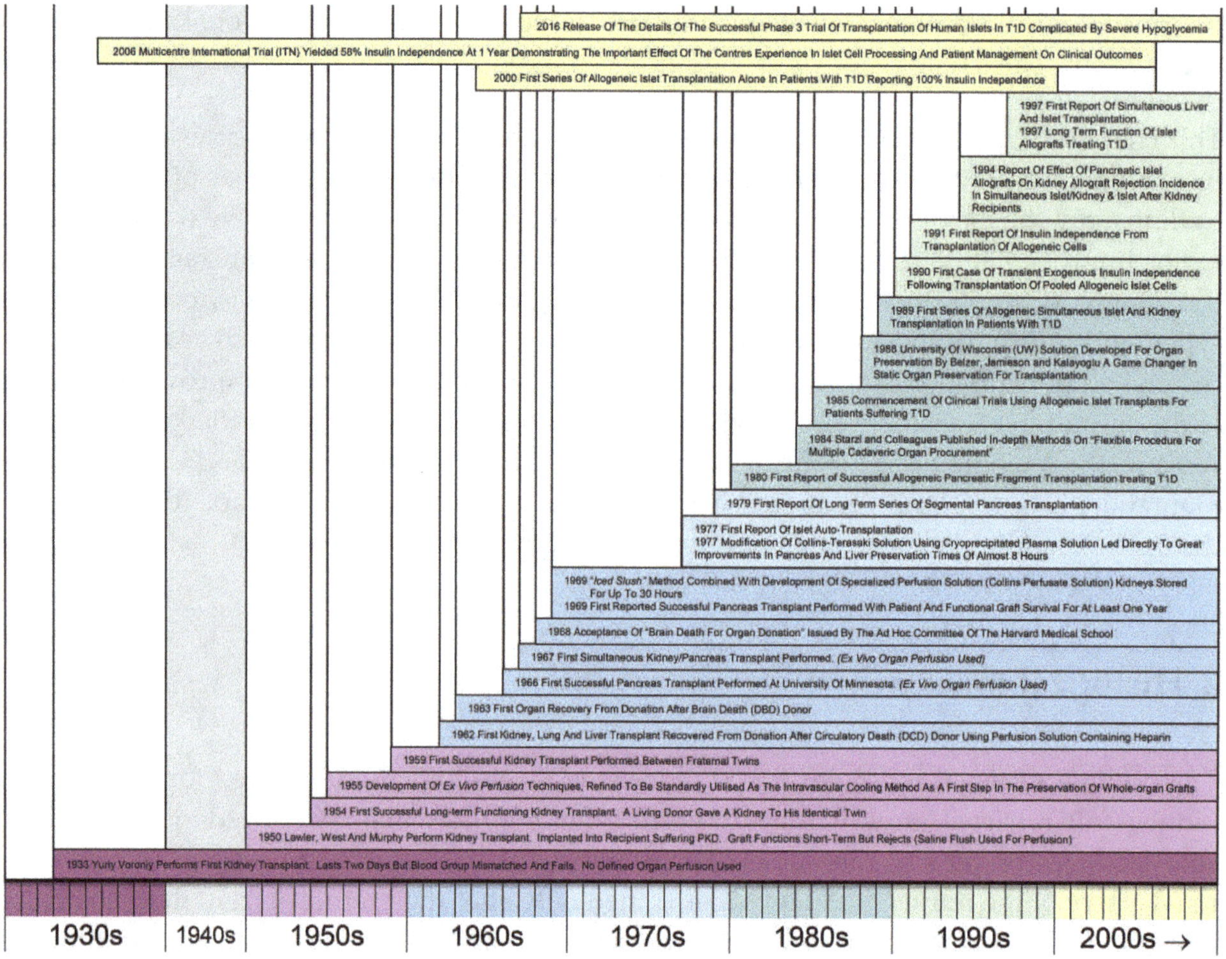

Figure 1. A time line in the significant development of transplantation over the years with focus on the techniques used for whole pancreas and islet cell transplantation.

and colleagues developed a relatively simple technique (infusion of mannitol, phenoxybenzamine, and their Collins perfusate) providing good preservation in kidneys stored for up to 30 hours [17]. Other perfusates, such as Ringer's lactate and 10% invert-sugar solutions, gave inferior results. The new perfusate solution and technique extended the time of simple ice storage from 12 hours to 30 hours. Continuous hypothermic perfusion saw further additions by Ackerman and Snell [18] and Merkel, Jonasson, and Bergan [19] who following many organ donor studies developed the widely accepted and much more simplified core cooling. These utilized cold perfusion solutions with the infusion of the fluids being performed directly to the vascular bed of all the organs via the distal aorta and demonstrated significant improvement for the pancreas but they were still less than ideal for this most sensitive organ. However, the development of these techniques used throughout the 70's meant that organs could generally be removed without causing issues when retrieving multiple organs, which included the liver and sometimes pancreas. Kidney preservation became more feasible along with the other abdominal organs seeing times of 1 to 2 days, long enough to allow tissue matching and sharing of organs between hospital units even interstate or in Europe between countries. However, these were purely focused still on the kidneys rather than the other abdominal organs and as such a number of groups undertook experiments focusing on other organs including the pancreas and liver; landmark papers included those by Benichou et al. [20], using the Collins-Terasaki solution, and de Gruyl et al. [21] using cryoprecipitated plasma perfusion preservation of duct-ligated pancreatic allografts, along with Wall et al. [22] using similar plasma-like solution. This led directly to great improvements in pancreas and liver preservation and allowed organ sharing amongst transplant centers, although the preservation period was still limited to less than 8 hours.

The development of University of Wisconsin (UW) solution for organ preservation by Belzer, Jamieson, and Kalayoglu in the 1980s was a game changer in static organ preservation for transplantation [23]. This new flushout solution for preservation of the pancreas was tested in the dog model of segmental pancreas autotransplantation. The solution has an osmolality of 320 mOsm/L ($K+ = 120$ mM, $Na + = 30$ mM), and contains lactobionate, and raffinose as impermeants. The role of hydroxyethyl starch (HES), the colloid component of UW solution, was shown to be particularly important for pancreas preservation, in comparison to the liver and kidney [24]. UW perfusate solution preservation almost tripled the time of safe preservation of the various organs, including the pancreas, making national sharing of most organs a viable and practical process [25].

However, despite significant success the preservation or extended preservation of the pancreas still required further refinement, and significant research using animal models of static perfusion were pursued, in particular for use in islet cell transplantation. Along with perfusion fluids a number of standardly used retrieval techniques became more readily adopted [19]. However, until 1981 transplantation of the extra-renal organs was an unusual event such that the focus of perfusion only really focused on kidneys. By the mid-1980s, it became apparent that multiple organs would start to become transplanted in earnest, with liver, pancreas and thoracic organ transplant procedures becoming more widely accepted. A safe and effective method for multi-organ procurement and preservation was required by which the abdominal organs, kidneys, liver, and pancreas, could all be suitably retrieved using the same solution. At this stage Starzl and colleagues published an in-depth method on their "flexible procedure for multiple cadaveric organ procurement" [26], which was adopted by many centers worldwide.

However, even at this point the pancreas was often over-looked with the focus on the kidneys and liver as the principal organs to be retrieved. Starzl's publication stated "*If the whole pancreas is transplanted as we recommend, the combination of liver and pancreas removal is incompatible*" and it was often the case when surgical teams were procuring the liver and pancreas together that there were issues relating to the suitable separation of their vasculature [27]. At this time, our own surgical team also retrieved the pancreas with the liver, but always removed liver to the back-table before the pancreas and kidneys. The major perceived reason for this was the need for the life-saving liver to take priority. Furthermore, as the portal vein and the branches of the celiac trunk, drain or supply both organs, preference was given to sacrificing the pancreas' vessels instead of the liver. It was a number of years before this routine surgical practice would change.

Whole organ research utilized canine models as the dog pancreas is more anatomically similar to humans in comparison to the tri-lobed porcine pancreas. These models allowed replication of the clinical situation and further refinement of the retrieval and transplant procedures [28, 29]. From these came the widespread implementation of newer perfusion fluids such as UW solution, and the utilization of vascular extension grafts to the pancreatic vasculature helped resolve the situation of shortened pancreatic inflow and outflow conduits due to preference to the liver in combined retrievals [30]. The other major change to the procedure was the adoption of an *en bloc* liver pancreas retrieval technique, where both organs were rapidly removed in a bloodless field post perfusion, then separated on the back-table. Furthermore, the sharing of organs from a common donor by recipient teams from different units became routine by the early-1990s, in particular due to the use of UW solution, which had clearly been shown to be a real advantage in pancreas retrieval both experimentally and clinically [31].

In the 1990's the focus on research and advances relating to the retrieval process started to shift, with attention once again shifting to the perfusate solutions, which were thought to be especially impactful for islet cell transplantation. A number of groups also investigated additives to the perfusate solutions such as the use of antibodies to reduce inflammation and further improve graft outcomes, although this was met with limited success [32]. In the 2000's it became generally accepted this was achieved via cannulation of the aorta alone, with or without additional access to the portal venous system with variations that have been seen specifically in relation to multiorgan retrieval where some groups chose to perform 'dual' perfusion technique which are all discussed in greater detail later in this chapter [33, 34].

3. Use of the pancreas for whole organ or cellular transplantation—donor selection

Underpinning the entire transplantation process, regardless of whether the donor is for whole pancreas or islet cell transplantation, is appropriate donor selection such that the donor organ is of a suitable size and quality to allow for use in either type of therapy. In order to be utilized in clinical transplantation, it is imperative that the donor be appropriately screened to ensure the organ to be retrieved is free from any disease that may subsequently manifest in the donor, including cancer, and infections with viruses, bacteria, fungi, or prions [9]. It is paramount that we avoid the more commonly occurring diseases when screening the donor before accepting the pancreas for organ donor retrieval and subsequent clinical transplantation. Infectious risk factors depend on the history of patient, any underlying disease of the organ donor, and the immunosuppressive treatment administered to the recipient [35]. Transmission of most pathogens is possible, but their frequency varies according to the endemic population from the transplanted organ, the selected immunosuppressive therapy and prophylaxis utilized in the recipient, and also at the donor procedure [36]. Obviously, there are many more variables with regards to organ donor selection criteria, and these will be discussed in more detail in the following sections.

4. Pancreas retrieval

4.1. Surgical techniques

Pancreas retrieval for both whole organ and cellular transplantation necessitates meticulous surgical technique. In comparison to the liver and kidneys, the pancreas is more commonly damaged at retrieval, which subsequently results in non-utilization of a significant proportion of procured pancreata [37]. The organ must be procured without any parenchymal and/or capsular breach, and its arterial inflow and venous outflow vessels must be clearly identified (tagged) and maintained for subsequent back-table reconstruction when used for whole pancreas [38]. The extent of organ and vascular dissection depends upon whether the retrieval is from a brain-dead (DBD) or circulatory death (DCD) donor; a large proportion of pancreas dissection can be undertaken in the warm phase for DBD donors, whilst pursuit of the DCD pathway necessitates wholly cold-phase dissection, which is potentially more difficult as appropriate anatomy is harder to identify.

4.1.1. Anatomical considerations

The pancreas is situated in the retroperitoneum, nestled within the curvature of the duodenum. Important relations are both kidneys posteriorly, the spleen laterally and attached to the pancreas via its pedicle contained within the lienorenal ligament, the superior mesenteric vessels, bile duct, and portal vein in the region of the pancreatic head/neck, the inferior vena cava (IVC) deep to the head and portal vein, and the aorta, left suprarenal gland and left renal vein deep to the body. Pancreatic blood supply is primarily derived from the celiac artery in origin via the splenic and superior mesenteric arteries (via the inferior pancreaticoduodenal artery), and also the gastroduodenal artery (via the superior pancreaticoduodenal artery). The celiac trunk gives off the splenic artery, which emerges at the upper pancreatic border and runs along this border in a tortuous fashion until turning towards the splenic hilum within the lienorenal ligament. The superior mesenteric artery (SMA) emerges from the aorta inferior to the celiac trunk, and is directed inferiorly on the posterior aspect of the pancreatic neck, to then lie on the uncinate process and then the 3rd part of the duodenum prior to entering the root of the mesentery. Venous drainage occurs via the splenic vein for a large part of the pancreas, whilst the superior and inferior pancreaticoduodenal veins drain the head into the superior mesenteric vein (SMV) and portal vein confluence. It is the shared vasculature of the pancreas with the liver that often causes retrieval issues as the origin of the splenic artery is from the celiac, and the outflow of the splenic vein is through the portal vein, necessitating delicate surgical dissection and care in separation to ensure shared and usable vasculature for both organs [39].

4.1.2. DBD retrievals—pancreas-specific considerations

Pancreas retrieval in the DBD donor is a controlled process that allows significant preliminary organ and vascular pedicle dissection. The Cattell-Braasch maneuver is utilized to expose the aorta and IVC distally, with the proximal extent of dissection limited by the SMA overlying the left renal vein; this maneuver will incorporate mobilization of the small bowel mesentery and pancreatic head/duodenum [40]. Our approach to exposure and dissection of the remaining pancreas [41] is to access the lesser sac by mobilization of the greater curvature of the stomach; the greater omentum is detached at its origin using ultrasonic shears (Harmonic Scalpel) as per **Figure 2**. The short gastric vessels are also detached using this method at the upper portion of the greater curvature. The splenic flexure of the large bowel can thence be mobilized onto the lower pole of the spleen. Once the spleen is free of its surrounding attachments, it can be lifted and used as a handle to mobilize the tail and body of the pancreas without directly handling the pancreas itself. The Harmonic Scalpel is also very useful in the dissection of the superior and inferior pancreatic borders, particularly the relatively vascular splenic flexure of the colon. The posterior surface of the pancreas can be mobilized with standard electrocautery in a relatively bloodless plane. The SMA/SMV pedicle inferior to the pancreas needs to be skeletonized such that it can be divided using a vascular stapler prior to pancreas removal in the cold phase. Superiorly, the bile duct is ligated and transected proximal to the point of ligation; residual bile is flushed out its open proximal end using saline instilled into the gallbladder. We will also free attachments around the gastroduodenal junction and duodenojejunal flexure, which are then identified with circumferential vessel loops for stapled division later in the cold phase. The inferior mesenteric vein is ligated *in situ* post perfusion as subsequent retraction of the divided vessel may make it difficult to identify on the back-table. Diluted povidone-iodine solution is instilled into the duodenum via a nasogastric tube as a decontamination step, and is subsequently removed through the same route. Some authors report concerns with subsequent duodenal mucosal toxicity related to instillation of povidone-iodine, and

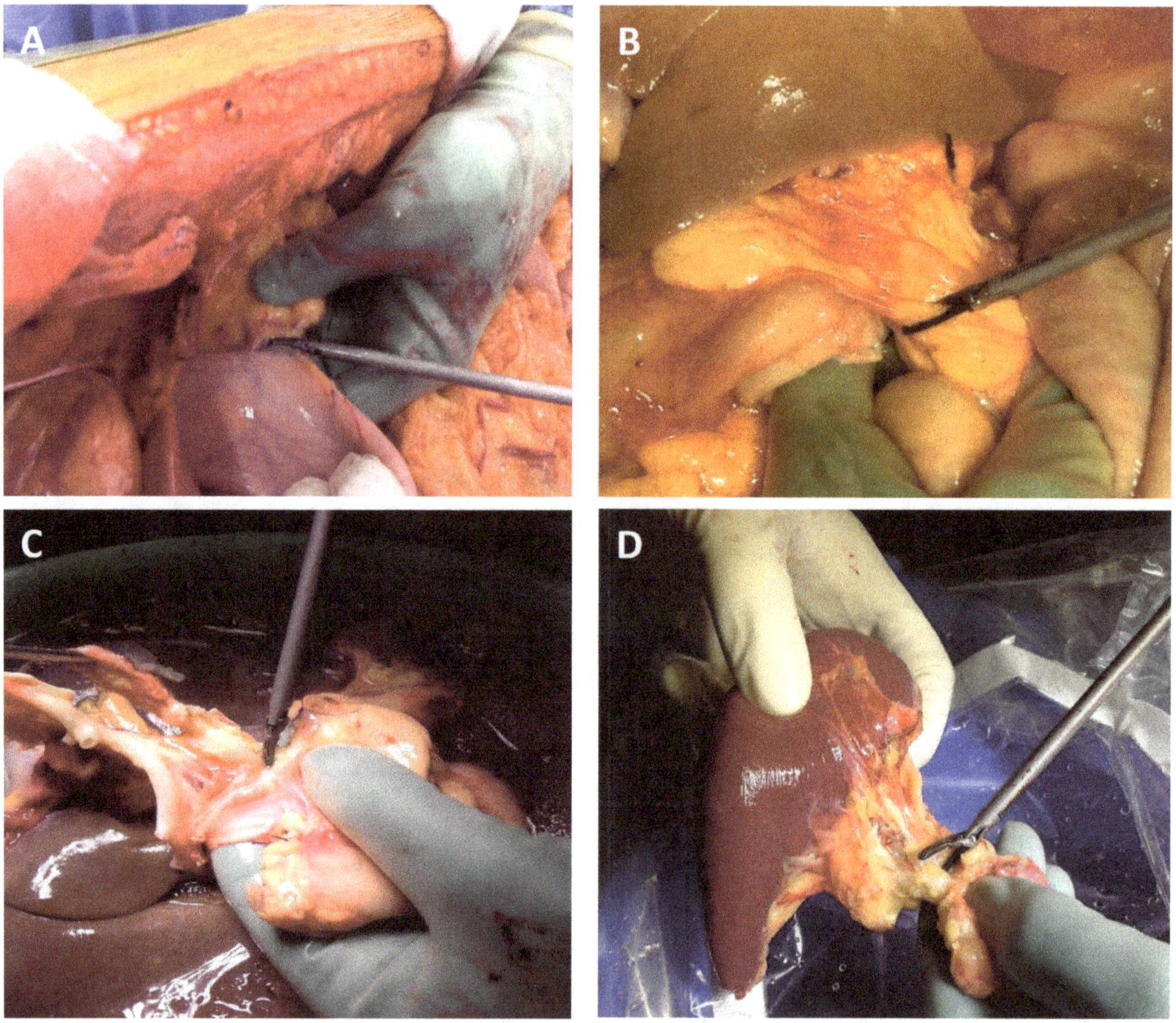

Figure 2. The harmonic scalpels utilization during pancreas procurement. (A) Mobilization of the greater curvature of the stomach, (B) creation of the superior mesenteric pedicle (cold phase), and back-table separation of (C) the liver-pancreas block, and (D) the pancreas and spleen.

suggest additional back-table flushing of the duodenum with an alternate solution [42, 43]. Alternatively, duodenal decontamination can be completed using an antibiotic solution, such as amphotericin [40]. However, the most important factor is to utilize a decontamination procedure to reduce the potential risk of cross infection to the recipient. Our own unit has utilized povidone-iodine solution instilled into the duodenum via a nasogastric tube as a decontamination step in more than 500 SPK transplants at our own center with no duodenal mucosal toxicity identified [44]. In the cold phase the duodenum is then divided above and below the pancreatic head with a linear cutting stapler, after carefully withdrawing the nasogastric tube from the duodenum into the body of the stomach. Any remaining superior mesenteric pedicle dissection is also completed, and a vascular (cutting) stapler is utilized to divide this pedicle. It is of paramount importance that the pancreas is not injured during this step as this will cause serious issues in both whole organ and islet cell transplantation. Furthermore, if the mesenteric pedicle is divided too close to the pancreas, or includes part of the uncinate process, there is a risk that blood supply to the pancreatic head via the inferior pancreaticoduodenal branch of the SMA will be compromised, creating a significant problem for whole organ transplantation [40, 45, 46]. Additionally, for the whole organ transplant an arterial and venous conduit should be retrieved for back-table pancreatic vascular reconstruction. This usually consists of a segment of the external iliac vein for use as a portal vein extension graft if required, and the common iliac artery bifurcation, including a length of the internal and external iliac arteries, to fashion a Y-graft connecting the native SMA and splenic artery. It is essential that the common iliac bifurcation is not damaged during this process [45]. Like a number of other major units our center preferentially retrieves the pancreas *en bloc* with the liver, with separation of both organs performed on the back-table (see below) [47].

4.1.3. DCD retrievals

DCD pancreas retrieval is technically feasible, and can achieve excellent outcomes in selected donors certainly in the whole organ arena (see Outcomes, below). In contrast to DBD procurement, the first step in all DCD retrievals after a rapid laparotomy is cannulation and cold perfusion via the aorta [48, 49]. Venous venting is conducted via the IVC. Alternatively, if local laws allow, an *in situ* flush can be achieved using femoral cannulae inserted prior to the withdrawal of life support [49, 50]. Ante-mortem interventions including heparinization have been shown to also provide significant improvements to pancreas retrieval outcomes in the DCD setting [51]. Standard pancreas retrieval can then be undertaken as described for DBD donors, although donor hemostasis is no longer a concern and therefore sharp dissection is commonly utilized. The use of energy devices such as the Harmonic Scalpel at this stage may help minimize recipient bleeding however, as described in the DBD setting.

4.1.4. Pancreas retrieval and multi-organ donors

Pancreas retrieval is almost never undertaken in isolation, but rather it is usually procured in the context of a multi-organ retrieval, often in the presence of multiple retrieval teams. Meticulous retrieval technique therefore needs to be maintained and balanced in the presence of these competing factors, especially in the presence of concomitant liver procurement, which is still given preference owing to the critical requirement of liver transplant recipients.

Pancreas-alone donors are uncommon in this day and age due to developments in procurement and preservation techniques. Some authors raised concerns that combined liver-pancreas retrieval, in contrast to pancreas retrieval alone, resulted in significant "flush" injury to the pancreas owing to a higher volume of perfusion solution and the utilization of dual aorto-portal cannulation in the combined donors [52]. However, other studies clearly demonstrated that multi-organ retrieval, including combined liver-pancreas retrieval, was not detrimental to pancreas transplantation outcomes [53–58]. Another factor that previously precluded combined liver-pancreas procurement was aberrant hepatic arterial anatomy, in particular the presence of an aberrant or accessory right hepatic artery originating from the superior mesenteric artery [58]. Abandoning retrieval of the pancreas due to this situation is now rare, as a preserved length of the right hepatic artery originating from the SMA stump can effectively be anastomosed to the GDA as part of a back-table reconstructive procedure [45, 46]. It is only when the right hepatic artery is within the substance of the pancreas that whole pancreas retrieval should be precluded in favor of the liver [59] but the pancreas can still be retrieved for islet cell isolation as the pancreas can still be readily perfused, and on the back table the vessels readily separated, including if necessary taking them from the body of the pancreas [9]. However, if this is undertaken then care should be taken to not damage the parenchyma of the pancreas as this makes the distension of the pancreas with collagenase for digestion more difficult [9]. Over the last 25 years and more than 1000 retrievals the authors have never found any anatomical vascular anomaly to prevent an *en bloc* liver-pancreas retrieval, although this is cited as a common reason to decline pancreas retrieval worldwide.

4.1.5. Back-table separation of the liver-pancreas block and further back-table preparation of the pancreas

The combined liver-pancreas block is taken to the back-table for separation. The aortic segment is divided such that the proximal portion of the SMA remains with the pancreas, whilst the celiac axis remains in continuity with the liver. Superior to the pancreatic head, the portal vein is divided approximately 1 cm from the pancreas, whilst the splenic artery is divided closer to its emergence from the celiac axis [45, 46]. The GDA is ligated and divided prior to entering the pancreas; a longer length remains with the liver. The splenic artery and portal vein associated with the pancreas should be marked with a prolene suture to facilitate identification at the transplant center. The spleen is also routinely removed at the donor hospital, in addition to skeletonization of the pancreas prior to transportation. The Harmonic Scalpel is once again a useful tool that facilitates all pancreas-related back-table work if the graft is to be used for whole pancreas transplantation [41]. Limited back-table perfusion of the pancreas with UW solution is employed to ensure no blood is left within the organ or its vessels, whilst minimizing the risk of graft pancreatitis or edema.

In pancreas retrievals for islet cell isolation, the author's use a similar en bloc technique, with careful mobilization of the pancreas prior to aortic cannulation as per **Figure 3**. However, there is no need for meticulous hemostasis post perfusion and it is not necessary to remove the bulk of the tissues as this can be performed at the islet isolation facility. At the isolation center, the duodenum, spleen, and connective, extracapsular and vascular tissues are removed from the pancreas prior to it being cannulated to allow infusion of the digestive collagenase enzyme for

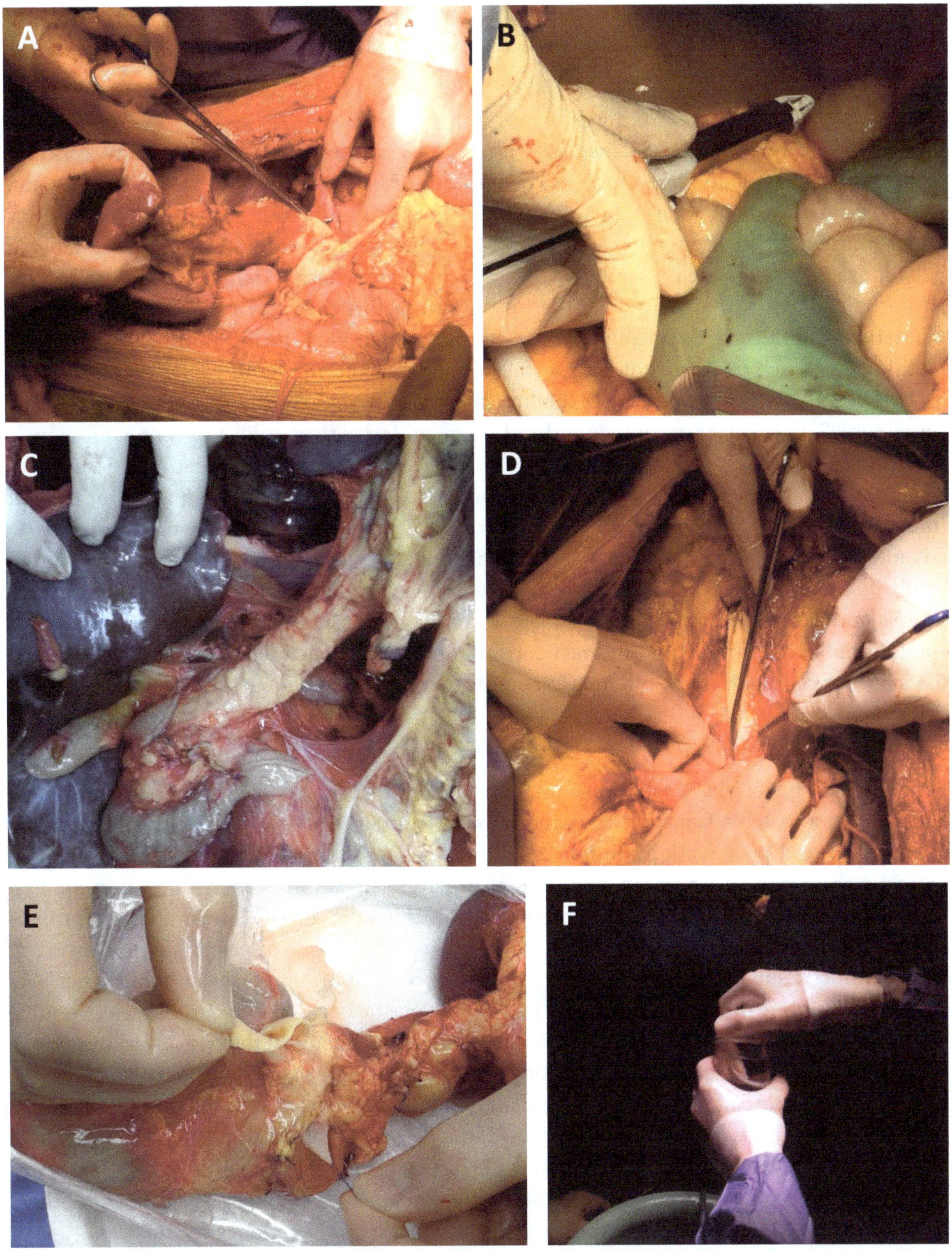

Figure 3. Procurement of the DBD pancreas. (A) Skeletonization of the pancreas, using the spleen as a handle, (B) stapled division of the superior mesenteric pedicle, (C) liver and pancreas ready for en bloc removal, (D) division of the aorta, (E) pancreas appearance after back-table preparation (n.b. Portal vein and superior mesenteric artery), and (F) back-table packing of iliac conduits in preservation solution.

islet cell isolation [9]. As such there is also no need for preservation of pancreas vasculature, which can be given wholly to the liver when separated on the back-table.

4.1.6. Pancreatic inspection and graft assessment

The pancreas must be closely inspected during the retrieval process, and any concerns regarding organ quality and/or integrity should be fully conveyed to the implanting surgeon. Graft assessment should include qualities inherent to the donor pancreas, in addition to any retrieval-related damage, and should be made both *in situ* and on the back-table as per **Figure 3**. The pancreas should be assessed for parenchymal damage, capsular breach, and/or hematoma(s). Furthermore, other important factors that may preclude further transplantation individually or in combination should be identified, including fibrosis, mass(es), high intra-parenchymal fat content, calcification, edema, and/or significantly diseased arteries [40, 46, 59]. It is important to note that much of this assessment is highly subjective, and an "acceptable" pancreatic appearance and/or texture will vary from center-to-center. Obviously some of the co-factors such as high intra-parenchymal fat content, calcification, edema, and/or significantly diseased arteries do not preclude the pancreas from being used for cellular transplantation. As an example, high intra-parenchymal fat content has been shown to be an advantage when performing islet isolation. Additionally, calcification, edema, and/or significantly diseased arteries do not affect the pancreas when used for islet cell isolation as all blood vessels and extraneous tissues are stripped from the pancreas prior to its use. The pancreas should not be discarded without direct consultation with the recipient team and exploration of its use for cellular transplantation if precluded from whole organ transplantation [9].

4.1.7. Packaging the organ for transport

Following perfusion, back-table dissection, and final inspection, the pancreas can then be packed into a suitable transport container along with perfusate solution to ensure ongoing exposure to cold preservation solution. Our unit uses the sterile triple plastic bag technique whereby the organ and a suitable volume of organ perfusion fluid is instilled into the first sterile plastic bag, without dilution from iced slush. All air is removed from the bag, prior to sealing it with a zip-tie or heavy tie. This bag is then placed inside a second sterile plastic bag filled with iced slush, ensuring close and adequate cooling of the perfusate-filled inner bag. These two bags are then placed inside a third sterile plastic bag that is securely sealed, double tied, and appropriately labeled to identify the organ and contents of the bags. Additional vessels retrieved for back-table reconstruction of the whole pancreas may also be packed into the triple sterile plastic bag set with the pancreas, or alternatively are placed inside a sterile vessel jar filled with preservation solution as per **Figure 3**, which is then double-bagged in sterile plastic bags, the first of which contains iced slush. The sealed pancreas and vessels are thence transported in a suitable, insulated iced shipping container. The container is labeled with its contents along with the contact details for both the donor and recipient coordinators.

4.2. In situ perfusion and cold static preservation

The function of *in situ* perfusion of the pancreas, as with other organs, is to achieve rapid removal of residual blood, whilst simultaneously cooling the organ and exposing it to preservation fluid media for subsequent cold static storage (CS).

4.2.1. Perfusion route

In order to achieve adequate *in situ* pancreatic perfusion during abdominal organ perfusion as a whole, the aorta must be securely cannulated and flushed using pressure such that perfusion media can flow into the pancreas via the superior mesenteric, gastroduodenal, and splenic arteries. Once perfusion fluid has traversed the pancreas, it must be allowed to exit the donor's vasculature via the systemic and/or portal routes to prevent graft edema. Aortic-only perfusion is routinely performed by our center, and subsequent venous venting is usually undertaken via the IVC in the thorax. In the event that dual aorto-portal perfusion is employed for combined liver-pancreas retrievals, portal venous access via an inferior mesenteric cannula can impede pancreatic outflow, and reduce the physiologic arterial-portal pressure difference that is required for pancreatic perfusion/flow [42, 60]. As such, in these cases, the portal vein may instead be accessed after dividing it superior to the pancreas, thereby also allowing unobstructed pancreatic venous drainage via the proximal aspect of the transected portal vein [60, 61]. A further back-table flush of the pancreas at the donor center is sometimes conducted via the splenic artery and SMA, although this step may be omitted [45, 62–65]. Evidence for or against either approach is currently lacking in both the case of whole pancreas and cellular transplantation. But preference in the cellular setting appears to favor not having any over-perfusion or edema as this can impede and dilute the infusion of the collagenase used for digestion of the pancreas in the isolation process [66].

4.2.2. Perfusion fluid types

In general, the same final fluid employed for the final *in situ* flush of the pancreas is then utilized for preservation of the organ in a bag of cold preservation fluid (CS). The preservation fluid utilized must maintain the organ at a hypothermic temperature (0–4°C), whilst simultaneously ameliorating the consequences of cold ischemia and prolonged organ immersion in fluid. As such, cold organ preservation fluids should ideally have the following properties that aim to minimize and/or reverse cellular and subcellular processes occurring within the pancreas during CS:

- Disrupted ionic pumps and ion accumulation and/or depletion, with subsequent downstream effects;
- Mitochondrial dysfunction, including reversal of the electron transport chain, and succinate accumulation;
- Altered redox potentials (RP);
- Cellular edema;
- Acidosis;
- Accumulation of reactive oxygen species (ROS);
- Adenosine triphosphate (ATP) depletion; and,
- Disruption in glycolytic pathways [67–69].

There are multiple preservation fluids currently in existence. These can be broadly classified as those that are intracellular and extracellular/intermediate in nature, based largely upon the solution's potassium content, or low viscosity compared to high viscosity solutions [70]. Common components include colloid and/or impermeants to counteract cellular edema, anti-oxidants for protection against ROS generation, ATP precursors to allow replenishment upon reperfusion, and buffers to retard the acidosis attendant with organ ischemia [70].

University of Wisconsin (UW) solution remains the most popular pancreatic preservation fluid, and was initially developed specifically for this purpose [71]. It is an intracellular solution with a high potassium content and high viscosity as it contains hydroxyethyl starch, a particularly important component for pancreas preservation [24]. UW contains other components that fulfill many ideal criteria that should be exhibited by preservation fluids, including the addition of impermeants such as raffinose, the ATP precursor adenosine, and anti-oxidants such as allopurinol. [68] Histidine-tryptophan-ketoglutarate (HTK) is another commonly utilized preservation fluid for the pancreas. In contrast to UW, HTK it is an "intermediate" solution with a significantly lower potassium and sodium concentration, thereby in effect preventing ongoing organ metabolism. HTK also has low viscosity, theoretically allowing higher flow rates, and the histidine component of HTK provides it with significant buffering capacity [68, 70]. The next most commonly studied and clinically utilized pancreas perfusion and preservation fluid is Celsior, which has similar potassium content to HTK in addition to containing histidine as a buffer. It differs from HTK in that it has much higher sodium content; furthermore, it incorporates some of the advantageous constituents of UW, including similar impermeants and one shared anti-oxidant [68, 70]. Most recently, the use of Institut Georges Lopez (IGL-1) solution has been reported in pancreatic transplantation [72]. This solution has similar constituents to UW, except the sodium and potassium concentrations are reversed such that it more closely resembles the extra-cellular environment [68]. A number of other more recently developed perfusion fluids have shown good effect in the preservation of pancreata for islet cell transplantation in particular the ET-Kyoto perfusion fluid. This fluid has a high sodium:low potassium ratio, and contains trehalose to protect the cell membrane against hypothermia and the nitric oxide donor nitroglycerin that facilitates vasodilatation [73].

National guidelines and/or protocols differ with respect to recommended perfusion and preservation fluids for the pancreas [45, 60, 74, 75]. UW and HTK solutions are the two most frequently recommended solutions for pancreas retrieval by such guidelines, although their utilization and volumes vary significantly. UK guidelines stipulate that *in situ* UW perfusion must be undertaken for pancreas retrieval, whilst Eurotransplant, German, and Australia/New Zealand guidelines allow for either UW or HTK. Furthermore, none of these guidelines preclude dual perfusion when the pancreas is being retrieved, although German standards stipulate portal venous perfusion via a catheter inserted directly into the portal vein above the pancreas/duodenum [45, 60, 74, 75]. The use of Celsior or IGL-1 solution has not yet been incorporated into major National or Regional guidelines, although both have been employed in the clinical context [64, 65, 72, 76].

A "pre-flush" is defined as a crystalloid fluid, such as Hartmann's solution, that is perfused *in situ* prior to the final flush/preservation fluid, such as UW. The pre-flush can be employed safely in pancreatic procurement, although it is not commonly utilized. The function of this pre-flush in the context of pancreas procurement is to potentially (1) reduce the amount of UW required, thereby reducing retrieval costs, and (2) to clear all blood from the vasculature such that any residual blood does not aggregate with the hydroxyethyl starch in UW [77, 78].

UW is traditionally perfused in much lower volumes in comparison to HTK, and this is also reflected in the various pancreas retrieval guidelines in existence. This is largely related to the higher viscosity of UW, in addition to the larger volume and time for HTK perfusion to achieve equilibration of electrolyte content with the extracellular milieu [79, 80]. Australian guidelines recommend a 2–4 L crystalloid/low viscosity solution *in situ* pre-flush, followed by a UW flush of at least 1–2 L; a volume range for HTK is not specified [45]. In contrast, UK guidelines state a UW flush of 50–70 ml/kg should be employed via the aorta, whilst Eurotransplant allows for 50–100 ml/kg UW or 150–300 ml/kg HTK [74, 75]. Published reports may deviate from this; perfusion volumes utilized in aortic-only perfusion range from 0.8–5.6 L, 4.9–9.7 L, and 0.8–7.9 L for UW, HTK, and Celsior respectively [81].

4.2.3. *Additive(s) to perfusate*

Heparin is a standard additive to the *in situ* perfusion fluid during DCD organ retrievals, including for the pancreas. Additionally, thrombolytics such as streptokinase or tissue plasminogen activator (tPA) can be added to the *in situ* perfusion fluid, or alternatively our approach is to directly inject tPA into the aorta before commencement of the cold *in situ* flush; the aim of this is to achieve a higher quality vascular flush through the clearance of microthrombi [82–84]. However no comparative evidence exists for or against the use of thrombolytics in DCD pancreas retrieval, although there is certainly enthusiasm for this approach [83, 85].

4.2.4. *Two-layer method*

Great focus has remained on improving the quality of pancreas transport to the islet transplant centers, including novel ways to provide oxygen rich media to the graft whilst in cold storage during shipping. In late 1988 Kuroda et al. was the first to report the use of the Two-Layer Method (TLM) for shipping of the pancreas prior to islet cell isolation [86]. The TLM uses a perfluorochemical (PFC) and the organ perfusion fluid; initially Euro-Collins' solution was used but was replaced by UW solution. The benefits of the use of the PFC are due to it being a biologically inert liquid that acts as an oxygen-supplying media. A pancreas preserved using the TLM is theoretically oxygenated through the PFC and substrates are supplied by the UW solution. This allows the pancreas preserved using the TLM to generate adenosine triphosphate during storage, prolonging the preservation time [87]. Strong debate still remains over its benefits, if any, when compared to the use of UW solution during CS [88, 89] and a recent publication of guidelines recommended against the use of the TLM for preservation of the pancreas preceding islet isolation [85].

5. Outcomes

5.1. Whole organ pancreas transplant outcomes

Vascularized pancreas transplantation outcomes have improved considerably over time. Although changes to immunosuppression and post-transplantation care can partly account for this, advances in retrieval surgery and organ preservation, in addition to better donor selection, are significant contributors [90, 91]. When exploring pancreas transplantation outcomes, it is paramount to account for the type of transplant performed, as these are associated with differential graft success and survival rates. More specifically, outcomes must be considered based on whether a simultaneous pancreas-kidney (SPK), pancreas after kidney (PAK) transplant, or pancreas transplant alone (PTA) was performed. An exploration of general pancreas transplantation outcomes is beyond the scope of this chapter, as the focus is on the specific impact of retrieval and preservation practices. Overviews investigating trends and recipient outcomes following pancreas transplantation have been published by others, including Dean et al., and Gruessner et al. [90–94]. In brief, the current expected 5-year graft and patient survival rates for pancreas (SPK) transplantation range from 73 to 82% and 89 to 93%, respectively, in the US, UK, Eurotransplant region, and Australia/New Zealand [91, 94–96]. Outcome differences are seen between SPKs, which have historically provided better results, and PTAs and PAKs, due to important variations in the type(s) of recipients for each transplant type, technical differences in the transplantation procedure, and a differential ability to diagnose and treat rejection episodes [91]. SPK transplantation is by far the most commonly performed type of pancreas transplant but islet cell transplantation has also seen a great increase in acceptance and success.

5.2. Islet cell transplant outcomes

Like its forebear, islet cell transplantation outcomes have improved considerably over time. The most impactful change was seen with advances in immunosuppression, clearly shown by the success of the Edmonton trial [97], one that revolutionized the progress of the cellular transplant. Other factors have also continued to impact the field, including post-transplantation care, advances in retrieval surgery and organ preservation, in addition to better donor selection. In brief, the most recent presentation from the Collaborative Islet transplant registry (CITR), presented the combined world islet cell transplant data where they reported that over 1055 allogeneic islet transplants have now been reported by 50 islet transplantation centers in Australia, Europe, North America, and Asia. Of these cases, islet transplant alone (ITA) was the most frequent procedure (n = 858) followed by islet after kidney (IAK) and simultaneous islet and kidney transplantation (SIK) (n = 197) [98]. More recently, according to outcomes of the Phase 3 Trial of Transplantation of Human Islets in Type 1 Diabetes Complicated by Severe Hypoglycemia, the primary end point of HbA1c < 7.0% was achieved by 87.5% of subjects at 1 year and by 71% at 2 years. The median HbA1c level was 5.6% at both 1 and 2 years. Hypoglycemia awareness was restored, with highly significant improvements in Clarke and HYPO scores (P > 0.0001). No study-related deaths or disabilities occurred [99]. This trial clearly demonstrated the significant improvements achieved in the outcomes of islet cell transplantation and its impact on those patients suffering from hypoglycemic unawareness.

5.3. The impact of procurement practices and techniques

Pancreas procurement techniques can significantly impact subsequent transplantation outcomes, and can also prove the difference between organ utilization and discard. In particular, there is ample evidence that factors such as *en bloc* retrieval, retrieval technique and graft handling, type(s) of instruments utilized, and perfusion routes are all important determinants of graft function and transplant-related morbidity. Ensuring that pancreas retrieval is performed by an experienced pancreatic transplant surgeon can significantly minimize such retrieval-related complications and risks [100].

Pancreatic damage during retrieval is not uncommon, and may deem the organ unusable certainly for whole organ transplant. Although the rates are different between centers and of course depends upon the level of training of the surgeons performing the retrievals, a large UK registry analysis showed a greater than 50% rate of surgical damage in retrieved pancreata; furthermore, approximately 10% of grafts were subsequently discarded due to damage sustained at retrieval in this analysis [37]. This was further seen as a significant loss as the grafts were also not utilized for islet cell transplantation due to extended cold ischemic times as a result of ongoing referrals. Within the same series, parenchymal and/or vascular (arterial) damage at procurement contributed to significantly higher rates of subsequent graft loss if the pancreas proceeded to transplantation [37]. In order to minimize surgical retrieval damage it is best to ensure that the staff performing the surgery are at a more senior level, and therefore our unit always sends a senior experienced surgeon to all pancreas retrieval surgeries to ensure adequate training of junior staff and optimize graft quality.

Graft thrombosis is the most important technical cause of whole organ pancreatic allograft loss. Pancreas retrieval and surgical technique is a significant etiologic factor in the incidence of graft thrombosis [101–104]. Graft pancreatitis, which in itself is a significant risk factor for graft thrombosis, is another potentially catastrophic complication associated with morbidity and graft loss that is partly attributable to retrieval technique [100]. Excessive graft handling and poor retrieval surgical technique, including damage to the inferior pancreaticoduodenal artery, are commonly accepted causes of graft pancreatitis in the recipient. [100] The same contributing factors also have an impact on the organs when they are used for islet cell isolation [9].

En bloc procurement of the liver and pancreas is associated with better recipient outcomes owing to faster organ retrieval and therefore shorter warm ischemia times [58, 100]. Interestingly, in the aforementioned UK registry analysis between 2008 and 2012, although the vast majority of liver and pancreas retrievals were not performed *en bloc*, there was a trend favoring the *en bloc* approach with respect to reduced pancreatic retrieval injury [37].

In situ perfusion routes, in particular the utilization of dual aorto-portal perfusion in preference to aortic-only perfusion, can impact both whole organ and cellular allograft outcomes. Dual perfusion is potentially associated with increased retrieval-related pancreatic injury through a combination of flush injury (increased perfusion volumes), and/or an obstruction of pancreatic portal venous outflow secondary to catheter placement within the inferior or superior mesenteric veins [52, 58]. This ultimately impacts on the pancreas that is retrieved for whole pancreas or cellular transplantation as it can cause a significant increase in edema, and may be associated with a higher rate of graft pancreatitis in whole organ, and poorer isolation results due to collagenase dilution in the islet isolation process. Importantly, an aortic-only perfusion technique does not seem to compromise hepatic allograft outcomes, especially in the standard criteria DBD donors from which pancreata are usually retrieved, and therefore should be considered by retrieval surgeons in these circumstances especially in centers that retrieve grafts for both whole and cellular transplantation [34, 58].

Furthermore, the specific instrument-type employed for pancreatic dissection is an important determinant of the amount of pancreatic bleeding upon reperfusion in the recipient [46]. We have shown that ultrasonic shear (e.g. Harmonic Scalpel) utilization during pancreas retrieval allows the sealing of peri-pancreatic vessels that are otherwise easily missed, thereby contributing to less bleeding and a reduced blood transfusion requirement after transplantation within the recipient [41].

5.4. The impact of perfusion and preservation fluids

Pancreas preservation by cold storage using University of Wisconsin solution has been the mainstay method used for pancreas transplantation over the past two decades. Other solutions, such as HTK, Celsior, and SCOT 15, struggled to demonstrate any advantage for short-term preservation periods. But the advent of clinical islet transplantation and the larger use of controlled DBD donors have prompted the transplantation community to develop methods for increasing pancreas graft quality while preventing ischemic reperfusion damage especially in the cellular arena. It has been thought that oxygenation by 1- or 2-layer methods during pancreas preservation, as well as the use of perfluorocarbons, may increase islet yield. Based on the former methods, there is a renewed interest in machine perfusion and oxygenation in pancreas preservation for pancreas transplantation and islet cell preparation [105].

A recent systematic review and meta-analysis by our group compared the outcomes of whole organ pancreas transplantation based on the *in situ* perfusion and subsequent preservation fluid utilized (UW, HTK, or Celsior) [81]. Ischemia-reperfusion injury of the pancreas, as reflected by post-operative peak lipase levels, was significantly lower when UW was employed as a perfusion/preservation fluid in comparison to HTK, but there was no significant difference in peak amylase. This pancreatic ischemia-reperfusion injury may translate to lower clinical graft pancreatitis rates when UW is used in comparison to HTK, although this is not a universal finding [106]. No significant disparity was observed in biochemical injury markers or graft pancreatitis rates between UW and Celsior [81].

As discussed above, post-transplantation graft thrombosis is a significant cause of graft loss. Thrombotic graft loss rates do not differ based on whether UW, HTK, or Celsior is used for *in situ* perfusion and preservation of the pancreas [81]. Furthermore, cumulative graft survival after first post-transplantation month does not favor UW over HTK, although a distinct trend favoring UW emerges at the 1-year mark [81, 106, 107]. A US registry analysis provided further evidence for this, showing a significant association between HTK perfusion/preservation and graft loss, in comparison to UW [108]. In comparison, the use of Celsior is associated with similar 1-year graft survival rates to UW [64, 76].

The comparative utility of each preservation fluid must also be considered in the context of additional donor and transplant-related factors. One important consideration when considering any possible superior preservation effects of UW is the expected pancreatic graft cold ischemic time (CIT). UW may especially be beneficial when CIT is greater than or equal to 12 hours [106, 108]. Furthermore, as already mentioned previously, pancreas retrieval is usually undertaken in the multi-organ donor setting. The perfusion/preservation fluid utilized must therefore not compromise any abdominal organ additionally procured, especially the liver. There is conflicting evidence regarding the relative efficacy of UW, HTK, Celsior, and IGL-1 for liver preservation. Some authors suggest that HTK results in inferior graft survival in comparison to UW, whilst others have reported similar survival but a reduction in post-liver transplantation biliary strictures when HTK is utilized [109, 110]. Overall, current cumulative evidence does not suggest a significant difference between these four fluids, and further research in this area is required [34].

5.5. Donation after circulatory death (DCD) vs. donation after brain death (DBD) transplantation and the importance of donor selection

With careful selection of donors, excellent whole organ pancreatic transplantation outcomes can be obtained even after DCD transplantation. The Pancreas Donor Risk Index (PDRI) is a tool that incorporates donor and preservation-related risk factors, including DCD donors, prolonged preservation time, and high body mass index (BMI), in a risk model for subsequent graft failure [111]. This model has been utilized in both the North American and European settings [111, 112]. It is important to note however that such models must not be used in isolation, and donor pancreata with one or more risk factors, including DCD donors, can still be used to achieve good outcomes. Indeed, our center's first DCD pancreas transplant was in 2007, and has been followed by a further six DCD pancreas transplants, all displaying good long-term graft function [84, 113]. Meta-analyses have shown equivalent graft and patient survival when comparing DBD and DCD pancreatic transplantation, although graft thrombosis rates are higher when DCD grafts are used [51, 114]. Importantly, this higher graft thrombosis rate can be abrogated when donor therapies such as systemic ante-mortem heparin administration are applied [51]. The use of younger donors, with a lower BMI, and low warm ischemic times, has contributed to the success of DCD whole organ pancreas transplantation [84, 115].

There has, however, been more reserved interest in DCD in pancreas for cellular transplantation as the perceived ischemic insult appears to have a much greater effect on the isolated islets for cellular transplantation than when the whole pancreas is transplanted. This is largely because the entire reserve of islets remains intact in the whole organ graft rather than being removed, and a smaller proportion is transplanted in the cellular graft [66, 99]. However, a number of encouraging studies have shown varying success. Albeit from a more advantageous DCD setting allowing earlier intervention including cannulation of the donor and antemortem heparin administration, which has, been shown to be a distinct advantage in this setting [51]. One such report from the Japanese Islet Registry reported their findings from 65 DCD islet isolations performed for 34 transplantations in 18 patients with T1DM. Despite the fact that all recipients remained free of severe hypoglycemia, only three patients achieved insulin independence for 14, 79, and 215 days. HbA1c levels and requirement of exogenous insulin were significantly improved in all patients [116]. In the more traditional DCD setting the Edmonton group have recently reported their findings comparing islet isolations from 15 DCD and 418 DBD donors performed between September 2008 and September 2014. Compared to DBD, pancreata from DCD were procured locally and donors required less vasopressive support ($P < 0.001$ and $P = 0.023$, respectively), but the other variables were similar between groups. The metabolic function was similar between DBD and DCD, as well as the mean decrease in insulin requirement at 1-month post-transplantation (DBD: 64.82%; DCD: 60.17% reduction, $P = 0.517$). These results support the broader use of DCD pancreata for islet isolation. However, a much larger DCD islet experience will be required to truly determine non-inferiority of both short and long-term outcomes [117].

6. Future perspectives

There has been considerable interest regarding the utility and advantages of dynamic preservation methods in comparison to CS alone for organs such as the liver, kidneys, heart, and lungs. The pancreas has not remained immune to attempts adapting such techniques during the post-procurement phase, although their current clinical success remains limited. Non-static methods of preservation can potentially:

- Reduce graft discard by allowing more accurate graft assessment after retrieval in comparison to current methods, which are largely subjective; and
- Improve organ quality by reducing ischemia-reperfusion-related damage, including by the targeted delivery of pharmacotherapies aimed against ischemia-reperfusion injury, and also gene therapies and stem cells, into the pancreas.

6.1. Machine perfusion

Machine (*ex vivo*) perfusion (MP) entails cannulation and mechanical perfusion of the pancreas via its inflow vessels; perfusion fluid is re-circulated through the circuit for the duration of perfusion. Broadly, MP can be hypothermic, subnormothermic or normothermic, pulsatile or non-pulsatile, and continuous or for a limited proportion of the preservation/transport phase (e.g. pre-implantation). Current pancreatic MP work is lacking in the sphere of clinical transplantation, and is limited to pre-clinical animal and discarded human pancreas studies; only the latter will be the focus of this section, with experimental animal work summarized in detail elsewhere [118–120].

There are certain pancreas-specific issues that need to be considered with respect to MP that do not apply to other organs such as the kidney. Most importantly, the pancreas is a low-flow organ, and even relatively low pressures in a MP setup can result in significant graft edema and weight gain [121]. Furthermore, higher perfusion pressures can contribute to vascular thrombosis secondary to endothelial damage [120]. However, especially if MP is undertaken at normal body temperature (normothermic), such risks must then be balanced against the need for adequate perfusion to sustain normal aerobic metabolism. An additional challenge during pancreatic MP is the need to adequately and safely account for the organ's exocrine output, which is stimulated during normothermic perfusion [122].

As a result of these issues, most pancreatic MP studies have been conducted in the field of islet cell transplantation rather than the whole pancreas [120, 123]. Graft edema, is disadvantageous for both whole organ and cellular transplantation. However some groups have studied its use as it theoretically facilitates the enzymatic digestion of pancreatic acinar tissue [124]. Hypothermic MP can potentially be employed to increase human islet yield, viability, and insulin secretion despite an extended CIT (> 12 hours), possibly increasing the number of pancreata that can be used for successful islet isolation [125]. Cases of human islet transplantation following MP are yet to be published, however. Whole organ pancreas MP has been investigated in the context of extended criteria organs that were not utilized for human transplantation. Some authors have shown 6 hours of oxygenated hypothermic MP using UW machine perfusion solution increases the ATP content of DCD pancreata to reach a level that is similar to DBD pancreata at baseline [126]. Graft edema can be kept to a minimum if low pressure hypothermic MP is utilized, even for as long as 24 hours [127]. Subsequent *ex vivo* normothermic perfusion can be used to simulate reperfusion at transplantation after initial hypothermic MP, and has been shown to demonstrate adequate insulin secretion by such pancreata [128].

Normothermic MP is an attractive alternative for whole pancreas preservation, and likely provides better graft viability assessment than hypothermic perfusion. Both endocrine and exocrine graft function can be assessed during perfusion by measuring C-peptide and/or insulin secretion and stimulation in response to glucose, and amylase and lipase release, respectively [122, 129]. Blood flow and resistance parameters can also be assessed using this technique, although this is also possible with hypothermic MP. However it is important to note that no defined cut-offs or validated protocols for human transplantation have been developed, and will require significantly more pre-clinical work.

6.2. Persufflation

Persufflation is a technique in which the pancreas is directly perfused with a humidified gas such as oxygen via the SMA and/or splenic arteries. Non-utilized human DBD pancreata have been perfused by this method, and subsequent graft assessment showed an increase in pancreatic ATP levels [130]. Porcine data from the same group showed significantly improved pancreatic histology after 24 hours of persufflation in comparison to utilization of the TLM [131]. Islet isolation after 24 hours of persufflation, including in human pancreata, is likely increased, compared to other methods such as the TLM [132]. This was confirmed in a later study, whereby islets of sufficient quantity and quality for transplantation were isolated from all five human pancreata that underwent persufflation using 40% humidified oxygen perfused at 10–25 mmHg [133]. Similar to MP however, pancreas persufflation has not yet been followed by clinical islet and/or whole organ pancreas transplantation although some research is now underway by a limited number of groups.

6.3. Normothermic regional perfusion

Normothermic Regional Perfusion (NRP) of the abdomen was initially utilized in Spain in the uncontrolled DCD setting, and has since been utilized in the controlled DCD setting in other European countries and Asia [134–138]. The donor's systemic arterial and venous systems are rapidly cannulated, and an *ex vivo* pump/oxygenator system is used to maintain an effective artificial circulation of the abdominal viscera. Cerebral and thoracic perfusion is avoided by clamping the supra-celiac aorta. This system reduces the organ's warm ischemic insult, and proposed benefits include facilitation of a more effective subsequent *in situ* cold flush, ATP replenishment, and reduced oxidative stress [139]. Current experience for NRP exists mainly in the sphere of kidney and liver transplantation. However, utilization of this technique for DCD pancreas preservation and transplantation is appealing, especially because DCD pancreata can have sustained, long-term graft function (as discussed above). Within the UK, five pancreata have been procured after initial NRP, resulting in two SPK transplants and one islet cell transplantation [136]. In Spain, one NRP pancreas has been transplanted in the context of a controlled DCD donor [140]. Future studies are required to more effectively classify evidence for this strategy, and define its comparative role or efficacy with respect to MP. In the DCD setting, NRP may prove to be a more feasible strategy than MP owing to the aforementioned difficulties of maintaining a pancreas on an *ex vivo* machine circuit, although no direct comparisons exist between the two methods.

7. Conclusions

This chapter outlines the numerous advances that have occurred over the past few decades in pancreas retrieval techniques for both whole organ and cellular transplantation. It clearly demonstrates the improved outcomes in both whole pancreas and islet cell transplantation from significant improvements to organ donor selection and management, and organ perfusion and retrieval surgery. We have seen insulin independence rates for more than 10 years post-transplant in both settings with minimal complications. Whole organ transplantation is obviously now a well-accepted clinical therapy for many patients worldwide. However, islet transplantation still has limited application to the broader population of patients with T1D due to its reliance on the availability of cadaveric donors and selection, isolation results and transplant engraftment, the side effects of immunosuppression and issues associated with the requirement for life-long immunosuppression. The future holds many interesting potential new therapies that may or may not yield appropriate and safe methods for treatment of type 1 diabetes. From what has been outlined in this chapter we can see that outcomes for patients have improved significantly. If, unfortunately, patients cannot be treated prior to the advent of their type 1 diabetes then they can still be treated by transplantation. Moving forward, researchers and clinicians have numerous fronts and multiple strategies arising at different stages of development in which to be able to offer patients treatments tailored to them and their disease. In the foreseeable future, transplantation and in particular the focus on organ retrieval and organ preservation will play a significant role in further improving outcomes, particularly with newer technologies such as machine perfusion and normothermic regional perfusion. Such technologies are hoped to increase both the number of suitable whole pancreata, as well as their quality, which will simultaneously lead to improved islet cell numbers and function in the cell therapy sphere of Diabetes care.

Acknowledgements

The authors wish to thank Callista Rainey for assistance with the figures in this chapter. The authors also wish to acknowledge support from the Royal Australasian College of Surgeons (Sir Roy McCaughey Surgical Research Fellowship).

Conflicts of interest

The authors declare no conflicts of interest.

Abbreviations

BMI	body mass index
CS	Celsior
CIT	cold ischemic time
DBD	donation after brain death
DCD	donation after circulatory death
PFC	perfluorochemical
T1D	type 1 diabetes
UW solution	University of Wisconsin
SPK	simultaneous pancreas and kidney
TLM	two-layer method
T1D	type 1 diabetes

Author details

Wayne J. Hawthorne[1,2,3]*, Ahmer Hameed[1,2,3] and Henry Pleass[1,3]

*Address all correspondence to: wayne.hawthorne@sydney.edu.au

1 Department of Surgery, Westmead Hospital, Sydney, Australia

2 Centre for Transplant and Renal Research, Westmead Institute for Medical Research, Sydney, Australia

3 Sydney Medical School, University of Sydney, Sydney, Australia

References

[1] Squifflet JP, Gruessner RW, Sutherland DE. The history of pancreas transplantation: Past, present and future. Acta Chirurgica Belgica. 2008;**108**:367-378

[2] Sutherland DE, Najarian JS. Transplantation of the pancreas. Transplantation Proceedings. 1979;**11**:1158-1162

[3] Barton FB, Rickels MR, Alejandro R, Hering BJ, Wease S, Naziruddin B, et al. Improvement in outcomes of clinical islet transplantation: 1999-2010. Diabetes Care. 2012;**35**:1436-1445. DOI: 10.2337/dc12-0063

[4] Squifflet JP. The history of transplantation at the Catholic University of Louvain-Belgium 1963-2003. Acta Chirurgica Belgica. 2003;**103**(Suppl 1):10-20. DOI: 10.1080/00015458.2003.11679382

[5] A definition of irreversible coma. Report of the ad hoc committee of the Harvard Medical School to examine the definition of brain death. Journal of the American Medical Association. 1968;**205**:337-340

[6] Bell MD. Non-heart beating organ donation: Old procurement strategy--new ethical problems. Journal of Medical Ethics. 2003;**29**:176-181

[7] Hawthorne WJ. Necessities for a clinical islet program. Advances in Experimental Medicine and Biology. 2016;**938**:67-88. DOI: 10.1007/978-3-319-39824-2_6

[8] O'Gorman D, Kin T, Murdoch T, Richer B, McGhee-Wilson D, Ryan E, et al. The standardization of pancreatic donors for islet isolation. Transplantation Proceedings. 2005;**37**:1309-1310. DOI: 10.1016/j.transproceed.2004.12.087

[9] Farney ACSD, Opara EC. Evolution of islet transplantation for the last 30 years. Pancreas. 2016;**45**:8-20. DOI: 10.1097/MPA.0000000000000391

[10] Bertuzzi FAB, Tosca MC, Galuzzi M, Bonomo M, Marazzi M, Colussi G. Islet transplantation in pediatric patients: Current indications and future perspectives. Endocrine Development. 2016;**30**:14-22. DOI: 10.1159/000439322

[11] Starzl TE. Experience in Renal Transplantation. Philadelphia: WB Saunders Co.; 1964

[12] Gwathmey O, Pierpont H. Stage occlusion and resection of the human aortic arch with hypothermia. The American Surgeon. 1955;**21**:827-834

[13] Owens JC, Prevedel AE, Swan H. Prolonged experimental occlusion of thoracic aorta during hypothermia. A.M.A. Archives of Surgery. 1955;**70**:95-97

[14] Marchioro TL, Huntley RT, Waddell WR, Starzl TE. Extracorporeal perfusion for obtaining postmortem homografts. Surgery. 1963;**54**:900-911

[15] Belzer FO, Ashby BS, Dunphy JE. 24-hour and 72-hour preservation of canine kidneys. Lancet. 1967;**2**:536-538

[16] Starzl TE. History of clinical transplantation. World Journal of Surgery. 2000;**24**:759-782

[17] Collins GM, Bravo-Shugarman M, Terasaki PI. Kidney preservation for transportation. Initial perfusion and 30 hours' ice storage. Lancet. 1969;**2**:1219-1222

[18] Ackermann JR, Snell ME. Cadaveric renal transplantation: A technique for donor kidney removal. British Journal of Urology. 1968;**40**:515-521

[19] Merkel FK, Jonasson O, Bergan JJ. Procurement of cadaver donor organs: Evisceration technique. Transplantation Proceedings. 1972;**4**:585-589

[20] Benichou J, Halgrimson CG, Weil R 3rd, Koep LJ, Starzl TE. Canine and human liver preservation for 6 to 18 hr by cold infusion. Transplantation. 1977;**24**:407-411

[21] de Gruyl J, Westbroek DL, Macdicken I, Ridderhof E, Verschoor L, van Strik R. Cryoprecipitated plasma perfusion preservation and cold storage preservation of duct-ligated pancreatic allografts. The British Journal of Surgery. 1977;**64**:490-493

[22] Wall WJ, Calne RY, Herbertson BM, Baker PG, Smith DP, Underwood J, et al. Simple hypothermic preservation for transporting human livers long distances for transplantation. Report of 12 cases. Transplantation. 1977;**23**:210-216

[23] Kalayoglu M, Sollinger HW, Stratta RJ, D'Alessandro AM, Hoffmann RM, Pirsch JD, et al. Extended preservation of the liver for clinical transplantation. Lancet. 1988;**1**:617-619

[24] Ploeg RJ, Boudjema K, Marsh D, Bruijn JA, Gooszen HG, Southard JH, et al. The importance of a colloid in canine pancreas preservation. Transplantation. 1992;**53**:735-741

[25] Belzer FO, Southard JH. Principles of solid-organ preservation by cold storage. Transplantation. 1988;**45**:673-676

[26] Starzl TE, Hakala TR, Shaw BW Jr, Hardesty RL, Rosenthal TJ, Griffith BP, et al. A flexible procedure for multiple cadaveric organ procurement. Surgery, Gynecology & Obstetrics. 1984;**158**:223-230

[27] Starzl TE, Miller C, Broznick B, Makowka L. An improved technique for multiple organ harvesting. Surgery, Gynecology & Obstetrics. 1987;**165**:343-348

[28] Deane SA, Ekberg H, Stewart GJ, Grierson JM, Williamson P, Hawthorne W, et al. Whole pancreas grafting with exocrine drainage into the bladder: Method of choice for clinical transplantation? Transplantation Proceedings. 1988;**20**:84-86

[29] Ekberg H, Deane SA, Allen RDM, Hawthorne WJ, Williamson P, Grierson JM, et al. Monitoring of canine pancreas allograft function with measurements of urinary amylase. ANZ Journal of Surgery. 1988;**58**:583-586. DOI: 10.1111/j.1445-2197.1988.tb06198.x

[30] Deane SA, Ekberg H, Stewart GJ, Grierson JM, Williamson P, Hawthorne WJ, et al. Canine whole pancreatic transplantation with exocrine drainage into the bladder. ANZ Journal of Surgery. 1989;**59**:659-664

[31] Griffin AD, Hawthorne WJ, Allen RD, Grierson JM, Jablonski P, Howden BO, et al. Twenty-four-hour preservation of canine pancreas allografts using low-cost, low-viscosity, modified University of Wisconsin cold storage solution. Transplantation Proceedings. 1993;**25**:1595-1596

[32] Wilson TG, Hawthorne WJ, Lau H, Williamson P, Chapman JR, Grierson JM, et al. Pretreatment of canine whole pancreas allografts with monoclonal antibodies does not prolong graft survival. Transplantation Proceedings. 1990;**22**:2163-2164

[33] Lam VW, Pleass HC, Hawthorne W, Allen RD. Evolution of pancreas transplant surgery. ANZ Journal of Surgery. 2010;**80**:411-418. DOI: 10.1111/j.1445-2197.2010.05309.x

[34] Hameed AM, Laurence JM, Lam VWT, Pleass HC, Hawthorne WJ. A systematic review and meta-analysis of cold in situ perfusion and preservation of the hepatic allograft: Working toward a unified approach. Liver Transplantation. 2017;**23**:1615-1627. DOI: 10.1002/lt.24829

[35] Greenwald MA, Kuehnert MJ, Fishman JA. Infectious disease transmission during organ and tissue transplantation. Emerging Infectious Diseases. 2012;**18**. DOI: 10.3201/eid1808.120277

[36] Martinez-Pourcher V. Infections in the transplant patient. La Revue du Praticien. 2015;**65**:1075-1078

[37] Ausania F, Drage M, Manas D, Callaghan CJ. A registry analysis of damage to the deceased donor pancreas during procurement. American Journal of Transplantation. 2015;**15**:2955-2962. DOI: 10.1111/ajt.13419

[38] Allen RD, Nankivell BJ, Hawthorne WJ, O'Connell PJ, Chapman JR. Pancreas and islet transplantation: An unfinished journey. Transplantation Proceedings. 2001;**33**:3485-3488

[39] Allen RD, Chapman JR, Hawthorne WJ, Pearl TA, Wilson TG, Lau H, et al. Advantages and disadvantages of pancreas transplantation. Transplantation Proceedings. 1992;**24**:171-172

[40] Fridell JA, Powelson JA, Kubal CA, Burke GW, Sageshima J, Rogers J, et al. Retrieval of the pancreas allograft for whole-organ transplantation. Clinical Transplantation. 2014;**28**:1313-1330. DOI: 10.1111/ctr.12459

[41] Hameed A, Yu T, Yuen L, Lam V, Ryan B, Allen R, et al. Use of the harmonic scalpel in cold phase recovery of the pancreas for transplantation: The westmead technique. Transplant International. 2016;**29**:636-638. DOI: 10.1111/tri.12777

[42] Forsythe JL. In: Garden OJ, Paterson-Brown S, editors. A Companion to Surgical Practice: Transplantation. 5th ed. Saunders Elsevier: Edinburgh; 2014

[43] Olson DW, Kadota S, Cornish A, Madsen KL, Zeng J, Jewell LD, et al. Intestinal decontamination using povidone-iodine compromises small bowel storage quality. Transplantation. 2003;**75**:1460-1462. DOI: 10.1097/01.tp.0000060871.02234.1b

[44] Thwaites SE, Lam VWT, Yao J, Kable K, Jenkins L, Chen C, et al. Surgical morbidity of simultaneous kidney and pancreas transplantation: A single-Centre experience in the Tacrolimus era. ISRN Transplantation. 2013;**2013**(6). DOI: 10.5402/2013/685850

[45] TSANZ. Guidance Document - Surgical Technique for Deceased Donor Abdominal Organ Procurement (ATCA-TSANZ Guidelines G003/2015). Sydney, Australia: TSANZ; 2015

[46] Oniscu GC, Forsythe JLR, Fung JJ. Abdominal Organ Retrieval and Transplantation Bench Surgery. Chichester, West Sussex: John Wiley & Sons; 2013

[47] Thwaites SE, Gurung B, Yao J, Kable K, Robertson P, Ryan BJ, et al. Excellent outcomes of simultaneous pancreas kidney transplantation in patients from rural and urban Australia: A national service experience. Transplantation. 2012;**94**:1230-1235. DOI: 10.1097/TP.0b013e3182708e04

[48] Jeon H, Ortiz JA, Manzarbeitia CY, Alvarez SC, Sutherland DE, Reich DJ. Combined liver and pancreas procurement from a controlled non-heart-beating donor with aberrant hepatic arterial anatomy. Transplantation. 2002;**74**:1636-1639. DOI: 10.1097/01.tp.0000038707.82035.75

[49] Reich DJ, Mulligan DC, Abt PL, Pruett TL, Abecassis MM, D'Alessandro A, et al. ASTS recommended practice guidelines for controlled donation after cardiac death organ procurement and transplantation. American Journal of Transplantation. 2009;**9**:2004-2011. DOI: 10.1111/j.1600-6143.2009.02739.x

[50] D'Alessandro AM, Hoffmann RM, Knechtle SJ, Eckhoff DE, Love RB, Kalayoglu M, et al. Successful extrarenal transplantation from non-heart-beating donors. Transplantation. 1995;**59**:977-982

[51] Shahrestani S, Webster AC, Lam VW, Yuen L, Ryan B, Pleass HC, et al. Outcomes from pancreatic transplantation in donation after cardiac death: A systematic review and meta-analysis. Transplantation. 2017;**101**:122-130. DOI: 10.1097/tp.0000000000001084

[52] Nghiem DD, Cottington EM. Pancreatic flush injury in combined pancreas-liver recovery. Transplant International. 1992;**5**:19-22

[53] Dunn DL, Morel P, Schlumpf R, Mayoral JL, Gillingham KJ, Moudry-Munns KC, et al. Evidence that combined procurement of pancreas and liver grafts does not affect transplant outcome. Transplantation. 1991;**51**:150-157

[54] D'Alessandro AM, Reed A, Hoffmann RM, Sollinger HW, Kalayoglu M, Knechtle SJ, et al. Results of combined hepatic, pancreaticoduodenal, and renal procurements. Transplantation Proceedings. 1991;**23**:2309-2311

[55] Conway MB, Saunders R, Munn SR, Perkins JD. Combined liver/pancreaticoduodenal procurement effect on allograft function. Transplantation Proceedings. 1990;**22**:429-430

[56] Spees EK, Orlowski JP, Temple DR, Kam I, Karrer IF. Efficacy of simultaneous cadaveric pancreas and liver recovery. Transplantation Proceedings. 1990;**22**:427-428

[57] Abu-Elmagd K, Fung J, Bueno J, Martin D, Madariaga JR, Mazariegos G, et al. Logistics and technique for procurement of intestinal, pancreatic, and hepatic grafts from the same donor. Annals of Surgery. 2000;**232**:680-687

[58] Brockmann JG, Vaidya A, Reddy S, Friend PJ. Retrieval of abdominal organs for transplantation. The British Journal of Surgery. 2006;**93**:133-146. DOI: 10.1002/bjs.5228

[59] Maglione M, Ploeg RJ, Friend PJ. Donor risk factors, retrieval technique, preservation and ischemia/reperfusion injury in pancreas transplantation. Current Opinion in Organ Transplantation. 2013;**18**:83-88. DOI: 10.1097/MOT.0b013e32835c29ef

[60] Wunderlich H, Brockmann JG, Voigt R, Rauchfuss F, Pascher A, Brose S, et al. DTG procurement guidelines in heart beating donors. Transplant International. 2011;**24**:733-757. DOI: 10.1111/j.1432-2277.2011.01266.x

[61] Sollinger HW, Vernon WB, D'Alessandro AM, Kalayoglu M, Stratta RJ, Belzer FO. Combined liver and pancreas procurement with Belzer-UW solution. Surgery. 1989;**106**:685-690 discussion 690-681

[62] Potdar S, Malek S, Eghtesad B, Shapiro R, Basu A, Patel K, et al. Initial experience using histidine-tryptophan-ketoglutarate solution in clinical pancreas transplantation. Clinical Transplantation. 2004;**18**:661-665. DOI: 10.1111/j.1399-0012.2004.00262.x

[63] Fridell JA, Mangus RS, Powelson JA. Histidine-tryptophan-ketoglutarate for pancreas allograft preservation: The Indiana University experience. American Journal of Transplantation. 2010;**10**:1284-1289. DOI: 10.1111/j.1600-6143.2010.03095.x

[64] Boggi U, Vistoli F, Del Chiaro M, Signori S, Croce C, Pietrabissa A, et al. Pancreas preservation with University of Wisconsin and Celsior solutions: A single-center, prospective, randomized pilot study. Transplantation. 2004;**77**:1186-1190

[65] Nicoluzzi J, Macri M, Fukushima J, Pereira A. Celsior versus Wisconsin solution in pancreas transplantation. Transplantation Proceedings. 2008;**40**:3305-3307. DOI: 10.1016/j.transproceed.2008.05.080

[66] Hawthorne WJ. Beta cell therapies for type 1 diabetes. In: Hardikar AA, editor. Pancreatic Islet Biology. Switzerland: Springer Press; 2016

[67] Churchill TA. Organ Preservation for Transplantation. Functional Metabolism. John Wiley & Sons, Inc.; 2005. pp. 529-555. DOI: 10.1002/047167558X.ch19

[68] Guibert EE, Petrenko AY, Balaban CL, Somov AY, Rodriguez JV, Fuller BJ. Organ preservation: Current concepts and new strategies for the next decade. Transfusion Medicine and Hemotherapy. 2011;**38**:125-142. DOI: 10.1159/000327033

[69] Chouchani ET, Pell VR, Gaude E, Aksentijevic D, Sundier SY, Robb EL, et al. Ischaemic accumulation of succinate controls reperfusion injury through mitochondrial ROS. Nature. 2014;**515**:431-435. DOI: 10.1038/nature13909

[70] Bon D, Chatauret N, Giraud S, Thuillier R, Favreau F, Hauet T. New strategies to optimize kidney recovery and preservation in transplantation. Nature Reviews. Nephrology. 2012;**8**:339-347. DOI: 10.1038/nrneph.2012.83

[71] Wahlberg JA, Love R, Landegaard L, Southard JH, Belzer FO. 72-hour preservation of the canine pancreas. Transplantation. 1987;**43**:5-8

[72] Chedid MF, Grezzana-Filho TJ, Montenegro RM, Leipnitz I, Hadi RA, Chedid AD, et al. First report of human pancreas transplantation using IGL-1 preservation solution: A case series. Transplantation. 2016;**100**:e46-e47. DOI: 10.1097/tp.0000000000001242

[73] Chen F, Nakamura T, Wada H. Development of new organ preservation solutions in Kyoto University. Yonsei Medical Journal. 2004;**45**:1107-1114. DOI: 10.3349/ymj.2004.45.6.1107

[74] Eurotransplant Foundation. Eurotransplant Manual. Leiden: Netherlands: Eurotransplant; 2016

[75] Zalewska K, Ploeg R. National Standards for Organ Retrieval from Deceased Donors (NORS Retrieval Standards). UK: Bristol; 2014

[76] Manrique A, Jimenez C, Herrero ML, Meneu JC, Abradelo M, Moreno A, et al. Pancreas preservation with the University of Wisconsin versus Celsior solutions. Transplantation Proceedings. 2006;**38**:2582-2584. DOI: 10.1016/j.transproceed.2006.08.058

[77] van der Plaats A, t Hart NA, Morariu AM, Verkerke GJ, Leuvenink HG, Ploeg RJ, et al. Effect of University of Wisconsin organ-preservation solution on haemorheology. Transplant International. 2004;**17**:227-233. DOI: 10.1007/s00147-004-0705-8

[78] Gonzalez AM, Filho GJ, Pestana JO, Linhares MM, Silva MH, Moura RM, et al. Effects of Eurocollins solution as aortic flush for the procurement of human pancreas. Transplantation. 2005;**80**:1269-1274

[79] Blech M, Hummel G, Kallerhoff M, Ringert RH. Electrolyte equilibration of human kidneys during perfusion with HTK-solution according to Bretschneider. Urological Research. 1997;**25**:331-335

[80] Troisi R, Meester D, Regaert B, Jacobs B, Van den Broucke C, Cuvelier C, et al. Physiologic and metabolic results of pancreatic cold storage with Histidine-tryptophan-Ketoglutarate-HTK solution (Custodiol) in the porcine autotransplantation model. Transplant International. 2000;**13**:98-105

[81] Hameed AM, Wong G, Laurence JM, Lam VWT, Pleass HC, Hawthorne WJ. A systematic review and meta-analysis of cold in situ perfusion and preservation for pancreas transplantation. HPB: The Official Journal of the International Hepato Pancreato Biliary Association. 2017;**19**:933-943. DOI: 10.1016/j.hpb.2017.07.012

[82] Fridell JA, Mangus RS, Thomas CM, Kubal CA, Powelson JA. Donation after circulatory arrest in pancreas transplantation: A report of 10 cases. Transplantation Proceedings. 2017;**49**:2310-2314. DOI: https://doi.org/10.1016/j.transproceed.2017.10.009

[83] Rathnasamy Muthusamy AS, Friend PJ, Dor FJM, Crane JS, Papalois V, Herbert P, et al. DCD pancreas transplantation meta-analysis: Ethical and technical considerations. Transplantation. 2017;**101**:e57. DOI: 10.1097/tp.0000000000001560

[84] Shahrestani S, Robertson P, Pleass HCC, Hawthorne WJ. The authors' reply. Transplantation. 2017;**101**:e58. DOI: 10.1097/tp.0000000000001561

[85] Berney T, Boffa C, Augustine T, Badet L, de Koning E, Pratschke J, et al. Utilization of organs from donors after circulatory death for vascularized pancreas and islet of Langerhans transplantation: Recommendations from an expert group. Transplant International. 2016;**29**:798-806. DOI: 10.1111/tri.12681

[86] Kuroda YKT, Suzuki Y, Fujiwara H, Yamamoto K, Saitoh Y. A new, simple method for cold storage of the pancreas using perfluorochemical. Transplantation. 1988;**46**:457-460

[87] Fujino Y. Two-layer cold storage method for pancreas and islet cell transplantation. World Journal of Gastroenterology. 2010;**16**:3235-3238. DOI: 10.3748/wjg.v16.i26.3235

[88] Hosgood SA, Nicholson ML. The role of perfluorocarbon in organ preservation. Transplantation. 2010;**89**:1169-1175. DOI: 10.1097/TP.0b013e3181da6064

[89] Iwanaga Y, Sutherland DE, Harmon JV, Papas KK. Pancreas preservation for pancreas and islet transplantation. Current Opinion in Organ Transplantation. 2008;**13**:135-141. DOI: 10.1097/MOT.0b013e3282f63942

[90] Gruessner AC, Sutherland DE, Gruessner RW. Long-term outcome after pancreas transplantation. Current Opinion in Organ Transplantation. 2012;**17**:100-105. DOI: 10.1097/MOT.0b013e32834ee700

[91] Dean PG, Kukla A, Stegall MD, Kudva YC. Pancreas transplantation. BMJ. 2017;**357**. DOI: 10.1136/bmj.j1321

[92] Dean PG, Kudva YC, Stegall MD. Long-term benefits of pancreas transplantation. Current Opinion in Organ Transplantation. 2008;**13**:85-90. DOI: 10.1097/MOT.0b013e3282f2fd7f

[93] Gruessner RWG, Gruessner AC. The current state of pancreas transplantation. Nature Reviews. Endocrinology. 2013;**9**:555-562. DOI: 10.1038/nrendo.2013.138

[94] Gruessner AC, Gruessner RW. Long-term outcome after pancreas transplantation: A registry analysis. Current Opinion in Organ Transplantation. 2016;**21**:377-385. DOI: 10.1097/mot.0000000000000331

[95] NHS Blood and Transplant. Annual Report on Pancreas and Islet Transplantation. UK: NHS; 2017

[96] ANZIPTR. ANZIPTR Report 2017 - Australia and New Zealand Islet and Pancreas Transplant Registry Data 1984-2016. Westmead: ANZIPTR; 2017

[97] Shapiro AM, Ricordi C, Hering BJ, Auchincloss H, Lindblad R, Robertson RP, et al. International trial of the Edmonton protocol for islet transplantation. The New England Journal of Medicine. 2006;**355**:1318-1330. DOI: 10.1056/NEJMoa061267

[98] Barton FB. CITR Update. Melbourne: IPITA/IXA/CTS Joint Congress; 2015

[99] Hering BJ, Clarke WR, Bridges ND, Eggerman TL, Alejandro R, Bellin MD, et al. Phase 3 trial of transplantation of human islets in type 1 diabetes complicated by severe Hypoglycemia. Diabetes Care. 2016;**39**:1230-1240. DOI: 10.2337/dc15-1988

[100] Nadalin S, Girotti P, Konigsrainer A. Risk factors for and management of graft pancreatitis. Current Opinion in Organ Transplantation. 2013;**18**:89-96. DOI: 10.1097/MOT.0b013e32835c6f0f

[101] Troppmann C, Gruessner AC, Benedetti E, Papalois BE, Dunn DL, Najarian JS, et al. Vascular graft thrombosis after pancreatic transplantation: Univariate and multivariate operative and nonoperative risk factor analysis. Journal of the American College of Surgeons. 1996;**182**:285-316

[102] Farney AC, Rogers J, Stratta RJ. Pancreas graft thrombosis: Causes, prevention, diagnosis, and intervention. Current Opinion in Organ Transplantation. 2012;**17**:87-92. DOI: 10.1097/MOT.0b013e32834ee717

[103] Patel SR, Hakim N. Prevention and management of graft thrombosis in pancreatic transplant. Experimental and Clinical Transplantation. 2012;**10**:282-289

[104] Troppmann C. Complications after pancreas transplantation. Current Opinion in Organ Transplantation. 2010;**15**:112-118. DOI: 10.1097/MOT.0b013e3283355349

[105] Squifflet JP, LeDinh H, de Roover A, Meurisse M. Pancreas preservation for pancreas and islet transplantation: A minireview. Transplantation Proceedings. 2011;**43**:3398-3401. DOI: 10.1016/j.transproceed.2011.09.052

[106] Alonso D, Dunn TB, Rigley T, Skorupa JY, Schriner ME, Wrenshall LE, et al. Increased pancreatitis in allografts flushed with histidine-tryptophan-ketoglutarate solution: A cautionary tale. American Journal of Transplantation. 2008;**8**:1942-1945. DOI: 10.1111/j.1600-6143.2008.02312.x

[107] Englesbe MJ, Moyer A, Kim DY, Granger DK, Pietroski R, Yoshida A, et al. Early pancreas transplant outcomes with histidine-tryptophan-ketoglutarate preservation: A multicenter study. Transplantation. 2006;**82**:136-139. DOI: 10.1097/01.tp.0000225764.21343.e3

[108] Stewart ZA, Cameron AM, Singer AL, Dagher NN, Montgomery RA, Segev DL. Histidine-tryptophan-ketoglutarate (HTK) is associated with reduced graft survival in pancreas transplantation. American Journal of Transplantation. 2009;**9**:217-221. DOI: 10.1111/j.1600-6143.2008.02449.x

[109] Stewart ZA, Cameron AM, Singer AL, Montgomery RA, Segev DL. Histidine-tryptophan-Ketoglutarate (HTK) is associated with reduced graft survival in deceased donor livers, especially those donated after cardiac death. American Journal of Transplantation. 2009;**9**:286-293. DOI: 10.1111/j.1600-6143.2008.02478.x

[110] Mangus RS, Fridell JA, Vianna RM, Milgrom MA, Chestovich P, Chihara RK, et al. Comparison of histidine-tryptophan-ketoglutarate solution and University of Wisconsin solution in extended criteria liver donors. Liver Transplantation. 2008;**14**:365-373. DOI: 10.1002/lt.21372

[111] Axelrod DA, Sung RS, Meyer KH, Wolfe RA, Kaufman DB. Systematic evaluation of pancreas allograft quality, outcomes and geographic variation in utilization. American Journal of Transplantation. 2010;**10**:837-845. DOI: 10.1111/j.1600-6143.2009.02996.x

[112] Blok JJ, Kopp WH, Verhagen MJ, Schaapherder AF, de Fijter JW, Putter H, et al. The value of PDRI and P-PASS as predictors of outcome after pancreas transplantation in a large European pancreas transplantation center. Pancreas. 2016;**45**:331-336. DOI: 10.1097/mpa.0000000000000485

[113] Suh N, Ryan B, Allen R, O'Connell P, Pleass H. Simultaneous pancreas and kidney transplantation from organ donation after cardiac death. ANZ Journal of Surgery. 2009;**79**:245-246. DOI: 10.1111/j.1445-2197.2009.04853.x

[114] van Loo ES, Krikke C, Hofker HS, Berger SP, Leuvenink HGD, Pol RA. Outcome of pancreas transplantation from donation after circulatory death compared to donation after brain death. Pancreatology. 2017;**17**:13-18. DOI: https://doi.org/10.1016/j.pan.2016.11.002

[115] Muthusamy AS, Mumford L, Hudson A, Fuggle SV, Friend PJ. Pancreas transplantation from donors after circulatory death from the United Kingdom. American Journal of Transplantation. 2012;**12**:2150-2156. DOI: 10.1111/j.1600-6143.2012.04075.x

[116] Saito T, Gotoh M, Satomi S, Uemoto S, Kenmochi T, Itoh T, et al. Islet transplantation using donors after cardiac death: Report of the Japan islet transplantation registry. Transplantation. 2010;**90**:740-747. DOI: 10.1097/TP.0b013e3181ecb044

[117] Andres A, Kin T, O'Gorman D, Livingstone S, Bigam D, Kneteman N, et al. Clinical islet isolation and transplantation outcomes with deceased cardiac death donors are similar to neurological determination of death donors. Transplant International. 2016;**29**:34-40. DOI: 10.1111/tri.12650

[118] Kuan KG, Wee MN, Chung WY, Kumar R, Mees ST, Dennison A, et al. Extracorporeal machine perfusion of the pancreas: Technical aspects and its clinical implications – A systematic review of experimental models. Transplantation Reviews. 2016;**30**:31-47. DOI: https://doi.org/10.1016/j.trre.2015.06.002

[119] Taylor MJ, Baicu SC. Current state of hypothermic machine perfusion preservation of organs: The clinical perspective. Cryobiology. 2010;**60**:S20-S35. DOI: 10.1016/j.cryobiol.2009.10.006

[120] Balfoussia D, Yerrakalva D, Hamaoui K, Papalois V. Advances in machine perfusion graft viability assessment in kidney, liver, pancreas, lung, and heart transplant. Experimental and Clinical Transplantation. 2012;**10**:87-100

[121] Hamaoui K, Gowers S, Sandhu B, Vallant N, Cook T, Boutelle M, et al. Development of pancreatic machine perfusion: Translational steps from porcine to human models. In: J Surg Res. 2018. DOI: 10.1016/j.jss.2017.11.052

[122] Barlow AD, Hamed MO, Mallon DH, Brais RJ, Gribble FM, Scott MA, et al. Use of ex vivo Normothermic perfusion for quality assessment of discarded human donor pancreases. American Journal of Transplantation. 2015;**15**:2475-2482. DOI: 10.1111/ajt.13303

[123] Barlow AD, Hosgood SA, Nicholson ML. Current state of pancreas preservation and implications for DCD pancreas transplantation. Transplantation. 2013;**95**:1419-1424. DOI: 10.1097/TP.0b013e318285558f

[124] Taylor MJ, Baicu S, Leman B, Greene E, Vazquez A, Brassil J. Twenty-four hour hypothermic machine perfusion preservation of porcine pancreas facilitates processing for islet isolation. Transplantation Proceedings. 2008;**40**:480-482. DOI: 10.1016/j.transproceed.2008.01.004

[125] Leeser DB, Bingaman AW, Poliakova L, Shi Q, Gage F, Bartlett ST, et al. Pulsatile pump perfusion of pancreata before human islet cell isolation. Transplantation Proceedings. 2004;**36**:1050-1051. DOI: 10.1016/j.transproceed.2004.04.041

[126] Leekmuil M, Engelse M, Ploeg RJ, de Koning E, Krikke C, Leuvenink HG, editors. Hypothermic Machine Perfusion Improves the Quality of Marginal Donor Pancreata [Abstract]. American Transplant Congress; 2015 Am J Transplant

[127] Cantarovich D, Renaudin K, Branchereau J, editors. Preservationof Human Pancreas with Hypothermic Machine Perfusion [Abstract]. Congress of the Transplantation Society. Hong Kong: Transplantation; 2016

[128] Hamaoui K, Gowers S, Sandhu B, Vallant N, Cook T, Boutelle M, et al. Development of pancreatic machine perfusion: Translational steps from porcine to human models. The Journal of Surgical Research. 2018. DOI: 10.1016/j.jss.2017.11.052

[129] Nassar A, Liu Q, Urcuyo D, Medearis S, El-Gazzaz G, Eghtesad B, et al. Establishing an ex-vivo pancreas perfusion model on discarded human grafts [abstract]. World transplant congress; 2014. Transplantation. 2014;**98**:376

[130] Scott WE, Weegman BP, Ferrer-Fabrega J, Stein SA, Anazawa T, Kirchner VA, et al. Pancreas oxygen Persufflation increases ATP levels as shown by nuclear magnetic resonance. Transplantation Proceedings. 2010;**42**:2011-2015. DOI: 10.1016/j.transproceed.2010.05.091

[131] Scott WE, O'Brien TD, Ferrer-Fabrega J, Avgoustiniatos ES, Weegman BP, Anazawa T, et al. Persufflation improves pancreas preservation when compared with the two-layer method. Transplantation Proceedings. 2010;**42**:2016-2019. DOI: 10.1016/j.transproceed.2010.05.092

[132] Scott WE, Rizzari MD, Stein ES, Avgoustiniatos ES, Suszynski TM, Weegman BP, et al., editors. Oxygen Persufflation of the Human Pancreas Increases ATP Levels and Improves Viable Islet Yields Compared with the two-Layer Method [Abstract]. Prague: IPITA; 2011

[133] Papas KK, Karatzas T, Purvis WG, Kitzmann JP, Gruessner A, O'Gorman D, et al., editors. Pancreas Oxygen Gas Perfusion (Persufflation) during Preservation Improves Clinical Islet Isolation Yields and Success Rates [Abstract]. Melbourne: IPITA; 2015

[134] Demiselle J, Augusto JF, Videcoq M, Legeard E, Dube L, Templier F, et al. Transplantation of kidneys from uncontrolled donation after circulatory determination of death: Comparison with brain death donors with or without extended criteria and impact of normothermic regional perfusion. Transplant International. 2016;**29**:432-442. DOI: 10.1111/tri.12722

[135] Butler AJ, Randle LV, Watson CJ. Normothermic regional perfusion for donation after circulatory death without prior heparinization. Transplantation. 2014;**97**:1272-1278. DOI: 10.1097/tp.0000000000000082

[136] Oniscu GC, Randle LV, Muiesan P, Butler AJ, Currie IS, Perera MT, et al. In situ normothermic regional perfusion for controlled donation after circulatory death--the United Kingdom experience. American Journal of Transplantation. 2014;**14**:2846-2854. DOI: 10.1111/ajt.12927

[137] Valero R, Cabrer C, Oppenheimer F, Trias E, Sanchez-Ibanez J, De Cabo FM, et al. Normothermic recirculation reduces primary graft dysfunction of kidneys obtained from non-heart-beating donors. Transplant International. 2000;**13**:303-310

[138] Lee JH, Hong SY, Oh C-K, Hong YS, Yim H. Kidney transplantation from a donor following cardiac death supported with extracorporeal membrane oxygenation. Journal of Korean Medical Science. 2012;**27**:115-119. DOI: 10.3346/jkms.2012.27.2.115

[139] Hessheimer AJ, Billault C, Barrou B, Fondevila C. Hypothermic or normothermic abdominal regional perfusion in high-risk donors with extended warm ischemia times: Impact on outcomes? Transplant International. 2015;**28**:700-707. DOI: 10.1111/tri.12344

[140] Minambres E, Suberviola B, Dominguez-Gil B, Rodrigo E, Ruiz-San Millan JC, Rodriguez-San Juan JC, et al. Improving the outcomes of organs obtained from controlled donation after circulatory death donors using abdominal Normothermic regional perfusion. American Journal of Transplantation. 2017;**17**:2165-2172. DOI: 10.1111/ajt.14214

5

Metabolic Drug Interactions with Immunosuppressants

Katalin Monostory

Abstract

Organ transplantation has become a routine clinical practice for patients with end-stage disease of liver, kidney, heart, or lung. Although improved immunosuppressant therapy substantially contributes to the success of transplantation, clinicians continue to face challenges because of wide interindividual variations in blood concentrations resulting in subtherapeutic or supratherapeutic levels. Many undesired side-effects or therapeutic failure of immunosuppressants as a consequence are the results of differences or changes in drug metabolism. Considering genetic and nongenetic factors, such as co-medication, can refine the immunosuppressant therapy, facilitating personalized treatments to individual recipients. This review provides an up-to-date summary of functional polymorphisms of enzymes involved in the metabolism of immunosuppressants with low molecular weight and of the clinical significance of metabolic drug interactions between immunosuppressive agents and other drugs in therapeutic regimens of transplant recipients.

Keywords: drug metabolism, genetic polymorphism, phenoconversion, calcineurin inhibitors, mTOR inhibitors, corticosteroids, inosine monophosphate dehydrogenase inhibitors

1. Introduction

Many undesired side-effects or therapeutic failures of drugs are the results of differences or changes in drug metabolism. A patient's drug metabolizing capacity, highly influenced by genetic variations or alterations in the expression and activities of drug-metabolizing enzymes, can substantially modify the pharmacokinetics of a drug and eventually its efficacy or toxicity [1]. Even if the routine clinical practice applies blood concentration guided dosing, the interindividual variability in drug metabolism calls for personalized medication primarily for drugs with narrow therapeutic index [2, 3]. The identification of genetic and nongenetic factors that can potentially affect the pharmacokinetics of a particular drug is a prerequisite of tailored pharmacotherapy [4, 5].

2. Genetic and nongenetic variations of drug-metabolizing cytochrome P450 (CYP) enzymes

CYP enzymes are the key players in the metabolism of most drugs; therefore, interindividual and intraindividual variations in CYP activities are of significant importance in clinical practice. The pharmacokinetic variability can divide the population into poor, intermediate, extensive, and ultra-rapid metabolizer phenotypes. The loss-of-function mutations in CYP genes result in permanent poor metabolism, whereas nongenetic (internal or environmental) factors can substantially modify the expression and activities of CYP enzymes, evoking transient poor or extensive/ultra-rapid metabolism [6, 7]. The clinical relevance for many CYP genetic variants, regarding drug efficacy, adverse drug reactions, or dose requirement, has been clearly evidenced [6–9]; however, the heritable genetic polymorphisms are not the only determinant factors in interindividual differences in drug metabolism. CYP genotype determines the potential for the expression of functional or nonfunctional enzymes; and nongenetic host factors (age, sex, and disease states) and environmental factors (nutrition, medication, smoking, and alcohol consumption) can alter the expression and activities of CYP enzymes [10]. Homozygous wild genotype, predicted to be translated to functional CYP enzyme, can be transiently switched into poor or extensive metabolizer phenotype, due to phenoconversion [1, 11]. Consequently, both the CYP genotype and the current CYP expression or activity should be considered for the estimation of a patient's drug-metabolizing capacity.

The prevalence of loss-of-function or gain-of-function alleles is generally 1–10%; however, the distribution of the common CYP variants varies among different ethnic populations. CYP3A enzymes, responsible for the metabolism of approximately 40% of the drugs on the market, including many immunosuppressant agents, display great genetic and nongenetic variations. For CYP3A5, substantial interethnic differences in allelic variants have been demonstrated. The prevalence of *CYP3A5*3* allele (6986A > G), resulting in splicing defect and nonfunctional CYP3A5 protein, is 88–97% in white (Caucasian), 66% in Asian, and 12–35% in African populations; consequently, a higher average proportion of functional CYP3A5 in the total hepatic CYP3A pool is expected in subjects of black origin [7, 12]. On the other hand, the enormous, even more than 100-fold interindividual variability in the expression and activity of CYP3A4 is attributed to nongenetic factors rather than genetic polymorphisms [13]. *CYP3A4*1B* allele, which has a frequency of 3–5% in white populations, but a much higher frequency in African population (50–82%) has been reported to result in increased transcription; however, the clinical significance of *CYP3A4*1B* to CYP3A4 function seems to be doubtful [14, 15]. *CYP3A4*22* allele with the prevalence of 2.5–8% in white and of 4% in Asian populations displays low hepatic CYP3A4 expression and results in decreased CYP3A4 activity [16]. Although the association between *CYP3A4* genotype and pharmacokinetic behavior of CYP3A-substrates has been extensively studied, no clear phenotype-genotype relationship has been described for CYP3A4.

Beside the genetic polymorphisms, one of the major sources of interindividual or intraindividual variability in drug metabolism is concomitant medication and co-morbidities, evoking phenoconversion, notably CYP induction and enzyme inhibition [17]. CYP induction leads to an increase in the expression and activity of CYP enzymes and contributes to the increased elimination of drugs metabolized by the particular enzyme. Several pathways involving the activation of various nuclear receptors (PXR pregnane X receptor, CAR constitutive androstane receptor, and glucocorticoid receptor) have been reported to enhance the transcription of CYP3A genes and to contribute to the complex regulation of CYP3A enzymes by drugs such as rifampicin, phenobarbital, carbamazepine, and synthetic or natural steroids [18–21]. Reduced drug concentration as a consequence of CYP3A induction leads to the lack of the pharmacological effect and drug failure. Phenoconversion converting genotypic extensive metabolism into phenotypic poor metabolism of drugs may occur during inflammation (sterile or infection-induced inflammation). Elevated release of proinflammatory cytokines (IL-6, IL-1β, TNF-α) has been associated with downregulation of several drug-metabolizing CYPs, including CYP3A enzymes. The mechanism of downregulation is the repression of PXR and CAR that are involved in transcriptional regulation of CYP3A expression [22–26]. As a consequence, transient poor metabolizer phenotype is developed, significantly increasing the risk of adverse drug reactions and impacting the clinical outcome [1, 27]. Likewise, co-medication can also give rise to poor metabolism. Several drugs or food components (e.g., bergamottin) are known to inhibit the function of drug-metabolizing CYPs; therefore, the concomitant treatment with a CYP inhibitor is expected to increase the exposure of those pharmacons that are metabolized by the particular enzyme. As a consequence of CYP inhibition, the risk of increased exposure and drug-induced adverse reactions can be anticipated, primarily for drugs with narrow therapeutic index, such as tacrolimus and ciclosporin.

By recognizing individual differences in drug metabolism, personalized drug therapy adjusted to the patient's drug-metabolizing capacity can help to avoid the potential side effects of drugs. The graft and recipient survival are highly influenced by drug-metabolizing capacity of the liver, and it is essential to predict potential drug-drug interactions and to tailor medication at both early and late postoperative periods.

3. Metabolism of immunosuppressants

In recent decades, transplantation (liver, kidney, heart, and lung) has become a routine procedure for patients with end stage disease. Advances in surgical techniques and postoperative therapy have led to increasing numbers of transplantation and extended survival among these patients. The final outcome of transplantation and the long-term graft function have been improved mainly due to the development of potent and specific immunosuppressive drugs. Immunosuppressants efficiently decrease the risk of rejection, blocking the recipient's immune system and protecting the transplanted organ. Because of the narrow therapeutic indexes and increased risk of adverse drug reactions, it is essential to apply personalized immunosuppressive therapy adjusted to patient's drug-metabolizing capacity.

Immunosuppressants are generally classified according to their molecular mode of action; however, in terms of metabolic drug interactions, two main categories must be distinguished

Immunosuppressant	Pharmacology	Adverse effects	Enzymes responsible for the metabolism
Calcineurin inhibitors:			
Ciclosporin	Selective inhibition of T-cell dependent immune response: Calcineurin inhibition, Inhibition of cytokine production	Nephrotoxicity, hepatotoxicity, Hyperlipidaemia, hypertension, Tremor, hyperkalaemia, hypomagnaesemia, Hypertrichosis, gingiva hyperplasia	CYP3A4/5
Tacrolimus	Selective inhibition of T-cell dependent immune response: Calcineurin inhibition, Inhibition of cytokine production	Nephrotoxicity, hypertension, diabetes, cholestasis, diarrhea, Tremor, hyperkalaemia, hypomagnaesemia	CYP3A4/5
mTOR inhibitors:			
Sirolimus	Inhibition of B- and T-cell proliferation	Thrombocytopenia, anaemia, leukopenia, lymphocele, pneumonitis Hyperlipidaemia, Stomatitis aphtosa, wound-healing complications	CYP3A4/5
Everolimus	Inhibition of B- and T-cell proliferation	Thrombocytopenia, anaemia, leukopenia, lymphocele, pneumonia Hyperlipidaemia, hypertonia, wound-healing complications	CYP3A4/5
Purine analogues:			
Azatioprin	Inhibition of purine metabolism	Bone marrow suppression, leukopenia, anaemia, thrombocytopenia, myeloid dysplasia, Cholestasis, hepatotoxicity	Thiopurine S-methyl-transferase, Xantine oxidase
Inosine monophosphate dehydrogenase inhibitors:			
Mycofenolate mofetil **Mycofenolate**	Selective inhibition of inosine monophosphate dehydrogenase, Inhibition of B- and T-cell proliferation	Vomiting, diarrhea, abdominal pain muscle weakness, Anaemia, leucopenia	UDP-glucuronyl transferase, CYP3A4/5
Corticosteroids:			
Prednisone **Methyl-prednisolone**	Inhibition of T-cell migration and production of T-cell lymphokines	Adrenal cortex suppression Hypercholesterolemia, diabetes, hypertension, osteoporosis, osteonecrosis, cataracta, skin atrophy	CYP3A4/5

Table 1. Immunosuppressants with low molecular weight.

according to their molecular weights (agents with low or high molecular weights). High-molecular-weight agents, such as polyclonal and monoclonal antibodies (e.g., thymoglobulin, basiliximab, belatacept), that are not substrates for drug-metabolizing enzymes, are metabolized in common protein degradation pathways (intracellular catabolism by endosomal-lysosomal system) [28]; therefore, they are not subjects of metabolic drug interactions and not subjects of this review. In the metabolism of immunosuppressants with low molecular weight, drug-metabolizing CYP enzymes are involved which may entail metabolic drug interactions (**Table 1**).

3.1. Calcineurin inhibitors

For solid organ transplant recipients, the mainstay of the immunosuppressive regimens is calcineurin inhibitor (CNI) therapy with ciclosporin or tacrolimus which selectively blocks several signaling processes, resulting in the inhibition of T-cell activation and proliferation (**Figure 1**) [29, 30]. These drugs effectively treat allograft rejection; however, they display large interindividual variability in their pharmacokinetics, requiring monitoring of blood concentrations for optimal safety and therapeutic efficacy.

Ciclosporin A is an 11-amino acid cyclopeptide that blocks the production of IL-2 by inhibition of calcineurin and, as a consequence, the activation of T-cells (**Figure 1**) [31]. Ciclosporin undergoes extensive metabolism by CYP3A enzymes, producing more than 30 metabolites. The major metabolic pathways are *N*-demethylation to 4-*N*-demethyl ciclosporin, hydroxylation at several positions (1-, 6-, 9-monohydroxy and 1,9- or 6,9-dihydroxy-metabolites), and oxidation to carboxylic acid [32]. Some of the metabolites (e.g., 1,9-dihydroxy-ciclosporin,

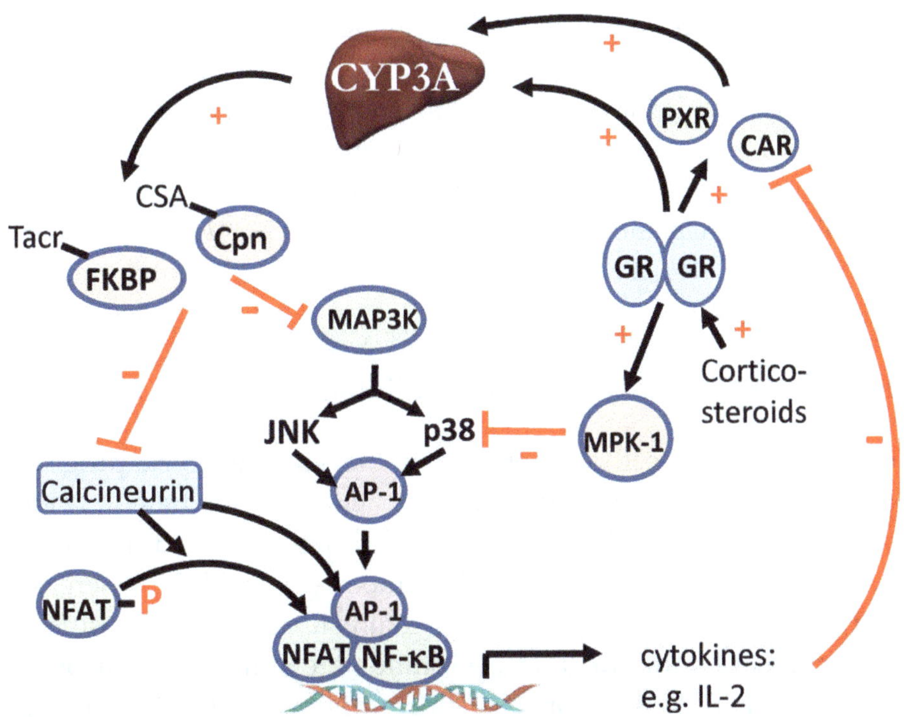

Figure 1. Molecular action of calcineurin inhibitors and corticosteriods. AP-1 activator protein 1, CAR constitutive androstane receptor, CSA ciclosporin, FKBP tarcolimus binding protein, GR glucocoticoid receptor, IL-2 interleukin 2, JNK c-Jun N-terminal kinase, MAP3K mitogen-activated protein 3 kinase, MPK-1 mitogen-activated protein kinase 1, NFAT nuclear factor of activated T-cells, PXR pregnane X receptor, Tacr tacrolimus.

1c9-dihydroxy-ciclosporin, 1-carboxy-ciclosporin) are toxic contributing to the nephrotoxic and hepatotoxic properties of the parent compound [33, 34]. Consequently, high CYP3A activity increases the rate of ciclosporin metabolism and decreases the immunosuppressive effect, which requires dose modification [35]. However, high CYP3A activity also increases the toxic metabolite formation and the risk of nephrotoxicity and hepatotoxicity. Therefore, immunosuppressive strategy must consider the blood concentrations of both ciclosporin and the toxic metabolites, especially if they are accompanied with symptoms indicating nephrotoxicity or hepatotoxicity.

Immunosuppressive properties of tacrolimus are similar to ciclosporin; however, for the same pharmacological effect, significantly lower blood concentration of tacrolimus is required than that of ciclosporin. Tacrolimus, the 23-membered macrocyclic lactone, is converted by demethylation, hydroxylation, and ring rearrangement to at least 15 metabolites, and only a minor proportion of tacrolimus dose is eliminated as unchanged parent drug [36]. Metabolism of tacrolimus leads to the inactivation of the molecule, except for the major 13-*O*-demethyl and the minor 31-*O*-demethyl metabolites. The 13-*O*-demethyl-tacrolimus possesses some immunosuppressive effect; however, it is about one tenth as active as tacrolimus, whereas the 31-*O*-demethyl metabolite displays an immunosuppressive activity comparable to tacrolimus [37, 38]. On the other hand, high blood concentration of 15-*O*-demethyl-tacrolimus metabolite has been reported to be associated with nephrotoxicity and myelotoxicity and with higher incidence of infections [39]. Similarly to ciclosporin, tacrolimus is metabolized by CYP3A enzymes, anticipating great interindividual and intraindividual differences in pharmacokinetics of tacrolimus: (1) CYP3A activity of enterocytes contributes to the first-pass metabolism of tacrolimus; (2) substantial interindividual differences in hepatic CYP3A activity result in great variability in the rate of tacrolimus metabolism, which requires continuous drug monitoring and dose modification primarily in the early postoperative period; (3) concomitant treatment with CYP3A inhibitors is the potential source of metabolic drug interactions; (4) genetic polymorphisms of CYP3A5 also contribute to the high interindividual variability. Since the relative contribution of CYP3A5 to tacrolimus biotransformation is significantly higher than that of CYP3A4 [40], the recipients carrying wild type *CYP3A5*1* allele or transplanted with liver grafts carrying *CYP3A5*1* are able to metabolize tacrolimus more rapidly than CYP3A5 nonexpressers [35, 41].

3.2. mTOR (mammalian target of rapamycin) inhibitors

The mTOR inhibitors prevent cell proliferation by blocking cell cycle progression from the G1-phase to the S-phase. The immunosuppressive activity is mediated *via* blocking mTOR protein kinases, resulting in inhibition of growth factor–mediated T-cell proliferation in response to IL-2 trigger [42]. Sirolimus is a 31-membered macrolide, whereas everolimus is a sirolimus derivative having a 2-hydroxyethyl chain substitution at position 40. Although the chemical structures of sirolimus and everolimus are similar to that of tacrolimus, the mechanism of action of mTOR inhibitors is distinct from calcineurin inhibitors, which allows the application of combination regimens. Additionally, the main advantages of mTOR inhibitors are their nonnephrotoxic properties; therefore, mTOR inhibitors in combination with reduced dose calcineurin inhibitors can augment the calcineurin inhibitor–induced nephrotoxicity [43–45].

The structural similarities can explain some common metabolic pathways of mTOR inhibitors and tacrolimus, such as *O*-dealkylation and hydroxylation at several positions [42]. Sirolimus is primarily metabolized by CYP3A enzymes and by CYP2C8 at lower extent, producing hydroxylated and *O*-demethylated metabolites (e.g., 12-hydroxy-, 16-*O*-demethyl-, 39-*O*-demethyl-, 27–39-*O*-didemethyl- and dihydroxy-sirolimus as major metabolites) [46, 47]. The metabolism of sirolimus leads to inactivation, despite the fact that some metabolites display some pharmacological activity less than one tenth of the parent drug. Everolimus is also metabolized by CYP3A and CYP2C8 enzymes; however, the elimination rate of everolimus is more rapid than sirolimus (with 30 h *vs.* 62 h elimination half-lives, respectively). Everolimus is *O*-demethylated and hydroxylated at several positions (forming both mono- and dihydroxy-metabolites); furthermore, a ring-opened metabolite is also formed from everolimus [46]. Everolimus-induced adverse effects are associated with the exposure rather to the parent compound than to its metabolites.

3.3. Antimetabolite purine analogues

One of the oldest agents with immunosuppressive activity introduced for kidney transplant recipients was the purine analogue 6-mercaptopurine, which acts by inhibiting purine nucleotide synthesis and, as a consequence, cell proliferation. The prodrug of 6-mercaptopurine, azathioprine with more favorable side-effect profile was later introduced to prevent rejection. Azathioprine is converted to 6-mercaptopurine by nonenzymatic cleavage of the thioether in enterocytes and hepatocytes or in erythrocytes. The major active metabolites, 6-thioguanine nucleotides, are formed *via* 6-thioinosine monophosphate in natural purine synthetic pathways. Inhibition of cell proliferation is mediated by incorporation of the thiopurine nucleotide analogues into DNA (and RNA), causing DNA damage [48]. 6-Mercaptopurine, independently from either direct administration or production from azathioprine, undergoes metabolic inactivation by xanthine oxidase and thiopurine S-methyl transferase and is excreted in the urine, leaving less parent compound available to form thiopurine nucleotides [49]. Due to genetic polymorphism, the thiopurine S-methyl transferase activity is highly variable in patients; namely, those subjects who carry one or two nonfunctional thiopurine S-methyl transferase alleles are unable to tolerate normal doses of azathioprine and can experience serious myelosuppression [50]. Therefore, genotyping assay is recommended before starting azathioprine therapy to identify high-risk patients, and dosage reduction or alternative therapy is recommended for these patients.

3.4. Inosine monophosphate dehydrogenase inhibitors

Mycophenolic acid is a selective inhibitor of inosine monophosphate dehydrogenase, which is responsible for *de novo* biosynthesis of guanosine monophosphate, one of the building blocks of DNA. Depletion of the guanosine pool in the cell arrests the lymphotic cell proliferation and suppresses the subsequent immune response triggered by allogenic transplanted organ [51]. In several rapidly dividing cells (e.g. enterocytes), an alternative salvage pathway exists for purine synthesis in addition to *de novo* synthetic pathway; however, lymphocytes seem to be dependent on the *de novo* pathway. Consequently, mycophenolic acid is able to selectively block proliferation of T- and B-cells. Mycophenolic acid is available as enteric-coated mycophenolate sodium and as mycophenolate mofetil ester prodrug that is extensively hydrolyzed to the active metabolite mycophenolic acid by carboxylesterases.

Mycophenolic acid is primarily metabolized by UDP-glucuronyl transferases (UGT1A7/8/9, UGT2B7), forming the major 7-*O*-mycophenolic glucuronide that is pharmacologically inactive and to the minor acil-glucuronide that has pharmacological activity comparable to the mycophenolic acid [52, 53]. The major proportion of the glucuronide conjugates is excreted in urine, whereas a smaller proportion that is eliminated *via* bile is metabolized by bacteria in the gut, and the deconjugated mycophenolic acid can be reabsorbed (enterohepatic circulation) [54]. Furthermore, in patients' blood and urine, a minor demethylated metabolite (6-*O*-demethyl-mycophenolic acid) was also detected that was proved to be produced by CYP3A enzymes.

3.5. Corticosteroids

At the beginning of transplantation history, glucocorticosteroids were the primary immunosuppressive agents in the rejection prophylaxis strategy, and nowadays, they are still the first-line agents for treatment of graft rejection. The high-dose glucocorticoids given in peritransplantation are tapered to low doses in the maintenance phase, aiming the steroid-free immunosuppression regimens because of serious adverse effects of glucocorticoids developing in long-term therapy. Acute rejection is generally treated with methylprednisolone, whereas the maintenance therapy applies either methylprednisolone or prednisone. Corticosteroids activate the cytosolic glucucorticoid receptor and modulate several cellular functions, including transcription of genes involved in proliferative and inflammatory processes. The activated receptor inhibits the transcription of NF-kB and activator protein 1 dependent genes, including proinflammatory cytokines (**Figure 1**). This process leads to the depletion of T-cells and macrophage dysfunction [55].

Regioselective and stereospecific hydroxylation of corticosteroids at several positions (at carbon 2, 6, 7, 15, 16, and 21) are catalyzed by CYP3A enzymes. Additionally, dual effect of corticosteroids on CYP3A enzymes has been demonstrated: (1) corticosteroids can competitively inhibit the function of CYP3A [56], and (2) they can induce CYP3A transcription. Activated glucocorticoid receptor upregulates the expression of nuclear receptors (PXR and CAR) that are involved in transcriptional regulation of CYP3A genes. Moreover, the proximal promoter region of CYP3A4 gene contains glucocorticoid responsive element, which directly binds activated glucocorticoid receptor [18, 57]. As a consequence of increased expression and activity of CYP3A enzymes, metabolic drug interactions can be expected upon concomitant treatment with drugs that require CYP3A activity for their metabolism.

3.6. Novel investigational immunosuppressant agents

Although calcineurin inhibitor–based immunosuppression efficiently prevents rejection, adverse reactions of ciclosporin and tacrolimus, primarily nephrotoxicity, prompt the discovery of novel agents with immunosuppressive activity [58]. Two investigational agents with low molecular weight should be mentioned: voclosporin and sotrastaurin. Voclosporin, a next-generation calcineurin inhibitor, is an analogue of ciclosporin with a single carbon extension added to the amino acid-1 of ciclosporin. Voclosporin displays higher binding affinity to cyclophillin A than ciclosporin leading to more potent inhibition of calcineurin [59]. Furthermore, it has a favorable safety property that it appears to be less toxic than currently available calcineurin inhibitors. Similarly to ciclosporin, voclospiron is a substrate for CYP3A enzymes, anticipating pharmacokinetic/metabolic drug interactions with those agents that interact with ciclosporin as well [60]. However, voclosporin is no longer pursed in transplantation. Sotrastaurin is protein kinase C inhibitor that effectively inhibits IL-2 production with the mechanism different from calcineurin or mTOR inhibition. Although sotrastaurin displayed some potential in preventing allograft rejection in animal studies, high efficacy and safety failure rate were observed in clinical trials involving kidney and liver transplant patients [61, 62]. Therefore, further development of sotrastaurin in transplantation has been halted.

4. Significant metabolic drug interactions with immunosuppressants

4.1. Combined immunosuppressive therapy

Transplant recipients' immunosuppressive therapy is often a multidrug therapy, primarily in the early postoperative period, which constitutes a challenge for clinicians to consider the complexity of drug interactions. Due to the fact that the metabolism of immunosuppressants with low molecular weight is catalyzed by the same enzymes (CYP3A4 and CYP3A5), the blood concentrations, elimination half-lives, and consequently, the efficacy or toxicity of certain immunosuppressant agents are expected to be modified during concomitant treatment. Therefore, during multidrug therapy or during withdrawal of any of the immunosuppressive drugs, special attention is required for optimal dosing for therapeutic concentrations. Each modification in immunosuppressive regimens can lead to changes in blood concentration of a drug (**Table 2**).

Calcineurin inhibitors are often applied in combination with mTOR inhibitors. Since both mTOR inhibitors and calcineurin inhibitors are substrates of CYP3A enzymes and can inhibit CYP3A activities, reduction of calcineurin inhibitor doses is recommended. Standard doses of ciclosporin were observed to decrease the clearance of sirolimus or everolimus more substantially than the doses of tacrolimus [45]. The major drawback of calcineurin inhibitor therapy is the risk of nephrotoxicity which appears to be dose dependent. The combination of low calcineurin inhibitor doses with mTOR inhibitors was found to be beneficial regarding retaining low rejection rates and lowering the risk of nephrotoxicity [44, 63]. To avoided renal dysfunction, the complete substitution of calcineurin inhibitors for mTOR inhibitors was attempted; however, the substitution showed an increase in graft failure in patients treated with merely mTOR inhibitors [64].

Corticosteroids have been demonstrated to induce the expression of the efflux pump transporter ABCB1 (P-glycoprotein) playing a main role in intestinal drug absorption and of CYP3A enzymes responsible for the metabolism of the majority of drugs [18, 65]. Therefore, the concomitant treatment of calcineurin inhibitors or mTOR inhibitors with corticosteroids can be expected to decrease the blood concentrations of tacrolimus/ciclosporin or of sirolimus/everolimus. Although the evidence for clinically significant interactions between corticosteroids and ciclosporin or mTOR inhibitors is limited, clear clinical effect of corticosteroids on tacrolimus exposure has been demonstrated [66, 67]. This also implies that dose reduction or cessation of corticosteroids leads to an increase in blood concentrations of tacrolimus, requiring dose

Immunosuppressant	Drug interactions	Consequences
Ciclosporin Tacrolimus	sirolimus, everolimus	Increased blood levels of ciclosporin and mTOR inhibitors; increased risk of nephrotoxicity
	prednisolone	Decreased blood levels due to enhanced metabolism of ciclosporin/tacrolimus, increased risk of rejection
	Antifungals:	
	ketoconazole	Increased blood levels of ciclosporin/tacrolimus; replacement of ketoconazole to other azole derivatives
	fluconazole, voriconazole, itraconazole	Inhibition of CYP3A4; dose reduction of ciclosporin, tacrolimus is necessary
	Antibiotics:	
	clarithromycin, erythromycin, azithromycin	Irreversible inhibition of CYP3A4; increased blood levels of ciclosporin/tacrolimus
	rifampicin	CYP3A4 induction; enhanced metabolism of ciclosporin, tacrolimus; increased risk of rejection
	Antiviral agents:	
	ritonavir	Irreversible inhibition of CYP3A4; increased blood levels of ciclosporin/tacrolimus
	Lipid-lowering agents:	
	fluvastatin, simvastatin, atorvastatin	Increased statin exposure by ciclosporin; incrased risk of myopathy and rhabdomyolysis
	Antihypertensive agents:	
	diltiazem, verapamil, amlodipine	Irreversible inhibition of CYP3A4, formation of metabolic intermediate complex; Increased blood levels of ciclosporin / tacrolimus
	nifedipine	Reversible, competitive inhibition CYP3A4
	carvedilol	Inhibition of ABCB1 transporter; increase absorption of oral ciclosporin
	Antidiabetic agents:	
	troglitazone, rosiglitazone	CYP3A4 induction; enhanced metabolism of ciclosporin/tacrolimus; increased risk of rejection
	Psychopharmacons:	
	carbamazepine, valproic acid	CYP3A4 induction; enhanced metabolism of ciclosporin/tacrolimus; increased risk of rejection
	fluvoxamine	Inhibition of CYP3A4; contraindicated
	Herbs:	
	St John's wort	CYP3A4 induction; enhanced metabolism of ciclosporin/tacrolimus; increased risk of rejection
	grapefruit, pomelo	Irreversible inhibition of CYP3A4; increased blood levels of ciclosporin/tacrolimus

Immunosuppressant	Drug interactions	Consequences
Sirolimus Everolimus	ciclosporin	Increased blood levels of ciclosporin and mTOR inhibitors; increased risk of nephrotoxicity
	prednisolone	Decreased blood levels due to enhanced metabolism of sirolimus/everolimus, increased risk of rejection
	Antifungals:	
	ketoconazole	Increased blood levels of mTOR inhibitors; replacement of ketoconazole to other azole derivatives
	fluconazole, voriconazole, itraconazole	Inhibition of CYP3A4; dose reduction of sirolimus, everolimus is necessary; voriconazole – sirolimus combination is contraindicated
	Antibiotics:	
	clarithromycin, erythromycin, azithromycin	Irreversible inhibition of CYP3A4; increased blood levels of sirolimus/everolimus
	rifampicin	CYP3A4 induction; enhanced metabolism of sirolimus/everolimus; increased risk of rejection
	Antiviral agents:	
	ritonavir	Irreversible inhibition of CYP3A4; increased blood levels of sirolimus/everolimus
	Antihypertensive agents:	
	diltiazem, verapamil, amlodipine	Irreversible inhibition of CYP3A4, formation of metabolic intermediate complex; Increased blood levels of sirolimus/everolimus; verapamil-sirolimus combination is associated with increased blood levels of verapamil
	Antidiabetic agents:	
	troglitazone, rosiglitazone	CYP3A4 induction; enhanced metabolism of sirolimus/everolimus; increased risk of rejection
	Psychopharmacons:	
	carbamazepine, valproic acid	CYP3A4 induction; enhanced metabolism of sirolimus/everolimus; increased risk of rejection
	Herbs:	
	St John's wort	CYP3A4 induction; enhanced metabolism of sirolimus/everolimus; increased risk of rejection
	grapefruit, pomelo	Irreversible inhibition of CYP3A4; increased blood levels of sirolimus/everolimus
6-mercaptopurine Azathioprine	allopurinol	Inhibition of xantine oxidase; myelotoxicity
Mycophenolate	Ciclosporin	Inhibition of enterohepatic circulation, decrease in blood levels of mycophenolic acid

Immunosuppressant	Drug interactions	Consequences
	Antiviral agents:	
	ganciclovir, valganciclovir	Mycophenolate-glucuronide inhibits renal tubular secretion of ganciclovir; increased blood levels of ganciclovir and increased risk of toxicity (nephrotoxicity, neutropenia, leukopenia)
Prednisolone Methylprednisolone	*Antifungals*:	
	ketoconazole, fluconazole, voriconazole, itraconazole	Increased blood levels of corticosteroids Inhibition of CYP3A4
	Antibiotics:	
	rifampicin	CYP3A4 induction; enhanced metabolism of corticosteroids
	Antiviral agents:	
	ritonavir	Irreversible inhibition of CYP3A4; increased blood levels of corticosteroids

Table 2. Clinically relevant pharmacokinetic drug interactions with immunosuppressants.

adjustment [68]. Interestingly, CYP3A5 nonexpressers with *CYP3A5*3/*3* genotype are more susceptible to glucocorticoid induction than *CYP3A5*1* carriers [69]; thus, more pronounced increase in tacrolimus exposure can be expected in CYP3A5 nonexpressers after glucocorticoid withdrawal.

Clinically significant interaction between mycophenolic acid, the active metabolite of mycophenolate mofetil, and ciclosporin has been reported [70]. The mycophenolate-glucuronide metabolite eliminated into bile undergoes enterohepatic cycling because of intestinal bacterial metabolism and reabsorption of mycophenolic acid. The enterohepatic circulation, contributing to overall pharmacokinetics of mycophenolic acid by 37% in human, is inhibited by concomitant administration of ciclosporin but does not interfere with tacrolimus or sirolimus [71, 72]. In ciclosporin-mycophenolate combination therapy, the reduced blood concentration of mycophenolic acid is necessary to ameliorate by increasing dose of mycophenolate mofetil. Furthermore, special attention on optimal dosing is required during switching ciclosporin-mycophenolate to tacrolimus-mycophenolate therapy and *vice versa*.

4.2. Metabolic drug interactions between immunosuppressants and post-transplant medication

4.2.1. Treatment and prevention of infections

Environmental circumstances and immune deficiencies due to immunosuppression therapy make recipients susceptible for infections that are one of the leading complications after organ transplantation; therefore, prevention and management of infections is a major task primarily in the early postoperative period. Since fungal infections are a threatening cause of morbidity and mortality, the antifungal prophylaxis is an important element of posttransplant medication. The antifungal azole-derivatives are potent (some of them are very strong) CYP3A inhibitors, predicting potential metabolic drug interactions with calcineurin inhibitors, mTOR inhibitors, or corticosteroids. The most potent CYP3A inhibitor is ketoconazole, able to increase blood concentrations (AUC) of ciclosporin (> 4-fold), tacrolimus (> 2-fold), sirolimus (11-fold), everolimus (15-fold), and methylprednisolone (> 2-fold) [73, 74]. Because of the substantial increase in blood concentrations of several immunosuppressants that can be avoided by drastic reduction of immunosuppressant doses and because of other adverse effects of ketoconazole, the concomitant medication is discouraged. Fluconazole, itraconazole, and voriconazole are alternative regimens for antifungal therapy or prophylaxis; however, all three drugs are azole derivatives and have the capability to inhibit CYP3A function, albeit at a lower extent than ketoconazole [75–77]. Although the continuous immunosuppressant monitoring is highly recommended and dose adjustment (reduction) is generally required, the antifungal treatment with fluconazole, itraconazole, or voriconazole can be safely applied except for voriconazole-sirolimus combination [78]. Because of an extreme (7-fold) increase of sirolimus blood concentrations as a consequence of concomitant use of voriconazole, this combination is contraindicated. Amphotericin B, the nonazole type antifungal agent, does not influence CYP activities; therefore, no metabolic drug interactions can be expected in concomitant treatment with immunosuppressants. However, the widespread use of amphotericin B is limited because of its toxicity profile, primarily because its nephrotoxic side-effect can contribute to the renal injury by ciclosporin or tacrolimus.

Organ transplant patients are at high risk for developing bacterial infections that occur in 20–40% of transplants. Potential sources of infection are from hospital and community exposures, as well as from endogenous flora of patients. Among the antibiotics used for treatment of infections, the macrolide erythromycin and clarithromycin have been reported to interact with immunosuppressive agents. These macrolides are CYP3A substrates and bind to CYP3A4 enzymes, leading to a complex formation that completely inactivates CYP3A4 enzyme [79–82]. The *in vitro* findings were confirmed by clinical observations that blood concentrations of ciclosporin/tacrolimus or sirolimus/everolimus increased as a consequences of concomitant treatment with erythromycin or clarithromycin [73, 83–86]. Page et al. [87] and Mori et al. [88] have reported some potential of azithromycin for drug interaction with ciclosporin and tacrolimus; however, *in vitro* experiments demonstrated that azithromycin poorly interfere with CYP3A4 [89]. When concomitant therapy with these macrolides is necessary, blood concentrations of calcineurin inhibitors or mTOR inhibitors should be carefully monitored, and the immunosuppressant doses should be adjusted. In contrast, the macrolide rifampicin is a potent CYP3A4 inducer and can activate PXR, resulting in a substantial increase in CYP3A4 expression [90]. The increased CYP3A4 activity consequently enhances the metabolism and elimination of calcineurin inhibitors, mTOR inhibitors, and corticosteroids [91–93]. However, blood concentration–guided dose-adjustment of immunosuppressants should be applied carefully because increased metabolism can evoke elevation of toxic metabolite formation (e.g., ciclosporin).

A significant cause of graft failure still remains viral infections, which are acquired as new infection or reactivation of latent viruses. After transplantation, cytomegalovirus (CMV) is the most common viral infection in recipients, primarily in those CMV-seronegative patients who were transplanted with graft from CMV-seropositive donors, resulting in viral reactivation. For prophylaxis and treatment of CMV infection, aciclovir, ganciclovir, and valganciclovir (the prodrug of ganciclovir) are generally applied. None of these antiviral drugs influences the function of drug-metabolizing CYPs or UDP-glucuronyl transferases, and consequently, they do not modify the pharmacokinetic properties of immunosuppressants. Aciclovir and ganciclovir are eliminated primarily in the urine as unchanged compounds. Increased risk of nephrotoxicity and leukopenia has been reported in patients who were co-medicated with a drug that can reduce renal clearance of aciclovir or ganciclovir. During co-administration with mycophenolate or mycophenolate-mofetil, mycophenolate-glucuronide and aciclovir or ganciclovir can significantly compete for renal tubular secretion, resulting in an increase in aciclovir/ganciclovir and mycophenolate-glucuronide exposure, as well as the risk of nephrotoxicity or leukopenia [94–96]. Management of potent metabolic drug interactions between antiviral protease inhibitors and immunosuppressants is a major challenge because most of the protease inhibitors are clinically significant CYP3A4 inhibitors. Ritonavir-boosted therapies require substantial reduction of immunosuppressant doses (to 5–20% for ciclosporin; to 1–3.5% for tacrolimus) with continuous monitoring of blood concentrations [97–101].

4.2.2. Treatment of dyslipidemia

Dyslipidemia is often developed as an adverse impact of immunosuppressive therapy [102]. Ciclosporin, mTOR inhibitors, and prednisone are mainly implicated in lipid alterations. For treatment of hypercholesterolemia, the basic guidelines for dyslipidemia recommend diet and HMG-CoA reductase (hydroxymethyl-glutaryl-CoA reductase) inhibitor statins with special considerations for transplant patients. Although both ciclosporin and most statins (atorvastatin, fluvastatin, simvastatin, lovastatin) are primarily metabolized by CYP3A4 and metabolic drug interactions are likely occur, statins do not evoke increased ciclosporin exposure [103–106]. In contrast, ciclosporin induces significant elevation of statin blood concentrations which can be explained by the ten-fold higher molar concentrations of ciclosporin than statins. In combination with ciclosporin, the blood levels are increased in a statin-dependent manner, e.g., lovastatin is increased to a much greater extent than atorvastatin [104, 107]. Dose reduction of lipid-lowering agents is recommended to avoid myopathy or rhabdomyolysis. The blood concentrations of macrolide immunosuppressants (tacrolimus, sirolimus, and everolimus) are similar to that of statins [108, 109]; therefore, the lack of clinically relevant interactions between macrolides and statins is not unexpected.

4.2.3. Antihypertensive agents

Organ transplantation and immunosuppressive therapy (e.g., ciclosporin, prednisone) frequently trigger hypertension or worsen the preexisting disease in patients. While most of the antihypertensive agents (β-adrenoceptor blockers, α1-adrenergic receptor antagonists, central α2-adrenergic receptor agonists, angiotensin-converting enzyme inhibitors, and angiotensin II receptor blockers) are not expected to influence the pharmacokinetics of immunosuppressants, medication with diltiazem, verapamil, or amlodipine requires special consideration and frequent monitoring of immunosuppressant blood concentrations. The metabolism of all three Ca-channel blockers is primarily catalyzed by CYP3A4, anticipating potential drug interactions with immunosuppressants. Furthermore, significant inhibition of CYP3A4 by diltiazem, verapamil, and amlodipine has been demonstrated with an additional inhibitory property of metabolite intermediate complex formation that catalytically inactivates CYP3A4 and CYP3A5 enzymes [79, 80, 82, 110–114]. The inactivation of CYP3A enzymes by comedication with these antihypertensive drugs consequently leads to a permanent increase in blood concentrations of calcineurin inhibitors or mTOR inhibitors [115–122]. In transplant recipients comedicated with sirolimus and verapamil, an increase of blood concentrations of both sirolimus and verapamil was observed [123]. Furthermore, in patients carrying wild-type *CYP3A5*1* allele, concomitant treatment with amlodipine significantly decreased tacrolimus clearance, and along with the changes in tacrolimus pharmacokinetics, an increase in amlodipine blood concentrations was also observed [124]. The metabolism of the Ca-channel blocker nifedipine is catalyzed almost exclusively by CYP3A enzymes, and competition for the active site of CYP3As may be expected if nifedipine and CYP3A substrate calcineurine inhibitors or mTOR inhibitors are concomitantly applied. In contrast, no evidence for pharmacokinetic drug interactions has been provided in transplant recipients treated with nifedipine and ciclosporin/tacrolimus or sirolimus/everolimus. Carvedilol is often used for treatment of hypertension in transplant patients, and pharmacokinetic drug interaction between carvedilol and ciclosporin has been observed that required 10–20% reduction of ciclosporin doses to maintain the blood concentrations within the therapeutic range [125, 126]. The major metabolic pathways of carvedilol are catalyzed by CYP2D6 and CYP1A2 rather than by CYP3A4 [127]; however, inhibition of CYP3A enzymes by carvedilol does not account for pharmacokinetic drug interaction with ciclosporin. Carvedilol has been demonstrated to block the function of the ABCB1 transporter protein (ATP-binding cassette B1; previously called as Pgp) [128]. In the intestinal wall, ABCB1 transporter pumps pharmacons or other xenobiotics passed into the enterocytes back into the gut lumen. The inhibition of ABCB1-mediated transcellular transport in the intestine by carvedilol is responsible for the increased absorption of ciclosporin. Under careful monitoring of ciclosporin blood concentration, the ABCB1 inhibition by carvedilol can be beneficial in ciclosporin-sparing therapy for transplant patients. Since the absorption of tacrolimus and mTOR inhibitors is also mediated by ABCB1, similar pharmacokinetic drug interactions between these immunosuppressants and carvedilol are presumably developed as with ciclosporin.

4.2.4. Antihyperglycemic therapy

Hyperglycemia developing posttransplant diabetes mellitus is generally medication related. Corticosteroids can evoke reduction of glucose tolerance, whereas ciclosporin and tacrolimus directly block insulin-release by islet cells. The metabolism of the sulfonylurea type antidiabetic agents (e.g., tolbutamide, glipizide, glibenclamide, and glimepiride) is mediated by CYP2C9; therefore, metabolic drug interactions with immunosuppressants are not expected in patients treated with any of these oral hypoglycemic drugs. Although the thiazolidinedione type troglitazone and rosiglitazone are not CYP3A substrates, they can induce the expression of CYP3A enzymes by activation of the nuclear receptors, PXR and CAR [129–132]. Enhanced transcription results in an increase in CYP3A activities and the metabolism of calcineurin inhibitors, mTOR inhibitors and corticosteroids, increasing the risk of rejection [133]. Immunosuppressant dose adjustment is required to avoid subtherapeutic blood concentrations, and careful monitoring of immunosuppressant blood concentrations is recommended during withdrawal of troglitazone or rosiglitazone and during switching to other antihyperglycemic agent.

4.2.5. Psychiatric medication

The most common psychiatric disorders encountered in transplant patients are anxiety, depression, mood disorders, behavior problems, and insomnia that are reversible in most cases; however, they often require psychotherapy with antidepressants, mood stabilizers, anxiolytic agents, or even with antipsychotics. Many of these pharmacons are metabolized by enzymes other than CYP3A4 and do not influence the drug-metabolizing activities of CYP3A4; consequently, metabolic drug interactions with immunosuppressants cannot be expected. Nevertheless, the CYP3A4 inducing or inhibitory properties of some of these psychopharmacons should be considered. The mood stabilizer carbamazepine and valproic acid have been clearly evidenced to be able to activate CAR and PXR. The nuclear receptor activation leads to an increase in transcription of *CYP3A4* gene and CYP3A4 metabolic activity [134, 135], anticipating decrease of immunosuppressant blood concentrations [136]. To reduce the risk of organ rejection, adjustment (increase) of immunosuppressant doses is required with continuous monitoring of immunosuppressant blood levels. Furthermore, the CYP3A4 deinduction process can last for about 2 weeks after cessation of carbamazepine or valproic acid [137]; thus, careful monitoring of immunosuppressant blood concentrations during withdrawal is essential. The comedication with the antidepressant fluvoxamine is contraindicated because of its strong inhibitory properties for CYP3A4 substrates and potential drug interactions with ciclosporin/tacrolimus or with sirolimus/everolimus [80, 138, 139]. For psychotherapeutic agents that are CYP3A substrates (haloperidol, quetiapine, clonazepam, midazolam, alprazolam), continuous monitoring of immunosuppressant blood levels is highly recommended to avoid metabolic drug interactions.

4.2.6. Treatment of hyperuricemia

The metabolic drug interactions with ciclosporin/tacrolimus, sirolimus/everolimus, and corticosteroids are generally associated with reversible or irreversible inhibition of CYP3A activities, as well as with transcriptional induction of CYP3A4 and CYP3A5 expression. Clinically significant drug interaction occurs during simultaneous therapy with azathioprine (or 6-mercaptopurine) and allopurinol, the antihyperuricemic agent [140, 141]; however, it involves enzyme other than CYP3As. The metabolism of both 6-mercaptopurine and allopurinol is catalyzed by xantine oxidase, anticipating metabolic drug interactions and developing serious adverse reactions. As a consequence of inhibition of xantine oxidase by allopurinol, myelotoxicity is evoked by the accumulation of 6-thioguanine-nucleotide metabolites of azathioprine. The risk of bone marrow depletion is increased in patients with low thiopurine methyl-transferase activity. To avoid the serious myelosuppression during treatment of hyperuricemia and gout, substantial reduction of azathioprine dose (by at least 50%) is required when allopurinol is given concomitantly, or alternative agents other than allopurinol should be considered [142–144].

4.3. Metabolic drug interactions between immunosuppressants and herb components

Pharmacokinetic herb-drug interactions can also significantly influence the outcome of immunosuppressive therapy and long-term graft survival [145]. St John's wort (*Hypericum perforatum*) extract and grapefruit juice are well described as modifiers of pharmacokinetic properties of ciclosporin and tacrolimus [146–148]. St John's wort extract is a herbal product for treatment of symptoms of mild or moderate depression, including anxiety, fatigue, and sleeping problems. The extract contains a number of biologically active components, e.g., hyperforin of high interest. Hyperforin has a strong affinity for PXR and significantly increases the expression and activities of CYP3A4 enzyme, which is involved in metabolism of many drugs [149, 150]. Consequently, chronic consumption of St John's wort extract can decrease the blood concentrations of CYP3A substrates, such as calcineurin inhibitors, mTOR inhibitors, and corticosteroids [151–154]. In addition, St John's wort extract has been reported to induce the expression of ABCB1 transporter that reduces the absorption of ABCB1-ligand drugs from the gut. The hyperforin contents of commercially available St John's wort preparations are variables that appear to significantly affect the extent of pharmacokinetic interactions [150, 155]. Coadministration of ciclosporin with St John's wort extract has been reported to lead a 40–60% decrease of ciclosporin blood concentrations, increasing the risk of rejection; therefore, substantial dose adjustment is required [151, 152, 155–159]. Since clinicians are often unaware of concomitant consumption of herbal supplements, transplant patients should be informed about the drug interaction potential of St John's wort that can endanger the success of organ transplantation.

Concomitant intake of grapefruit (*Citrus paradisii*) or pomelo (*Citrus grandis*) has been demonstrated to increase the bioavailability of immunosuppressants [147, 160, 161]. Some components of these citrus fruits, bergamottin and naringenin responsible for the bitter taste, can inhibit the activities of CYP3A4 and CYP3A5 enzymes both in the intestinal wall and in the liver, resulting in significant reduction of first-pass metabolism of CYP3A substrates, including ciclosporin and tacrolimus [162–164]. Significant reduction of ciclosporin/tacrolimus doses is necessary to avoid the risk of nephrotoxicity or other adverse events associated with immunosuppressive therapy. The furanocoumarin bergamottin is a "suicide substrate," namely it is metabolized by CYP3A4 to an epoxid metabolite that covalently binds to and inactivates the enzyme [165]. The flavonoid naringenin was found to be a less-potent CYP3A4 inhibitor than bergamottin [166]; however, during consumption of grapefruit, the inhibitory effects of naringenin and bergamottin are added together. Since clear evidence of bergamottin content and CYP3A4 inhibitory potential of citruses other than grapefruit and pomelo was provided [167], the transplantation centers do not recommend citrus consumption for transplant patients during immunosuppressive therapy.

5. Concluding remarks

Although success of organ transplantation is continuously improving, several short- and long-term complications can adversely affect the outcome. One of the most significant factors influencing the long-term graft and patient survival is the appropriate immunosuppressive therapy. Subtherapeutic blood concentrations of immunosuppressive drugs can evoke acute or chronic graft injury mediated by immunological mechanisms, whereas overdosing leads to over-suppression of the immune system that consequently develops serious infections, as well as adverse and even life-threatening side effects. Because of the narrow therapeutic indexes, dosing of most of the immunosuppressive agents is applied under careful monitoring of their blood concentrations. The knowledge of the potential factors that can modify immunosuppressive therapy, as well as pharmacokinetic and metabolic drug interactions, can decrease the fluctuation of immunosuppressant blood concentrations, can facilitate to avoid the serious adverse events, can improve the therapeutic outcome for transplant patients, and can reduce the medical costs.

The appropriate and tailored immunosuppressive medication is a great challenge and requires careful and continuous attention, because unrecognized simple interactions can induce serious complications. As such during administratrion of clarithromycin or antifungal agents without dose reduction of calcineurin inhibitors or mTOR inhibitors, blood concentrations of immunosuppressants can substantially exceed the therapeutic range within some days. Without dose modification, a reverse outcome is expected during comedication with anticonvulsants (valproic acid and carbamazepine) or with rifampicin resulting in subtherapeutic blood concentrations of immunosuppressants and increasing the risk of organ rejection. The lack of mycophenolate dose reduction during cessation of ciclosporin or replacement of ciclosporin to another immunosuppressant can also evolve development of serious adverse reactions. It is anticipated that the special attention and the knowledge of potential drug interactions can prevent the majority of misdosing-induced adverse events.

Acknowledgements

This work was supported by MedInProt Synergy VIII program of the Hungarian Academy of Sciences and by the Society of Hungarian Toxicologists.

Author details

Katalin Monostory

Address all correspondence to: monostory.katalin@ttk.mta.hu

Institute of Enzymology, Research Centre for Natural Sciences, Hungarian Academy of Sciences, Budapest, Hungary

References

[1] Shah RR, Smith RL. Addressing phenoconversion: The Achilles' heel of personalized medicine. British Journal of Clinical Pharmacology. 2015;**79**:222-240. DOI: 10.1111/bcp.12441

[2] Squassina A, Manchia M, Manolopoulos VG, Artac M, Lappa-Manakou C, Karkabouna S, Mitropoulos K, Del Zompo M, Patrinos GP. Realities and expectations of pharmacogenomics and personalized medicine: Impact of translating genetic knowledge into clinical practice. Pharmacogenomics. 2010;**11**:1149-1167. DOI: 10.2217/pgs.10.97

[3] Gervasini G, Benítez J, Carrillo JA. Pharmacogenetic testing and therapeutic drug monitoring are complementary tools for optimal individualization of drug therapy. European Journal of Clinical Pharmacology. 2010;**66**:755-774. DOI: 10.1007/s00228-010-0857-7

[4] Shah RR, Shah DR. Personalized medicine: Is it a pharmacogenetic mirage? British Journal of Clinical Pharmacology. 2012;**74**:698-721. DOI: 10.1111/j.1365-2125.2012.04328.x

[5] Sim SC, Kacevska M, Ingelman-Sundberg M. Pharmacogenomics of drug-metabolizing enzymes: A recent update on clinical implications and endogenous effects. The Pharmacogenomics Journal. 2013;**13**:1-11. DOI: 10.1038/tpj.2012.45

[6] Zhou SF, Liu JP, Chowbay B. Polymorphism of human cytochrome P450 enzymes and its clinical impact. Drug Metabolism Reviews. 2009;**41**:89-295. DOI: 10.1021/tx0100439

[7] Zanger UM, Schwab M. Cytochrome P450 enzymes in drug metabolism: Regulation of gene expression, enzyme activities, and impact of genetic variation. Pharmacology & Therapeutics. 2013;**138**:103-141. DOI: 10.1016/j.pharmthera.2012.12.007

[8] Samer CF, Lorenzini KI, Rollason V, Daali Y, Desmeules JA. Applications of CYP450 testing in the clinical setting. Molecular Diagnosis & Therapy. 2013;**17**:165-184. DOI: 10.1007/s40291-013-0028-5

[9] Zhou ZW, Chen XW, Sneed KB, Yang YX, Zhang X, He ZX, Chow K, Yang T, Duan W, Zhou SF. Clinical association between pharmacogenomics and adverse drug reactions. Drugs. 2015;**75**:589-631. DOI: 10.1007/s40265-015-0375-0

[10] Rendic S, Guengerich FP. Update information on drug metabolism systems - 2009, part II: Summary of information on the effects of diseases and environmental factors on human cytochrome P450 (CYP) enzymes and transporters. Current Drug Metabolism. 2010;**11**:4-84. DOI: 10.2174/138920010791110917

[11] Shah RR, Gaedigk A, LLerena A, Eichelbaum M, Stingl J, Smith RL. CYP450 genotype and pharmacogenetic association studies: A critical appraisal. Pharmacogenomics. 2016;**17**:259-275. DOI: 10.2217/pgs.15.172

[12] Zhou Y, Ingelman-Sundberg M, Lauschke VM. Worldwide distribution of cytochrome P450 alleles: A meta-analysis of population-scale sequencing projects. Clinical Pharmacology and Therapeutics. 2017;**102**:688-700. DOI: 10.1002/cpt.690

[13] Temesvári M, Kóbori L, Paulik J, Sárváry E, Belic A, Monostory K. Estimation of drug-metabolizing capacity by cytochrome P450 genotyping and expression. The Journal of Pharmacology and Experimental Therapeutics. 2012;**341**:294-305. DOI: 10.1124/jpet.111.189597

[14] Amirimani B, Ning B, Deitz AC, Weber BL, Kadlubar FF, Rebbeck TR. Increased transcriptional activity of the *CYP3A4*1B* promoter variant. Environmental and Molecular Mutagenesis. 2003;**42**:299-305. DOI: 10.1002/em.10199

[15] García-Martín E, Martínez C, Pizarro RM, García-Gamito FJ, Gullsten H, Raunio H, Agúndez JA. *CYP3A4* variant alleles in white individuals with low CYP3A4 enzyme activity. Clinical Pharmacology and Therapeutics. 2002;**71**:196-204. DOI: 10.1067/mcp.2002.121371

[16] Okubo M, Murayama N, Shimizu M, Shimada T, Guengerich FP, Yamazaki H. CYP3A4 intron 6 C>T polymorphism (CYP3A4*22) is associated with reduced CYP3A4 protein level and function in human liver microsomes. The Journal of Toxicological Sciences. 2013;**38**:349-354. DOI: 10.2131/jts.38.349

[17] Zhou SF. Drugs behave as substrates, inhibitors and inducers of human cytochrome P450 3A4. Current Drug Metabolism. 2008;**9**:310-322. DOI: 10.2174/138920008784220664

[18] Monostory K, Dvorak Z. Steroid regulation of drug-metabolizing cytochromes P450. Current Drug Metabolism. 2011;**12**:154-172. DOI: 10.2174/138920011795016854

[19] Hukkanen J. Induction of cytochrome P450 enzymes: A view on human in vivo findings. Expert Review of Clinical Pharmacology. 2012;**5**:569-585. DOI: 10.1586/ecp.12.39

[20] Sinz MW. Evaluation of pregnane X receptor (PXR)-mediated CYP3A4 drug-drug interactions in drug development. Drug Metabolism Reviews. 2013;**45**:3-14. DOI: 10.3109/03602532.2012.743560

[21] Matoulková P, Pávek P, Malý J, Vlček J. Cytochrome P450 enzyme regulation by glucocorticoids and consequences in terms of drug interaction. Expert Opinion on Drug Metabolism & Toxicology. 2014;**10**:425-435. DOI: 10.1517/17425255.2014.878703

[22] Aitken AE, Morgan ET. Gene-specific effects of inflammatory cytokines on cytochrome P450 2C, 2B6 and 3A4 mRNA levels in human hepatocytes. Drug Metabolism and Disposition. 2007;**35**:1687-1693. DOI: 10.1124/dmd.107.015511

[23] Dickmann LJ, Patel SK, Rock DA, Wienkers LC, Slatter JG. Effects of interleukin-6 (IL-6) and an anti-IL-6 monoclonal antibody on drug-metabolizing enzymes in human hepatocyte culture. Drug Metabolism and Disposition. 2011;**39**:1415-1422. DOI: 10.1124/dmd.111.038679

[24] Dickmann LJ, Patel SK, Wienkers LC, Slatter JG. Effects of interleukin 1β (IL-1β) and IL-1β/interleukin 6 (IL-6) combinations on drug metabolizing enzymes in human hepatocyte culture. Current Drug Metabolism. 2012;**13**:930-937. DOI: 10.2174/138920012802138642

[25] Ning R, Zhan Y, He S, Hu Y, Zhu Z, Hu G, Yan B, Yang J, Liu W. Interleukin-6 induces DEC1, promotes DEC1 interaction with RXRα and suppresses the expression of PXR, CAR and their target genes. Frontiers in Pharmacology. 2017;**8**:866. DOI: 10.3389/fphar.2017.00866

[26] Shah RR, Smith RL. Inflammation-induced phenoconversion of polymorphic drug metabolizing enzymes: Hypothesis with implications for personalized medicine. Drug Metabolism and Disposition. 2015;**43**:400-410. DOI: 10.1124/dmd.114.061093

[27] Shah RR. Pharmacogenetics and precision medicine: Is inflammation a covert threat to effective genotype-based therapy? Therapeutic Advances in Drug Safety. 2017;**8**:267-272. DOI: 10.1177/2042098617712657

[28] Ryman JT, Meibohm B. Pharmacokinetics of monoclonal antibodies. CPT: Pharmacometrics & Systems Pharmacology. 2017;**6**:576-588. DOI: 10.1002/psp4.12224

[29] Penninga L, Wettergren A, Chan AW, Steinbrüchel DA, Gluud C. Calcineurin inhibitor minimisation versus continuation of calcineurin inhibitor treatment for liver transplant recipients. Cochrane Database of Systematic Reviews. 2012;**3**:CD008852. DOI: 10.1002/14651858.CD008852.pub2

[30] Choudhary NS, Saigal S, Shukla R, Kotecha H, Saraf N, Soin AS. Current status of immunosuppression in liver transplantation. Journal of Clinical and Experimental Hepatology. 2013;**3**:150-158. DOI: 10.1016/j.jceh.2013.04.005

[31] Azzi JR, Sayegh MH, Mallat SG. Calcineurin inhibitors: 40 years later, can't live without. Journal of Immunology. 2013;**191**:5785-5791. DOI: 10.4049/jimmunol.1390055

[32] Christians U, Sewing KF. Cyclosporin metabolism in transplant patients. Pharmacology & Therapeutics. 1993;**57**:291-345. DOI: 10.1016/0163-7258(93)90059-M

[33] Christians U, Kohlhaw K, Budniak J, Bleck JS, Schottmann R, Schlitt HJ, Almeida VM, Deters M, Wonigeit K, Pichlmayr R, Sewing KF. Ciclosporin metabolite pattern in blood and urine of liver graft recipients. I. Association of ciclosporin metabolites with nephrotoxicity. European Journal of Clinical Pharmacology. 1991;**41**:285-290

[34] Christians U, Kohlhaw K, Sürig T, Bader A, Schottmann R, Linck A, Ringe B, Sewing KF. Parallel blood concentrations of second-generation cyclosporine metabolites and bilirubin in liver graft recipients. Therapeutic Drug Monitoring. 1995;**17**:487-498. DOI: 10.1097/00007691-199510000-00009

[35] Monostory K, Tóth K, Kiss Á, Háfra E, Csikány N, Paulik J, Sárváry E, Kóbori L. Personalizing calcineurin inhibitor therapy by adjusting to donor CYP3A-status in liver transplant patients. British Journal of Clinical Pharmacology. 2015;**80**:1429-1437. DOI: 10.1111/bcp.12747

[36] Iwasaki K. Metabolism of tacrolimus (FK506) and recent topics in clinical pharmacokinetics. Drug Metabolism and Pharmacokinetics. 2007;**22**:328-335. DOI: 10.2133/dmpk.22.328

[37] Iwasaki K, Shiraga T, Nagase K, Tozuka Z, Noda K, Sakuma S, Fujitsu T, Shimatani K, Sato A, Fujioka M. Isolation, identification, and biological activities of oxidative metabolites of FK506, a potent immunosuppressive macrolide lactone. Drug Metabolism and Disposition. 1993;**21**:971-977

[38] Iwasaki K, Shiraga T, Matsuda H, Nagase K, Tokuma Y, Hata T, Fujii Y, Sakuma S, Fujitsu T, Fujikawa A, Shimatani K, Sato A, Fujioka M. Further metabolism of FK506 (tacrolimus). Identification and biological activities of the metabolites oxidized at multiple sites of FK506. Drug Metabolism and Disposition. 1995;**23**:28-34

[39] Zegarska J, Hryniewiecka E, Zochowska D, Samborowska E, Jazwiec R, Borowiec A, Tszyrsznic W, Chmura A, Nazarewski S, Dadlez M, Paczek L. Tacrolimus metabolite M-III may have nephrotoxic and myelotoxic effects and increase the incidence of infections in kidney transplant recipients. Transplantation Proceedings. 2016;**48**:1539-1542. DOI: 10.1016/j.transproceed.2015.12.133

[40] Kamdem LK, Streit F, Zanger UM, Brockmöller J, Oellerich M, Armstrong VW, Wojnowski L. Contribution of CYP3A5 to the in vitro hepatic clearance of tacrolimus. Clinical Chemistry. 2005;**51**:1374-1381. DOI: 10.1373/clinchem.2005.050047

[41] Provenzani A, Notarbartolo M, Labbozzetta M, Poma P, Vizzini G, Salis P, Caccamo C, Bertani T, Palazzo U, Polidori P, Gridelli B, D'Alessandro N. Influence of CYP3A5 and ABCB1 gene polymorphisms and other factors on tacrolimus dosing in Caucasian liver and kidney transplant patients. International Journal of Molecular Medicine. 2011;**28**: 1093-1102. DOI: 10.3892/ijmm.2011.794

[42] Moes DJ, Guchelaar HJ, de Fijter JW. Sirolimus and everolimus in kidney transplantation. Drug Discovery Today. 2015;**20**:1243-1249. DOI: 10.1016/j.drudis.2015.05.006

[43] Jacquet A, Francois H, Frangie C, Ahmad L, Charpentier B, Durrbach A. Prevention of calcineurin inhibitor nephrotoxicity in renal transplantation. Transplant Immunology. 2008;**20**:29-31. DOI: 10.1016/j.trim.2008.09.002

[44] Kacar S, Gurkan A, Karaca C, Varılsuha C, Tilif S. Low-dose calcineurin inhibitor regimen combined with mammalian target of rapamycin inhibitors preserves kidney functions in renal transplant recipients without allograft nephropathy. Transplantation Proceedings. 2010;**42**:3513-3516. DOI: 10.1016/j.transproceed.2010.08.043

[45] Shihab F, Christians U, Smith L, Wellen JR, Kaplan B. Focus on mTOR inhibitors and tacrolimus in renal transplantation: Pharmacokinetics, exposure–response relationships, and clinical outcomes. Transplant Immunology. 2014;**31**:22-32. DOI: 10.1016/j.trim.2014.05.002

[46] Jacobsen W, Serkova N, Hausen B, Morris RE, Benet LZ, Christians U. Comparison of the in vitro metabolism of the macrolide immunosuppressants sirolimus and RAD. Transplantation Proceedings. 2001;**33**:514-515. DOI: 10.1016/S0041-1345(00)02116-3

[47] Mahalati K, Kahan BD. Clinical pharmacokinetics of sirolimus. Clinical Pharmacokinetics. 2001;**40**:573-585. DOI: 10.2165/00003088-200140080-00002

[48] Maltzman JS, Koretzky GA. Azathioprine: Old drug, new actions. The Journal of Clinical Investigation. 2003;**111**:1122-1224. DOI: 10.1172/JCI18384

[49] Rowland K, Lennard L, Lilleyman JS. In vitro metabolism of 6-mercaptopurine by human liver cytosol. Xenobiotica. 1999;**29**:615-628. DOI: 10.1080/004982599238434

[50] Relling MV, Gardner EE, Sandborn WJ, Schmiegelow K, Pui CH, Yee SW, Stein CM, Carrillo M, Evans WE, Hicks JK, Schwab M, Klein TE. Clinical Pharmacogenetics implementation consortium. Clinical pharmacogenetics implementation consortium guidelines for thiopurine methyltransferase genotype and thiopurine dosing: 2013 update. Clinical Pharmacology and Therapeutics. 2013;**93**:324-325. DOI: 10.1038/clpt.2013.4

[51] Staatz CE, Tett SE. Pharmacology and toxicology of mycophenolate in organ transplant recipients: An update. Archives of Toxicology. 2014;**88**:1352-1389. DOI: 10.1007/s00204-014-1247-1

[52] Picard N, Ratanasavanh D, Prémaud A, Le Meur Y, Marquet P. Identification of the UDP-glucuronosyltransferase isoforms involved in mycophenolic acid phase II metabolism. Drug Metabolism and Disposition. 2005;**33**:139-146. DOI: 10.1124/dmd.104.001651

[53] Staatz CE, Tett SE. Clinical pharmacokinetics and pharmacodynamics of mycophenolate in patients with autoimmune disease. Clinical Pharmacokinetics. 2007;**46**:13-58. DOI: 10.2165/00003088-200746010-00002

[54] Lamba V, Sangkuhl K, Sanghavi K, Fish A, Altman RB, Klein TE. PharmGKB summary: Mycophenolic acid pathway. Pharmacogenetics and Genomics. 2014;**24**:73-79. DOI: 10. 1097/FPC.0000000000000010

[55] Rhen T, Cidlowski JA. Antiinflammatory action of glucocorticoids--new mechanisms for old drugs. The New England Journal of Medicine. 2005;**353**:1711-1723. DOI: 10.1056/ NEJMra050541

[56] Pichard L, Fabre I, Daujat M, Domergue J, Joyeux H, Maurel P. Effect of corticosteroids on the expression of cytochromes P450 and on cyclosporin a oxidase activity in primary cultures of human hepatocytes. Molecular Pharmacology. 1992;**41**:1047-1055

[57] Pascussi JM, Gerbal-Chaloin S, Drocourt L, Maurel P, Vilarem MJ. The expression of CYP2B6, CYP2C9 and CYP3A4 genes: A tangle of networks of nuclear and steroid receptors. Biochimica et Biophysica Acta. 2003;**1619**:243-253. DOI: 10.1016/S0304-4165(02) 00483-X

[58] Wong TC, Lo CM, Fung JY. Emerging drugs for prevention of T-cell mediated rejection in liver and kidney transplantation. Expert Opinion on Emerging Drugs. 2017;**22**: 123-136. DOI: 10.1080/14728214.2017.1330884

[59] Kuglstatter A, Mueller F, Kusznir E, Gsell B, Stihle M, Thoma R, Benz J, Aspeslet L, Freitag D, Hennig M. Structural basis for the cyclophilin a binding affinity and immunosuppressive potency of E-ISA247 (voclosporin). Acta Crystallographica. Section D, Biological Crystallography. 2011;**67**:119-123. DOI: 10.1107/S0907444910051905

[60] Ling SY, Huizinga RB, Mayo PR, Larouche R, Freitag DG, Aspeslet LJ, Foster RT. Cytochrome P450 3A and P-glycoprotein drug-drug interactions with voclosporin. British Journal of Clinical Pharmacology. 2014;**77**:1039-1050. DOI: 10.1111/bcp.12309

[61] Tedesco-Silva H, Kho MM, Hartmann A, Vitko S, Russ G, Rostaing L, Budde K, Campistol JM, Eris J, Krishnan I, Gopalakrishnan U, Klupp J. Sotrastaurin in calcineurin inhibitor-free regimen using everolimus in de novo kidney transplant recipients. American Journal of Transplantation. 2013;**13**:1757-1768. DOI: 10.1111/ajt.12255

[62] Pascher A, De Simone P, Pratschke J, Salamé E, Pirenne J, Isoneimi H, Bijarnia M, Krishnan I, Klupp J. Protein kinase C inhibitor sotrastaurin in de novo liver transplant recipients: A randomized phase II trial. American Journal of Transplantation. 2015;**15**:1283-1292. DOI: 10.1111/ajt.13175

[63] van Gelder T, Fisher L, Shihab F, Shipkova M. Optimizing everolimus exposure when combined with calcineurin inhibitors in solid organ transplantation. Transplantation Reviews (Orlando, Fla.). 2017;**31**:151-157. DOI: 10.1016/j.trre.2017.02.007

[64] Sharif A, Shabir S, Chand S, Cockwell P, Ball S, Borrows R. Meta-analysis of calcineurin-inhibitor-sparing regimens in kidney transplantation. Journal of the American Society of Nephrology. 2011;**22**:2107-2118. DOI: 10.1681/ASN.2010111160

[65] Martin P, Riley R, Back DJ, Owen A. Comparison of the induction profile for drug disposition proteins by typical nuclear receptor activators in human hepatic and intestinal cells. British Journal of Pharmacology. 2008;**153**:805-819. DOI: 10.1038/sj.bjp.0707601

[66] Hesselink DA, Ngyuen H, Wabbijn M, Gregoor PJ, Steyerberg EW, van Riemsdijk IC, Weimar W, van Gelder T. Tacrolimus dose requirement in renal transplant recipients is significantly higher when used in combination with corticosteroids. British Journal of Clinical Pharmacology. 2003;**56**:327-330. DOI: 10.1046/j.0306-5251.2003.01882.x

[67] Anglicheau D, Flamant M, Schlageter MH, Martinez F, Cassinat B, Beaune P, Legendre C, Thervet E. Pharmacokinetic interaction between corticosteroids and tacrolimus after renal transplantation. Nephrology, Dialysis, Transplantation. 2003;**18**:2409-2414. DOI: 10. 1093/ndt/gfg381

[68] van Duijnhoven EM, Boots JM, Christiaans MH, Stolk LM, Undre NA, van Hooff JP. Increase in tacrolimus trough levels after steroid withdrawal. Transplant International. 2003;**16**:721-725. DOI: 10.1007/s00147-003-0615-1

[69] Roberts PJ, Rollins KD, Kashuba AD, Paine MF, Nelsen AC, Williams EE, Moran C, Lamba JK, Schuetz EG, Hawke RL. The influence of CYP3A5 genotype on dexamethasone induction of CYP3A activity in African Americans. Drug Metabolism and Disposition. 2008;**36**:1465-1469. DOI: 10.1124/dmd.107.020065

[70] Naito T, Shinno K, Maeda T, Kagawa Y, Hashimoto H, Otsuka A, Takayama T, Ushiyama T, Suzuki K, Ozono S. Effects of calcineurin inhibitors on pharmacokinetics of mycophenolic acid and its glucuronide metabolite during the maintenance period following renal transplantation. Biological & Pharmaceutical Bulletin. 2006;**29**:275-280. DOI: 10.1248/bpb.29.275

[71] Cattaneo D, Merlini S, Zenoni S, Baldelli S, Gotti E, Remuzzi G, Perico N. Influence of co-medication with sirolimus or cyclosporine on mycophenolic acid pharmacokinetics in kidney transplantation. American Journal of Transplantation. 2005;**5**:2937-2944. DOI: 10.1111/j.1600-6143.2005.01107.x

[72] Dalal P, Shah G, Chhabra D, Gallon L. Role of tacrolimus combination therapy with mycophenolate mofetil in the prevention of organ rejection in kidney transplant patients. International Journal of Nephrology and Renovascular Disease. 2010;**3**:107-115. DOI: 10.2147/IJNRD.S7044

[73] Kovarik JM, Beyer D, Schmouder RL. Everolimus drug interactions: Application of a classification system for clinical decision making. Biopharmaceutics & Drug Disposition. 2006;**27**:421-426. DOI: 10.1002/bdd.524

[74] Lu C, Hatsis P, Berg C, Lee FW, Balani SK. Prediction of pharmacokinetic drug-drug interactions using human hepatocyte suspension in plasma and cytochrome P450 phenotypic data. II. In vitro-in vivo correlation with ketoconazole. Drug Metabolism and Disposition. 2008;**36**:1255-1260. DOI: 10.1124/dmd.107.018796

[75] Lu C, Berg C, Prakash SR, Lee FW, Balani SK. Prediction of pharmacokinetic drug-drug interactions using human hepatocyte suspension in plasma and cytochrome P450 phenotypic data. III. In vitro-in vivo correlation with fluconazole. Drug Metabolism and Disposition. 2008;**36**:1261-1266. DOI: 10.1124/dmd.107.019000

[76] Yamazaki H, Nakamoto M, Shimizu M, Murayama N, Niwa T. Potential impact of cytochrome P450 3A5 in human liver on drug interactions with triazoles. British Journal of Clinical Pharmacology. 2010;**69**:593-597. DOI: 10.1111/j.1365-2125.2010.03656.x

[77] Zhang S, Pillai VC, Mada SR, Strom S, Venkataramanan R. Effect of voriconazole and other azole antifungal agents on CYP3A activity and metabolism of tacrolimus in human liver microsomes. Xenobiotica. 2012;**42**:409-416. DOI: 10.3109/00498254.2011.631224

[78] Saad AH, DePestel DD, Carver PL. Factors influencing the magnitude and clinical significance of drug interactions between azole antifungals and select immunosuppressants. Pharmacotherapy. 2006;**26**:1730-1744. DOI: 10.1592/phco.26.12.1730

[79] Galetin A, Burt H, Gibbons L, Houston JB. Prediction of time-dependent CYP3A4 drug-drug interactions: Impact of enzyme degradation, parallel elimination pathways, and intestinal inhibition. Drug Metabolism and Disposition. 2006;**34**:166-175. DOI: 10.1124/dmd/105.006874

[80] Watanabe A, Nakamura K, Okudaira N, Okazaki O, Sudo K. Risk assessment for drug-drug interaction caused by metabolism-based inhibition of CYP3A using automated in vitro assay systems and its application in the early drug discovery process. Drug Metabolism and Disposition. 2007;**35**:1232-1238. DOI: 10.1124/dmd.107.015016

[81] Aueviriyavit S, Kobayashi K, Chiba K. Species differences in mechanism-based inactivation of CYP3A in humans, rats and mice. Drug Metabolism and Pharmacokinetics. 2010;**25**:93-100. DOI: 10.2133/dmpk.25.93

[82] Kosaka M, Kosugi Y, Hirabayashi H. Risk assessment using cytochrome P450 time-dependent inhibition assays at single time and concentration in the early stage of drug discovery. Journal of Pharmaceutical Sciences. 2017;**106**:2839-2846. DOI: 10.1016/j.xphs.2017.04.077

[83] Westphal JF. Macrolide - induced clinically relevant drug interactions with cytochrome P-450A (CYP) 3A4: An update focused on clarithromycin, azithromycin and dirithromycin. British Journal of Clinical Pharmacology. 2000;**50**:285-295. DOI: 10.1046/j.1365-2125.2000.00261.x

[84] Rubinstein E. Comparative safety of the different macrolides. International Journal of Antimicrobial Agents. 2001;**18**(Suppl 1):S71-S76. DOI: 10.1016/S0924-8579(01)00397-1

[85] Capone D, Palmiero G, Gentile A, Basile V, Federico S, Sabbatini M, Potenza M, Perfetti A, Pieri M, Tarantino G. A pharmacokinetic interaction between clarithromycin and sirolimus in kidney transplant recipient. Current Drug Metabolism. 2007;**8**:379-381. DOI: 10. 2174/138920007780655405

[86] Pea F, Cojutti P, Tursi V, Livi U, Baraldo M. Everolimus overexposure in a heart transplant patient receiving clarithromycin for the treatment of pneumonia. Transplant Infectious Disease. 2015;**17**:926-928. DOI: 10.1111/tid.12446

[87] Page RL 2nd, Ruscin JM, Fish D, Lapointe M. Possible interaction between intravenous azithromycin and oral cyclosporine. Pharmacotherapy. 2001;**21**:1436-1443. DOI: 10.1592/ phco.21.17.1436.34434

[88] Mori T, Aisa Y, Nakazato T, Yamazaki R, Ikeda Y, Okamoto S. Tacrolimus-azithromycin interaction in a recipient of allogeneic bone marrow transplantation. Transplant International. 2005;**18**:757-758. DOI: 10.1111/j.1432-2277.2005.00135.x

[89] Polasek TM, Miners JO. Quantitative prediction of macrolide drug-drug interaction potential from in vitro studies using testosterone as the human cytochrome P4503A substrate. European Journal of Clinical Pharmacology. 2006;**62**:203-208. DOI: 10.1007/ s00228-005-0091-x

[90] Monostory K, Pascussi J-M. Regulation of drug-metabolizing human cytochrome P450s. Acta Chimica Slovenica. 2008;**55**:20-37

[91] Hebert MF, Fisher RM, Marsh CL, Dressler D, Bekersky I. Effects of rifampin on tacrolimus pharmacokinetics in healthy volunteers. Journal of Clinical Pharmacology. 1999;**39**:91-96. DOI: 10.1177/00912709922007499

[92] Bhaloo S, Prasad GV. Severe reduction in tacrolimus levels with rifampin despite multiple cytochrome P450 inhibitors: A case report. Transplantation Proceedings. 2003;**35**: 2449-2451. DOI: 10.1016/j.transproceed.2003.08.019

[93] Lee YT, Hwang S, Lee SG, Kim KW, Choi NK, Park GC, Yu YD, Yoo JW, Kim WS, Shim TS. Living-donor liver transplantation in patients with concurrent active tuberculosis at transplantation. The International Journal of Tuberculosis and Lung Disease. 2010;**14**:1039-1044

[94] Gimenez F, Foeillet E, Bourdon O, Weller S, Garret C, Bidault R, Singlas E. Evaluation of pharmacokinetic interactions after oral administration of mycophenolate mofetil and valaciclovir or aciclovir to healthy subjects. Clinical Pharmacokinetics. 2004;**43**:685-692. DOI: 10.2165/00003088-200443100-00004

[95] Brum S, Nolasco F, Sousa J, Ferreira A, Possante M, Pinto JR, Barroso E, Santos JR. Leukopenia in kidney transplant patients with the association of valganciclovir and mycophenolate mofetil. Transplantation Proceedings. 2008;**40**:752-754. DOI: 10.1016/j. transproceed.2008.02.048

[96] Mohammadpoor AH, Nazemian F, Khayyat MH, Naghibi M, Bahrami A, Kazemi M. Effect of ganciclovir on pharmacokinetics of mycophenolic mofetil, in kidney transplant patients. Iranian Journal of Basic Medical Sciences. 2008;**10**:233-238

[97] Sheikh AM, Wolf DC, Lebovics E, Goldberg R, Horowitz HW. Concomitant human immunodeficiency virus protease inhibitor therapy markedly reduces tacrolimus metabolism and increases blood levels. Transplantation. 1999;**68**:307-309. DOI: 10.1097/00007890-199907270-00027

[98] Vogel M, Voigt E, Michaelis HC, Sudhop T, Wolff M, Türler A, Sauerbruch T, Rockstroh JK, Spengler U. Management of drug-to-drug interactions between cyclosporine a and the protease-inhibitor lopinavir/ritonavir in liver-transplanted HIV-infected patients. Liver Transplantation. 2004;**10**:939-944. DOI: 10.1002/lt.20165

[99] Teicher E, Vincent I, Bonhomme-Faivre L, Abbara C, Barrail A, Boissonnas A, Duclos-Vallée JC, Taburet AM, Samuel D, Vittecoq D. Effect of highly active antiretroviral therapy on tacrolimus pharmacokinetics in hepatitis C virus and HIV co-infected liver transplant recipients in the ANRS HC-08 study. Clinical Pharmacokinetics. 2007;**46**:941-952. DOI: 10.2165/00003088-200746110-00002

[100] Mertz D, Battegay M, Marzolini C, Mayr M. Drug-drug interaction in a kidney transplant recipient receiving HIV salvage therapy and tacrolimus. American Journal of Kidney Diseases. 2009;**54**:e1-e4. DOI: 10.1053/j.ajkd.2009.01.268

[101] Pulzer A, Seybold U, Schönermarck U, Stangl M, Habicht A, Bogner JR, Franke J, Fischereder M. Calcineurin inhibitor dose-finding before kidney transplantation in HIV patients. Transplant International. 2013;**26**:254-258. DOI: 10.1111/tri.12020

[102] Mathis AS, Davé N, Knipp GT, Friedman GS. Drug-related dyslipidemia after renal transplantation. American Journal of Health-System Pharmacy. 2004;**61**:565-585

[103] Christians U, Jacobsen W, Floren LC. Metabolism and drug interactions of 3-hydroxy-3-methylglutaryl coenzyme a reductase inhibitors in transplant patients: Are the statins mechanistically similar? Pharmacology & Therapeutics. 1998;**80**:1-34. DOI: 10.1016/S0163-7258(98)00016-3

[104] Asberg A. Interactions between cyclosporin and lipid-lowering drugs: Implications for organ transplant recipients. Drugs. 2003;**63**:367-378. DOI: 10.2165/00003495-200363040-00003

[105] Neuvonen PJ, Backman JT, Niemi M. Pharmacokinetic comparison of the potential over-the-counter statins simvastatin, lovastatin, fluvastatin and pravastatin. Clinical Pharmacokinetics. 2008;**47**:463-474. DOI: 10.2165/00003088-200847070-00003

[106] Causevic-Ramosevac A, Semiz S. Drug interactions with statins. Acta Pharmaceutica. 2013;**63**:277-293. DOI: 10.2478/acph-2013-0022

[107] Gertz M, Cartwright CM, Hobbs MJ, Kenworthy KE, Rowland M, Houston JB, Galetin A. Cyclosporine inhibition of hepatic and intestinal CYP3A4, uptake and efflux transporters: Application of PBPK modeling in the assessment of drug-drug interaction potential. Pharmaceutical Research. 2013;**30**:761-780. DOI: 10.1007/s11095-012-0918-y

[108] Christians U, Jacobsen W, Benet LZ, Lampen A. Mechanisms of clinically relevant drug interactions associated with tacrolimus. Clinical Pharmacokinetics. 2002;**41**:813-851. DOI: 10.2165/00003088-200241110-00003

[109] Lemahieu WP, Hermann M, Asberg A, Verbeke K, Holdaas H, Vanrenterghem Y, Maes BD. Combined therapy with atorvastatin and calcineurin inhibitors: No interactions with tacrolimus. American Journal of Transplantation. 2005;**5**:2236-2243. DOI: 10.1111/j.1600-6143.2005.01005.x

[110] Ma B, Prueksaritanont T, Lin JH. Drug interactions with calcium channel blockers: Possible involvement of metabolite-intermediate complexation with CYP3A. Drug Metabolism and Disposition. 2000;**28**:125-130

[111] Wang YH, Jones DR, Hall SD. Prediction of cytochrome P450 3A inhibition by verapamil enantiomers and their metabolites. Drug Metabolism and Disposition. 2004;**32**:259-266. DOI: 10.1124/dmd.32.2.259

[112] Wang YH, Jones DR, Hall SD. Differential mechanism-based inhibition of CYP3A4 and CYP3A5 by verapamil. Drug Metabolism and Disposition. 2005;**33**:664-671. DOI: 10.1124/dmd/104.001834

[113] Zhao P, Lee CA, Kunze KL. Sequential metabolism is responsible for diltiazem-induced time-dependent loss of CYP3A. Drug Metabolism and Disposition. 2007;**35**:704-712. DOI: 10.1124/dmd.106.013847

[114] Krasulova K, Holas O, Anzenbacher P. Influence of amlodipine enantiomers on human microsomal cytochromes P450: Stereoselective time-dependent inhibition of CYP3A enzyme activity. Molecules. 2017;**22**:E1879. DOI: 10.3390/molecules22111879

[115] Crocker JF, Renton KW, LeVatte TL, McLellan DH. The interaction of the calcium channel blockers verapamil and nifedipine with cyclosporin a in pediatric renal transplant patients. Pediatric Nephrology. 1994;**8**:408-411. DOI: 10.1007/BF00856514

[116] Campana C, Regazzi MB, Buggia I, Molinaro M. Clinically significant drug interactions with cyclosporin. An update. Clinical Pharmacokinetics. 1996;**30**:141-179. DOI: 10.2165/00003088-199630020-00004

[117] Yildiz A, Sever MS, Türkmen A, Ecder T, Türk S, Akkaya V, Ark E. Interaction between cyclosporine a and verapamil, felodipine, and isradipine. Nephron. 1999;**81**:117-118

[118] Hebert MF, Lam AY. Diltiazem increases tacrolimus concentrations. The Annals of Pharmacotherapy. 1999;**33**:680-682. DOI: 10.1345/aph.18356

[119] Böttiger Y, Säwe J, Brattström C, Tollemar J, Burke JT, Häss G, Zimmerman JJ. Pharmacokinetic interaction between single oral doses of diltiazem and sirolimus in healthy volunteers. Clinical Pharmacology and Therapeutics. 2001;**69**:32-40. DOI: 10.1067/mcp.2001.112513

[120] Jones TE, Morris RG. Pharmacokinetic interaction between tacrolimus and diltiazem: Dose-response relationship in kidney and liver transplant recipients. Clinical Pharmacokinetics. 2002;**41**:381-388

[121] Kovarik JM, Beyer D, Bizot MN, Jiang Q, Allison MJ, Schmouder RL. Pharmacokinetic interaction between verapamil and everolimus in healthy subjects. British Journal of Clinical Pharmacology. 2005;**60**:434-437. DOI: 10.1111/j.1365-2125.2005.02434.x

[122] Bernard E, Goutelle S, Bertrand Y, Bleyzac N. Pharmacokinetic drug-drug interaction of calcium channel blockers with cyclosporine in hematopoietic stem cell transplant children. The Annals of Pharmacotherapy. 2014;**48**:1580-1584. DOI: 10.1177/1060028014550644

[123] Zimmerman JJ. Exposure-response relationships and drug interactions of sirolimus. The AAPS Journal. 2004;**6**:e28. DOI: 10.1208/aapsj060428

[124] Zuo XC, Zhou YN, Zhang BK, Yang GP, Cheng ZN, Yuan H, Ouyang DS, Liu SK, Barrett JS, Li PJ, Liu Z, Tan HY, Guo R, Zhou LY, Xie YL, Li ZJ, Li J, Wang CJ, Wang JL. Effect of CYP3A5*3 polymorphism on pharmacokinetic drug interaction between tacrolimus and amlodipine. Drug Metabolism and Pharmacokinetics. 2013;**28**:398-405. DOI: 10.2133/dmpk.DMPK-12-RG-148

[125] Kaijser M, Johnsson C, Zezina L, Backman U, Dimény E, Fellström B. Elevation of cyclosporin a blood levels during carvedilol treatment in renal transplant patients. Clinical Transplantation. 1997;**11**:577-581

[126] Bader FM, Hagan ME, Crompton JA, Gilbert EM. The effect of beta-blocker use on cyclosporine level in cardiac transplant recipients. The Journal of Heart and Lung Transplantation. 2005;**24**:2144-2147. DOI: 10.1016/j.healun.2005.05.002

[127] Oldham HG, Clarke SE. Vitro identification of the human cytochrome P450 enzymes involved in the metabolism of R(+)- and S(−)-carvedilol. Drug Metabolism and Disposition. 1997;**25**:970-977

[128] Amioka K, Kuzuya T, Kushihara H, Ejiri M, Nitta A, Nabeshima T. Carvedilol increases ciclosporin bioavailability by inhibiting P-glycoprotein-mediated transport. The Journal of Pharmacy and Pharmacology. 2007;**59**:1383-1387. DOI: 10.1211/jpp.59.10.0008

[129] Ramachandran V, Kostrubsky VE, Komoroski BJ, Zhang S, Dorko K, Esplen JE, Strom SC, Venkataramanan R. Troglitazone increases cytochrome P-450 3A protein and activity in primary cultures of human hepatocytes. Drug Metabolism and Disposition. 1999;**27**:1194-1199

[130] Sahi J, Black CB, Hamilton GA, Zheng X, Jolley S, Rose KA, Gilbert D, LeCluyse EL, Sinz MW. Comparative effects of thiazolidinediones on in vitro P450 enzyme induction and inhibition. Drug Metabolism and Disposition. 2003;**31**:439-446. DOI: 10.1124/dmd.31.4.439

[131] Sinz M, Kim S, Zhu Z, Chen T, Anthony M, Dickinson K, Rodrigues AD. Evaluation of 170 xenobiotics as transactivators of human pregnane X receptor (hPXR) and correlation to known CYP3A4 drug interactions. Current Drug Metabolism. 2006;**7**:375-388. DOI: 10.2174/138920006776873535

[132] Elbarbry FA, Marfleet T, Shoker AS. Drug-drug interactions with immunosuppressive agents: Review of the in vitro functional assays and role of cytochrome P450 enzymes. Transplantation. 2008;**85**:1222-1229. DOI: 10.1097/TP.0b013e31816fc03b

[133] Kaplan B, Friedman G, Jacobs M, Viscuso R, Lyman N, DeFranco P, Bonomini L, Mulgaonkar SP. Potential interaction of troglitazone and cyclosporine. Transplantation. 1998;**65**:1399-1400. DOI: 10.1097/00007890-199805270-00021

[134] Oscarson M, Zanger UM, Rifki OF, Klein K, Eichelbaum M, Meyer UA. Transcriptional profiling of genes induced in the livers of patients treated with carbamazepine. Clinical Pharmacology and Therapeutics. 2006;**80**:440-456. DOI: 10.1016/j.clpt.2006.08.013

[135] Cerveny L, Svecova L, Anzenbacherova E, Vrzal R, Staud F, Dvorak Z, Ulrichova J, Anzenbacher P, Pavek P. Valproic acid induces CYP3A4 and MDR1 gene expression by activation of constitutive androstane receptor and pregnane X receptor pathways. Drug Metabolism and Disposition. 2007;**35**:1032-1041. DOI: 10.1124/dmd.106.014456

[136] Cooney GF, Mochon M, Kaiser B, Dunn SP, Goldsmith B. Effects of carbamazepine on cyclosporine metabolism in pediatric renal transplant recipients. Pharmacotherapy. 1995;**15**:353-356. DOI: 10.1002/j.1875-9114.1995.tb04373.x

[137] Punyawudho B, Cloyd JC, Leppik IE, Ramsay RE, Marino SE, Pennell PB, White JR, Birnbaum AK. Characterization of the time course of carbamazepine deinduction by an enzyme turnover model. Clinical Pharmacokinetics. 2009;**48**:313-320. DOI: 10.2165/00003088-200948050-00003

[138] Kashuba AD, Nafziger AN, Kearns GL, Leeder JS, Gotschall R, Rocci ML Jr, Kulawy RW, Beck DJ, Bertino JS Jr. Effect of fluvoxamine therapy on the activities of CYP1A2, CYP2D6, and CYP3A as determined by phenotyping. Clinical Pharmacology and Therapeutics. 1998;**64**:257-268. DOI: 10.1016/S0009-9236(98)90174-6

[139] Jones DR, Ekins S, Li L, Hall SD. Computational approaches that predict metabolic intermediate complex formation with CYP3A4 (+b5). Drug Metabolism and Disposition. 2007;**35**:1466-1475. DOI: 10.1124/dmd.106.014613

[140] Cummins D, Sekar M, Halil O, Banner N. Myelosuppression associated with azathioprine-allopurinol interaction after heart and lung transplantation. Transplantation. 1996;**61**:1661-1662. DOI: 10.1097/00007890-199606150-00023

[141] Weiler S, Aellig N, Fauchère I, Jetter A, Corti N. Treatment of gout in a renal transplant patient leading to severe thrombocytopenia. Journal of Clinical Pharmacy and Therapeutics. 2014;**39**:571-572. DOI: 10.1111/jcpt.12190

[142] Perez-Ruiz F, Gomez-Ullate P, Amenabar JJ, Zarraga S, Calabozo M, Herrero-Beites AM, Nolla JM. Long-term efficacy of hyperuricaemia treatment in renal transplant patients. Nephrology, Dialysis, Transplantation. 2003;**18**:603-606. DOI: 10.1093/ndt/18.3.603

[143] Trück J, Laube GF, von Vigier RO, Goetschel P. Gout in pediatric renal transplant recipients. Pediatric Nephrology. 2010;**25**:2535-2538. DOI: 10.1007/s00467-010-1599-6

[144] Stamp LK, Chapman PT. Gout and organ transplantation. Current Rheumatology Reports. 2012;**14**:165-172. DOI: 10.1007/s11926-012-0235-9

[145] Colombo D, Lunardon L, Bellia G. Cyclosporine and herbal supplement interactions. Journal of Toxicology. 2014;**2014**:145325. DOI: 10.1155/2014/145325

[146] Arayne MS, Sultana N, Bibi Z. Grape fruit juice-drug interactions. Pakistan Journal of Pharmaceutical Sciences. 2005;**18**:45-57

[147] Nowack R. Review article: Cytochrome P450 enzyme, and transport protein mediated herb-drug interactions in renal transplant patients: Grapefruit juice, St John's Wort - and beyond. Nephrology (Carlton, Vic.). 2008;**13**:337-347. DOI: 10.1111/j.1440-1797.2008.00940.x

[148] Wanwimolruk S, Prachayasittikul V. Cytochrome P450 enzyme mediated herbal drug interactions (part 1). EXCLI Journal. 2014;**13**:347-391. DOI: 10.17877/DE290R-15628

[149] Komoroski BJ, Zhang S, Cai H, Hutzler JM, Frye R, Tracy TS, Strom SC, Lehmann T, Ang CY, Cui YY, Venkataramanan R. Induction and inhibition of cytochromes P450 by the St. John's wort constituent hyperforin in human hepatocyte cultures. Drug Metabolism and Disposition. 2004;**32**:512-518. DOI: 10.1124/dmd.32.5.512

[150] Gödtel-Armbrust U, Metzger A, Kroll U, Kelber O, Wojnowski L. Variability in PXR-mediated induction of CYP3A4 by commercial preparations and dry extracts of St. John's wort. Naunyn-Schmiedeberg's Archives of Pharmacology. 2007;**375**:377-382. DOI: 10.1007/s00210-007-0172-8

[151] Barone GW, Gurley BJ, Ketel BL, Lightfoot ML, Abul-Ezz SR. Drug interaction between St. John's wort and cyclosporine. The Annals of Pharmacotherapy. 2000;**34**:1013-1016. DOI: 10.1345/aph.10088

[152] Mai I, Krüger H, Budde K, Johne A, Brockmöller J, Neumayer HH, Roots I. Hazardous pharmacokinetic interaction of Saint John's wort (*Hypericum perforatum*) with the immunosuppressant cyclosporin. International Journal of Clinical Pharmacology and Therapeutics. 2000;**38**:500-502. DOI: 10.5414/CPP38500

[153] Ruschitzka F, Meier PJ, Turina M, Lüscher TF, Noll G. Acute heart transplant rejection due to Saint John's wort. Lancet. 2000;**355**:548-549. DOI: 10.1016/S0140-6736(99)05467-7

[154] Hebert MF, Park JM, Chen YL, Akhtar S, Larson AM. Effects of St. John's wort (Hypericum Perforatum) on tacrolimus pharmacokinetics in healthy volunteers. Journal of Clinical Pharmacology. 2004;**44**:89-94. DOI: 10.1177/0091270003261078

[155] Mai I, Bauer S, Perloff ES, Johne A, Uehleke B, Frank B, Budde K, Roots I. Hyperforin content determines the magnitude of the St John's wort-cyclosporine drug interaction. Clinical Pharmacology and Therapeutics. 2004;**76**:330-340. DOI: 10.1016/j.clpt.2004.07.004

[156] Karliova M, Treichel U, Malago M, Frilling A, Gerken G, Broelsch CE. Interaction of *Hypericum perforatum* (St. John's wort) with cyclosporin a metabolism in a patient after liver transplantation. Journal of Hepatology. 2000;**33**:853-855. DOI: 10.1016/S0168-8278(00)80321-9

[157] Ernst E. St John's Wort supplements endanger the success of organ transplantation. Archives of Surgery. 2002;**137**:316-319. DOI: 10.1001/archsurg.137.3.316

[158] Alscher DM, Klotz U. Drug interaction of herbal tea containing St. John's wort with cyclosporine. Transplant International. 2003;**16**:543-544. DOI: 10.1007/s00147-003-0560-z

[159] Mai I, Störmer E, Bauer S, Krüger H, Budde K, Roots I. Impact of St John's wort treatment on the pharmacokinetics of tacrolimus and mycophenolic acid in renal transplant patients. Nephrology, Dialysis, Transplantation. 2003;**18**:819-822. DOI: 10.1093/ndt/gfg002

[160] Hermann M, Asberg A, Reubsaet JL, Sather S, Berg KJ, Christensen H. Intake of grapefruit juice alters the metabolic pattern of cyclosporin a in renal transplant recipients. International Journal of Clinical Pharmacology and Therapeutics. 2002;**40**:451-456. DOI: 10.5414/CPP40451

[161] Bailey DJ, Dresser G, Malcolm J, Arnold O. Grapefruit–medication interactions: Forbidden fruit or avoidable consequences? Canadian Medical Association Journal. 2013; **185**:309-316. DOI: 10.1503/cmaj.120951

[162] Lin HL, Kent UM, Hollenberg PF. The grapefruit juice effect is not limited to cytochrome P450 (P450) 3A4: Evidence for bergamottin-dependent inactivation, heme destruction, and covalent binding to protein in P450s 2B6 and 3A5. The Journal of Pharmacology and Experimental Therapeutics. 2005;**313**:154-164. DOI: 10.1124/jpet.104.079608

[163] Messer A, Raquet N, Lohr C, Schrenk D. Major furocoumarins in grapefruit juice II: Phototoxicity, photogenotoxicity, and inhibitory potency vs. cytochrome P450 3A4 activity. Food and Chemical Toxicology. 2012;**50**:756-760. DOI: 10.1016/j.fct.2011.11.023

[164] Burkina V, Zlabek V, Halsne R, Ropstad E, Zamaratskaia G. In vitro effects of the citrus flavonoids diosmin, naringenin and naringin on the hepatic drug-metabolizing CYP3A enzyme in human, pig, mouse and fish. Biochemical Pharmacology. 2016;**110-111**:109-116. DOI: 10.1016/j.bcp.2016.04.011

[165] Lin HL, Kenaan C, Hollenberg PF. Identification of the residue in human CYP3A4 that is covalently modified by bergamottin and the reactive intermediate that contributes to the grapefruit juice effect. Drug Metabolism and Disposition. 2012;**40**:998-1006. DOI: 10.1124/dmd.112.044560

[166] Ho PC, Saville DJ, Wanwimolruk S. Inhibition of human CYP3A4 activity by grapefruit flavonoids, furanocoumarins and related compounds. Journal of Pharmacy & Pharmaceutical Sciences. 2001;**4**:217-227

[167] Fujita T, Kawase A, Niwa T, Tomohiro N, Masuda M, Matsuda H, Iwaki M. Comparative evaluation of 12 immature citrus fruit extracts for the inhibition of cytochrome P450 isoform activities. Biological & Pharmaceutical Bulletin. 2008;**31**:925-930. DOI: 10.1248/bpb.31.925

6

Anesthetic Considerations in Transplant Recipients for Nontransplant Surgery

Katarina Tomulić Brusich and Ivana Acan

Abstract

As solid organ transplantation increases and patient survival improves, it will become more common for these patients to present for nontransplant surgery. Recipients may present with medical problems unique to the transplant, and important considerations are necessary to keep the transplanted organ functioning. A comprehensive preoperative examination with specific focus on graft functioning is required. The anesthesiologist needs to pay close attention to considerations of immunosuppressive regimens, blood product administration, drug interactions as well as the risk and benefits of invasive monitoring in these immunosuppressed patients. This article reviews the post-transplant physiology and anesthetic considerations for patients after solid organ transplantation.

Keywords: anesthesia methods, intraoperative monitoring, organ transplantation physiology, perioperative care, solid organ transplantation

1. Introduction

The number of solid organ transplants performed worldwide is ever increasing. The improved survival rates are the result of well-established surgical techniques and effective immunosuppressive therapy. All this has led to an increase in number of patients who present for either elective or emergency non-transplant surgery [1, 2]. Laparotomy for small bowel obstruction, hip arthroplasty given the increased risk of fracture and avascular necrosis as a result of chronic steroid use causing bone demineralization and osteoporosis, lymph node excision and biopsy because of increased risk of lymphoproliferative disease, native nephrectomy in kidney transplant recipients, bronchoscopy in lung recipients, biliary tract interventions in liver recipients, and abscess drainage because of increased risk of infection are just a few of the increased surgical needs in this population. These patients cannot always return to the transplant facility for surgery, so it is incumbent on all anesthesiologists to review perioperative issues associated with transplantation.

Perioperative anesthetic management in majority of recipients is similar to the standard practice for any patient. However, we must bear in mind some essential considerations: problems of allograft denervation, the adverse effects of immunosuppression and its interaction with anesthetic drugs, the risk of infection, and the potential for organ rejection. When transplant recipients require nontransplant surgery, immune competence can be altered from the stress of surgery, acute illness, or disruption of the regimen by inexperienced providers [3].

Preoperative assessment of any transplant recipient undergoing non-cardiac surgery should focus on graft function and rejection, risks of infection, and function of other organs, particularly those that may be compromised due to either immunosuppressive therapy or dysfunction of the transplanted organ itself and drug interactions. There is no ideal anesthetic for use in organ transplant recipients. However, certain principles can be applied to all transplant patients who undergo anesthesia and surgery [4].

In this chapter, we will give an overview of immunosuppressive therapy and its interaction with anesthetic drugs as well as considerations regarding specific transplanted organs (heart, lungs, liver, kidney, pancreas, and intestine).

2. Immunosuppression

2.1. Immunosuppression protocol

Transplant patients are always under various regimens of immunosuppressive therapy (**Table 1**). Immunosuppression trends for solid organ transplantation have undergone a perceptible shift over the past decade. There are broad therapeutic patterns and numerous immunosuppressive protocols depending on transplanted organ, as well as the regional differences (country, hospital). However, some strategies are similar. We distinguish induction immunosuppressive therapy and maintenance of immunosuppressive therapy. Induction of immunosuppression begins immediately before the organ implantation. Antibodies are prescribed for the majority of kidney, pancreas, and intestine recipients and for just under half of thoracic organ recipients. It is extremely uncommon in liver transplantation [5]. Maintenance of immunosuppression involves one of the drugs from each group: calcineurin inhibitors (CNI), antimetabolites, and steroids.

The immunosuppressant strategy has been changing over the years. CNIs are still being used for the maintenance of immunosuppressive therapy, though shifting from cyclosporine to tacrolimus is being observed [6]. Modifications are also made among antimetabolites, from azathioprine to mycophenolate mofetil, and it is more common to decrease corticosteroid use or even implement steroid-free protocol in suitable transplant recipients [7, 8].

Most of the commonly used immunosuppressants have a narrow therapeutic index and display significant variability in blood concentrations between individuals. In transplant recipients,

General names	Generic names	Brand names
Corticosteroids	Prednisone	
	Methylprednisolone	
Calcineurin inhibitors	Tacrolimus (or FK-506)	Prograf
	Cyclosporine (or cyclosporine A)	Sandimmune, Neoral, Gengraf, Eon, SangCya, generic cyclosporine
Antimetabolites	Azathioprine	Imuran
	Cyclophosphamide	Cytoxan, Neosar
	Mycophenolate mofetil	CellCept
	Mycophenolate sodium	Myfortic
Polyclonal antibodies	Antithymocyte globulin (rabbit)	Thymoglobulin
	Antithymocyte globulin (equine)	ATGAM
	NRATG, NRATS, ALG	
Anti-CD3 monoclonal antibodies	Muromonab-CD3	Orthoclone OKT3
Anti-CD52 monoclonal antibodies	Alemtuzumab	Campath
Anti-IL-2 receptor monoclonal antibodies	Basiliximab	Simulect
	Daclizumab	Zenapax
TOR inhibitors (or rapamycin)	Sirolimus	Rapamune

Table 1. Most commonly used immunosuppressive drugs.

both supratherapeutic and subtherapeutic drug concentrations can have devastating results. Subtherapeutic levels increase the risk of transplant rejection, and supratherapeutic levels (overimmunosuppression) can lead to infection and/or drug-specific side effects. Importantly, the incidence of acute rejection has declined over the past decade. Treatments for acute rejection continue to include high-dose corticosteroid and antibody therapies [9].

2.2. Side effects and drug interactions

Chronic immunosuppressive therapy has its adverse effects such as lowered seizure threshold, diabetes, hypertension, hyperlipoproteinemia, decreased glomerular filtration, hyperkalemia, hypomagnesemia, increased risk of infection and tumors, pancytopenia, osteoporosis, and poor wound healing. This may have some impact on perioperative management and choice of anesthetic agents (**Table 2**) [10].

The blood level of both cyclosporine and tacrolimus must be kept within the indicated therapeutic range to get the desired effect. The perioperative fluctuation of the plasma level of these two drugs should be strictly monitored. There is a significant reduction of drug blood level by dilution with volume infusion or cardiopulmonary bypass in cardiac surgery [11]. Both these drugs are metabolized by cytochrome P-450 system of liver, and therefore many of the drugs administered perioperatively can affect their plasma levels [12, 13]. A better understanding of

CyA	Tac	Aza	Ster	MMF	ATG	OKT3	
Anemia	–	–	+	–	+	–	–
Leucopenia	–	–	++	–	+	+	+
Thrombocytopenia	–	–	–	–	+	–	–
Hypertension	++	+	–	+	–	–	–
Diabetes	+	++	–	++	–	–	–
Neurotoxicity	+	+	–	+	–	–	–
Renal insufficiency	+	++	–	–	–	–	–
Anaphylaxis	–	–	–	–	–	+	+
Fever	–	–	–	–	–	+	+

ATG = anti-thymocyte globulin; Aza = azathioprine; CyA = cyclosporine A; MMF = mycophenolate mofetil; OKT3 = monoclonal antibodies directed against CD-3 antigen on the surface of human T-lymphocytes; Ster = steroids; and Tac = tacrolimus.

Table 2. Side effects of immunosuppressive that have direct impact on anesthetic and perioperative management [1].

pharmacokinetics over the years, allows now days a reduction of immunosuppressant dose in elderly patients while maintaining the therapeutic level [14].

In the hospital settings, almost 3–5% of adverse drug reactions are due to drug-drug interactions. It is estimated that the percentage is even higher in solid organ transplant recipients dependent on immunosuppressive therapy. Reactions can be among two immunosuppressants or between the immunosuppressant and other drugs [15]. Due to the fact that the administration of cyclosporine (CyA) and tacrolimus (Tac) is ever increasing, we give an overview of their interaction with other drugs (**Table 3**).

During anesthesia, we provide a range of drugs from different groups, which increase the possibility of drug interaction and thus potentially endanger the patient in the perioperative period. One should keep in mind that many pharmacokinetic and pharmacodynamic interactions can occur among the drugs that patients take after transplantation, due to cytochrome P450 enzyme system induction or inhibition by another drug. There are few data concerning interaction between immunosuppressive drugs and anesthetic agents. Most of the evidence is based on clinical practice and occasional case reports or case studies. Large randomized controlled trials involving either general or regional anesthesia are still lacking. **Table 4** describes the effect of various anesthetic agents on immunosuppressant and vice versa.

Data on the effects of general anesthesia on cyclosporine or tacrolimus pharmacokinetics in humans are limited. Most of the inhalational anesthetic agents are well tolerated unless there is a significant heart failure. However, caution is advised in concurrent administration of oral cyclosporine and isoflurane anesthesia. Subtherapeutic blood levels have been reported in patients who received peroral drug form less than 4 hours preoperatively. It is probably due to a reduction in gastric emptying and absorption from the proximal small bowel, which can occur during isoflurane anesthesia [16]. Steady-state blood levels of cyclosporine and cyclosporine clearance are not altered by isoflurane/nitrous oxide anesthesia in animal model [17].

Drug class	Drug	Effect on blood level Adverse effect
Benzodiazepines	Diazepam, midazolam, alprazolam, flurazepam, clonazepam	↑ Benzodiazepines
Antibiotics	Erythromycin, metronidazole, norfloxacin, levofloxacin	↑ CyA and Tac level
Antimicrobial	Rifampicin	↓ CyA and Tac level
Antimalarial	Chloroquine, mefloquine	↑ CyA and Tac level
Antifungal	Ketoconazole, fluconazole, itraconazole, voriconazole, amphotericin B	↑ CyA and Tac level Renal dysfunction
Anti-retroviral	Ritonavir, atazanavir, darunavir, cobicistat, delaviridine	↑ CyA and Tac level
Cardiovascular drugs (antiarrhythmics and calcium channel blocker)	Amiodarone, lidocaine, quinidine, verapamil, diltiazem, amlodipine, felodipine	↑ CyA and Tac level QT prolongation by amiodarone and quinidine
Statins	Simvastatin, atorvastatin, lovastatin, pravastatin	↑ Statin concentration
Anticoagulants	Apixaban, dabigatran, rivaroxaban	↑ Anticoagulant concentration
Oral hypoglycemics	Sulfonylurea, biguanides	↑ CyA level
Gastrointestinal	Metoclopramide, omeprazole, lansoprazole, octreotide, cimetidine, ranitidine	↑ CyA and Tac level Renal dysfunction QT prolongation by octreotide with Tac
Analgesics	Nonsteroidal anti-inflammatory drugs	↑ CyA and Tac level Renal dysfunction
Antipsychotics	Haloperidol, desipramine, fluoxetine, trazodone, pimozide	↑ CyA and Tac level ↑ Pimozide level
Hormones	Estrogen and testosterone preparation	↑ CyA and Tac level
Others	Bosentan, carbamazepine	↓ CyA and Tac level

CyA = cyclosporine A; Tac = tacrolimus.

Table 3. Drugs that interact with cyclosporine A and tacrolimus.

Cyclosporine and tacrolimus increase blood level of benzodiazepines. Transplanted patients need dose modification [12, 13]. Propofol infusion does not modify the cyclosporine concentration. It is considered to be a suitable agent for intravenous anesthesia in cyclosporine-treated patients, provided a close postoperative monitoring of cyclosporine blood concentrations is maintained [18]. Cyclosporine tends to increase the analgesic effect produced by fentanyl, but the mechanism is unclear [19].

Most of relaxants can be used safely. Cyclosporine enhances the effects of muscle relaxants. Prolonged neuromuscular block in patients receiving cyclosporine after vecuronium and pancuronium administration has been described [20, 21]. Atracurium and cisatracurium

Anesthetic agent	Effect with immunosuppressive drugs
Isoflurane	↓ Clearance of oral CyA
Thiopental	Nil
Benzodiazepines	↑ Blood level of benzodiazepines
Propofol	Nil
Etomidate	Nil
Opioids	CyA ↑ analgesic effect produced by fentanyl
Muscle relaxants	Prolonged neuromuscular blockade
Neostigmine	Caution in heart transplant patients
Local anesthetics	Bupivacaine and ropivacaine can be safely used

Table 4. Effect of specific anesthetic agent on immunosuppressive drugs.

are preferred agents because their elimination is not affected by renal or hepatic function. Therefore, patients receiving cyclosporine as immunosuppressive therapy may require a smaller dose of nondepolarizing muscle relaxant and the recovery time may be prolonged [22]. Neostigmine can lead to bradycardia and cardiac arrest in patients with heart transplantation despite the concurrent use of an antimuscarinic agent [23]. Bupivacaine and ropivacaine can be safely used through regional routes without any side effects [24, 25].

3. Anesthesia and preoperative care

3.1. Preoperative assessment of transplant recipients

Many transplant recipients live relatively normal and productive lives, but often have limited physical reserves. A successful transplant abolishes the symptoms and replaces function of the failed organ, but often there are persistent abnormalities from the underlying or preexisting illness that may have caused the organ failure or chronic physiologic abnormalities resulting from the organ failure itself. The preoperative evaluation of transplant recipients undergoing non-transplant surgery should include graft function, signs of rejection, presence of infection, and function of other organs.

Allograft rejection may occur at any time during the post-transplant period, especially when discontinuing the use of immunosuppressants. Chronic rejection is the most significant medical obstacle to long-term morbidity-free allograft survival. The incidence is thought to progressively increase with time after transplantation, but after a period of 5 years, it affects about 10% of liver to around 60% of lung allograft recipients [26]. Chronic organ rejection results in a progressive deterioration of organ function (assessed trough laboratory tests) and is the main cause of late mortality in the transplant recipients. Mortality rate is high if rejection remains untreated before surgery [27]. Therefore, the presence of any degree of rejection should be ruled out and urgently managed preoperatively with increased immunosuppression.

Immunosuppressed patients are at risk of infections that may be bacterial, viral, fungal, or protozoan. Infection is a significant cause of morbidity and mortality after transplantation [28]. Its presence should also always be preoperatively ruled out (by obtaining laboratory, radiologic, and microbiology tests). It is imperative to emphasize that the immunosuppressed patient may not present the typical signs and symptoms of infection (i.e. fever, leukocytosis). Microbiology advice should be strongly sought for prevention as well as strict control of infection. Any infection should be treated preoperatively [29].

Although transplant patients are considered as risk hosts for infection because of their immune status, there is no evidence to suggest different bacteriology of surgical site infections than for the general population. Antimicrobial coverage need not be expanded to include atypical or opportunistic organisms as long as active infection with such an organism is not present or suspected [30]. Prophylaxis with broad spectrum antibiotic should be administered 1 hour before surgical incision (depending on hospital protocol) (**Table 5**).

Transplanted patients may also suffer from diabetes, hypertension, epilepsy, renal dysfunction, bone marrow suppression, lymphoproliferative disorders, and adrenal insufficiency as the side effects of chronic immunosuppressive therapy [31]. Hepatobiliary and pancreatic diseases are relatively common after transplantation, as well as the upper gastrointestinal bleeding secondary to peptic ulcer disease. Surgical stress, corticosteroids, and mycophenolate may contribute to gastrointestinal ulcers [32]. So, it is absolutely necessary to provide stress ulcer prophylaxis for transplanted patients.

The transplant patient population is considered as high-risk group for developing venous thromboembolism (VTE) given the fact that most of these patients have multiple identifiable risk factors [33]. However, the exact risk of developing VTEs in these patients is not clearly defined in the literature, nor there are clear guidelines regarding the appropriate use of thromboprophylaxis in transplant recipients [34]. In our opinion, VTE prophylaxis should be tailored to the patient's specific needs in accordance with current guidelines [35].

Operation	Recommended antibiotic prophylaxis
Cardiothoracic surgery	Cefazolin, cefuroxime, or cefamandole. If patient has a β-lactam allergy: vancomycin or clindamycin
Vascular surgery	Cefazolin or cefuroxime. If patient has a β-lactam allergy: vancomycin with or without gentamycin, or clindamycin
Colon surgery	Oral: neomycin plus erythromycin base, or neomycin plus metronidazole. Parenteral: cefoxitin or cefotetan, or cefazolin plus metronidazole
Hip or knee arthroplasty	Cefazolin or cefuroxime. If the patient has a β-lactam allergy: vancomycin or clindamycin
Vaginal or abdominal hysterectomy	Cefazolin, cefotetan, cefoxitin or cefuroxime

Table 5. Antimicrobial prophylaxis for selected surgical procedures [30].

3.2. Preoperative assessment and premedication

The transplant team as well as the attending anesthesiologist and surgeon should have a good coordination during perioperative period, especially if a major surgical procedure is planned. A comprehensive preoperative evaluation by the anesthesiologist should include: evaluation of the graft function, presence of infection, function of other organ systems, the presence of concomitant diseases as well as the preoperative performance or functional status. Adherence to the fundamental principles of preoperative evaluation along with a high level of vigilance is required. Information and medical history should be gathered from the medical records, interview with the patient and/or next of kin or guardian. If medical information is unavailable, attempts should be made to contact the transplant center for pertinent history. Other useful information from the transplant center includes their most recent evaluations and recent data on graft function and general health of the patient. Close communication with the transplant team may be the single most important step in preparing the patient for surgery and developing a perioperative anesthetic plan.

A thorough review of systems along with a physical examination is essential in this population. Findings such as recent weight gain, edema, dyspnea, sweats, malaise, fever, rashes, abdominal pain, abnormal breath sounds on auscultation, and changes in stool or urine output are some of the potential signs and symptoms of infection or rejection.

The following investigations should be available preoperatively.

1. Laboratory parameters:
    a. Complete blood count (to rule out bone marrow suppression)
    b. Electrolytes
    c. Renal function tests
    d. Liver function tests
    e. Coagulation tests
    f. Biomarkers (i.e. brain natriuretic peptide)
2. Chest radiograph
3. Electrocardiogram
4. Echocardiography
5. Miscellaneous: depending on the type of surgery and transplanted organ (i.e. coronary angiography, stress test, spirometry, biopsy)

Each preoperative evaluation and testing should be considered individually based on the target organ system(s) to be evaluated, the patient's medical history, and the inherent risks of the upcoming surgical procedure.

Cardiovascular disease is a major cause of mortality and morbidity among organ transplant recipients, especially in those with chronic kidney disease or previous heart transplant, making the risk of a perioperative cardiovascular event a legitimate concern. Many transplant recipients have undergone complete cardiac testing and in some cases, interventions, before their transplant surgery. Records of the testing and interventions can be easily obtained from the transplant center to be used for comparison and consideration before the upcoming surgery. We must also bear in mind that many of these patients may have asymptomatic coronary disease as a result of diabetes or the transplant itself [36].

If unexpected abnormal findings are identified on physical examination or laboratory testing, symptomatic changes outside the patient's baseline are documented, or suspicion for rejection or infection exists during the preoperative evaluation, it should be considered to postpone any surgery that is non-urgent or elective. The patient should also be expeditiously referred back to the transplant center, cardiologist, or other consulting physician as indicated.

Standard premedication may be used, as in non-transplant patients. However, dose adjustment for some drugs is needed (**Table 3**). Antibiotic, stress ulcer and VTE prophylaxis administration is recommended (as mentioned above). Supplemental steroids are not necessary for stress coverage except in post-transplant recipients in whom steroids are recently withdrawn [37].

Post-transplantation diabetes mellitus is a common metabolic consequence of the agents of immunosuppressive therapy agents [38]. It is imperative to institute a glycemic control plan before the surgery with closely managing intraoperative and postoperative glucose control.

The dose of immunosuppressive drugs should not be altered and should be continued postoperatively to reduce the risk of rejection. Daily monitoring of the steady-state blood level is recommended. Oral cyclosporine should be administered 4–6 h before surgery to maintain therapeutic blood levels. The alteration of dose of other immunosuppressive drugs dose is not required unless the route of administration needs to be changed from oral to intravenous [39].

3.3. General anesthetic considerations

There is no ideal anesthetic plan that can be used for all transplant recipients undergoing non-transplant surgery. A variety of anesthetic techniques have been successfully used in patients with a transplant history including general (inhalational, balanced, and total intravenous), neuraxial, and regional anesthesia.

3.3.1. Monitoring

Generally, invasive monitoring is not mandatory and anesthesia should be performed using standard European Society of Anesthesiology's monitoring guidelines [40]. The decision to use invasive hemodynamic monitors, placement of central venous access, pulmonary artery catheters, or other procedures such as transesophageal echocardiography should be made on a case-by-case basis. It should be guided by consideration of the patient's comorbidities, hemodynamic stability, the expertise of the anesthesiologist in placing the invasive devices, and by the type of surgery and anesthesia planned. Aseptic technique is of utmost importance to minimize exposure to infectious organisms and bacteremia when attempting any invasive procedures in this population [41].

3.3.2. *Airway management*

Airway management of transplant patients may pose a concern for several reasons. Many patients may have pre-existing diabetes mellitus before transplant or acquire diabetes after transplant. Diabetic patients can develop limitations in joint mobility caused by glycosylation of the connective tissue within their joints [38]. This population is also at increased risk for lymphoproliferative disorders secondary to immunosuppressant drugs, and lymphoproliferative growth may compromise any part of the airway or mediastinum and cause life-threatening airway obstruction during sedation and anesthesia [41]. Gingival hyperplasia is present at times in patients taking cyclosporine and it may lead to bleeding during airway manipulation. Aspiration risk may be increased in transplanted patients as a result of delayed gastric emptying and gastropathy [32]. These potential problems should all be taken into consideration when constructing the anesthetic plan for airway management.

Oral endotracheal intubation is preferred over nasal intubation because of the potential of infection caused by nasal flora [42]. The use of a laryngeal mask is acceptable (within its indications) [43]. Keep in mind that laryngoscopy and tracheal intubation may not produce a sympathetic response secondary to the loss of cardiac baroreceptor reflexes in heart transplanted patients [44]. Avoid hyperventilation in patients taking cyclosporine and tacrolimus because of a decrease in seizure threshold with these two drugs. Early postoperative extubation is preferred if possible to prevent the development of nosocomial or ventilator-associated pneumonia [45].

3.3.3. *General anesthesia*

All inhalational and intravenous anesthetics have been used with success in transplant recipients. The choice of anesthetics and adjunctive drugs should be determined by the type of surgery and condition of the patient. As a general guideline, if hepatic and renal functions are normal, all standard anesthetic medications and adjuncts may be used. Some special considerations for each type of organ transplant are discussed in the section on organ-specific considerations.

3.3.3.1. *Intravenous anesthetics*

The selection and administration of intravenous anesthetics should be guided by the patient's hemodynamic status, the drug's cardiovascular effects, and pharmacokinetic properties. Premedication with benzodiazepines is acceptable. Caution should be used in patients with hepatic or renal insufficiency as effects may be prolonged. Also, the dose of barbiturates should be adjusted in patients with hepatic insufficiency to avoid prolonged effects.

Propofol is extensively metabolized by the liver to inactive glucuronic acid metabolites that are excreted by the kidneys. Nevertheless, there seems to be no need for dose adjustments in patients with hepatic or renal failure indicating an extrahepatic route of elimination as well [46]. Caution should be used in patients with cardiovascular compromise as propofol can worsen cardiac contractility, compromise cardiac preload, cause bradycardia, and lower systemic vascular resistance culminating in diminished cardiac output and mean arterial pressure.

Etomidate does not have the cardiac depressant effect of barbiturates and propofol. Etomidate is metabolized rapidly by hydrolysis within the liver and by plasma esterases and also does not require dosage adjustment in renal or hepatic disease. One unique characteristic of etomidate is its ability to inhibit enzyme necessary for the synthesis of cortisol [47]. This may have clinical significance in patients who already have adrenal suppression as a result of exogenous corticosteroid use.

Ketamine is metabolized via the hepatic cytochrome P-450 system. Therefore, the clinical effects of ketamine are prolonged in the presence of hepatic insufficiency. The usual cardiac stimulating effects caused by central stimulation of the sympathetic system are not present in the denervated heart, but ketamine can still increase systemic vascular tone. Ketamine has neuroexcitatory effects and is known to cause myoclonic activity. It would be wisely to proceed with caution if the katamine is administered in patients who simultaneously take cyclosporin due to its potential for neurotoxicity.

3.3.3.2. Inhalational anesthetics

All inhaled anesthetics have been used in transplanted patients with success. Although halothane is nowadays rarely used, nevertheless it is necessary to mention its potential for hepatotoxicity and direct cardiac depressant effects. Most commonly used volatile anesthetics are isoflurane, sevoflurane, and desflurane. There does not seem to be a significant clinical advantage or disadvantage of one over the others. The choice of inhaled anesthetic can be dictated by the anesthesiologist's preference, experiences, and comfort with the anesthetic [48]. It is probably prudent to avoid prolonged use of N2O because of the potential risk of bone marrow suppression and the potential for altered immunologic response [49].

3.3.3.3. Opioids

Fentanyl is suitable and safe for short-term use during surgery. However, if used for long duration, the pharmacodynamic effects should be monitored due to accumulation effect. Reduced renal and liver function does not significantly alter the clearance and half-life of sufentanil. Tissue and blood esterases mainly metabolize remifentanil and its metabolite, excreted via kidneys, has low potency [50].

Among opioids used for postoperative pain treatment (morphine, codeine, oxycodone, and tramadol) have to be used with caution. Some of their active metabolites accumulate in renal failure and can mediate CNS and respiratory depression. Transdermal buprenorphine and methadone appear to be safe to use even in patients with renal dysfunction [51].

3.3.3.4. Neuromuscular blockade

The decision to use neuromuscular blockade should be based on the type of surgery and actual need for muscle relaxation during the procedure or the need to optimize intubating conditions. The choice of specific neuromuscular blocking agent should be dictated by length of surgery, underlying medical illnesses (i.e. myasthenia or other neuromuscular disorders), history of malignant hyperthermia, and the functional state of the patient's kidney and liver.

In the group of non-depolarizing drugs, it is preferable to use short-acting relaxants (mivacurium) or intermediate-acting agents independent of kidney and liver function (cisatracurium, atracurium). Vecuronium, rocuronium, and pancuronium can have prolonged effects in the face of hepatic or renal insufficiency. They require dose adjustments, close neuromuscular monitoring, and evidence of full reversal before extubation [52]. Some immunosuppressive drugs (i.e. azathioprine and cyclosporine) can prolong the action of the neuromuscular blocking agents [22].

Succinylcholine, the only depolarizing agent available, can be used in organ transplant recipients in the need for rapid sequence intubation and rapid airway control. It should be avoided only if there are other clinical reasons, such as hyperkalemia, muscular dystrophy, or history of malignant hyperthermia [53].

3.3.3.5. Anticholinesterase drugs

Most of the cholinesterase inhibitor drugs are eliminated through the kidneys (neostigmine, edrophonium, and pyridostigmine). Caution is advised in renal failure. Several reports described that neostigmine may produce a dose-dependent life-threatening bradycardia in heart transplant recipients, whereas another publication described the safe use of neostigmine [54]. Reversal of neuromuscular block with sugammadex is another possibility, but limited data exist in literature [55].

3.3.4. Regional and neuraxial anesthesia

The decision to perform a regional or neuraxial anesthetic technique in a previously transplanted patient must be made on an individual basis. We must carefully consider potential benefit and risks of these techniques as well as the anesthetic alternatives when constructing the anesthetic plan in this population. There may be several advantages to choosing a neuraxial or regional technique in this population. Superior analgesia over systemic opioids, especially in patients who may have narcotics tolerance as a result of long-term opioid use, reduced pulmonary complications, and decreased incidence of graft occlusion are just a few of the benefits of regional and neuraxial anesthesia [56]. Clinically relevant doses of bupivacaine and ropivacaine, which are commonly used local anesthetics for neuraxial anesthesia, do not seem to result in toxic levels or increased risk of toxic effects in renal and liver transplant recipients. However, it is important to be prepared for the risk of hypotension because of pre-existing autonomic neuropathy and cardiac denervation in this population. Cautious correction of hypovolemia before epidural or spinal anesthesia may help to attenuate the hypotension. Concurrent hemodynamic monitoring is imperative during the procedure. Direct and indirect-acting adrenergic agonists should be readily available along with emergency airway supplies.

The consideration of spinal or epidural anesthesia is appropriate in this population as long as there is no increased risk for bleeding complications. It is necessary to perform a total blood count to exclude bone marrow suppression, especially thrombocytopenia, and coagulation tests (PT, INR, APTT, and fibrinogen). Peripheral nerve blocks became popular anesthetic option due to hemodynamic stability and better postoperative analgesia. Some studies show no difference in duration of peripheral nerve blocks in patients after transplantation compared to the general surgical population [57, 58]. Nevertheless, large prospective randomized trials are still lacking.

Although the risk of infectious complications is very low, it is important to be highly vigilant when monitoring these patients after a neuraxial anesthesia as the attenuated inflammatory response may diminish the typical signs and symptoms of infection [59]. Again, aseptic technique and a mask should be considered essential when performing these procedures.

3.3.5. *Postoperative care management*

Regardless of the procedure performed, successful outcomes also depend on optimal postoperative care. Depending on the type of surgery, patients' comorbidities, and preoperative condition, patient is after surgery transferred either to intensive care unit (ICU) or post-anesthesia care unit (PACU). Adequate monitoring is tailored accordingly [60]. We reduce the delirium incidence by minimizing sedation, speed up extubation, and facilitate early ambulation and physical rehabilitation. Appropriate analgesia is essential component of postoperative surgical care. Opioids are the mainstay of analgesia in the early postoperative phase after major surgery. Parenteral paracetamol is an effective analgesic agent and may spare narcotics. There is no evidence of an increased risk of hepatotoxicity [61]. Once extubated, patient-controlled analgesia (PCA) devices are effective and well received by patients and nurses. Non-steroidal anti-inflammatory drugs should be avoided because of the risk of adverse interactions (e.g., gastrointestinal hemorrhage, nephrotoxicity, hepatic dysfunction). They augment nephrotoxicity of cyclosporine, as both drugs affect the renal microcirculation [62, 63].

Immunosuppressive therapy should be continued during the perioperative period and daily monitoring of steady-state cyclosporine or tacrolimus blood levels is recommended [64]. The dose of other immunosuppressive drugs should not be altered perioperatively unless the route of administration needs to be changed from oral to intravenous. In addition to the routine care as those for non-transplant recipients, increased attention should be paid to the preload status, renal function, and prevention of infection.

4. Specific anesthetic considerations

4.1. Heart transplant recipients

Transplanted heart is completely denervated, meaning it lacks neural regulating mechanisms [65]. Even though, it has the ability to adjust with compensatory mechanisms to the increased demands in stress returning the recipients to an active life. Transplanted heart has no sensory sympathetic and parasympathetic innervation. Therefore, it has a higher resting heart rate of 90–110 bpm secondary to the loss of vagal tone. The resting ECG is commonly altered showing two P waves: one is from the recipients' own SA node and the other is the donors' SA node. Patients are at higher risk of developing atrial flutter or atrial fibrillation. The transplanted heart is "preload dependent." Cardiac output becomes dependent on venous return. Therefore, it is important to maintain a sufficient systolic pressure and prevent hypovolemia [66].

Although the cardiac index of the transplanted heart is lower than that of normally innervated control hearts, it remains in the normal range. The catecholamine response is different from that of normal heart because intact sympathetic nerves are required for the normal uptake and metabolism of catecholamines. The receptor density, however, remains unchanged, and the transplanted heart can respond to direct-acting drugs (adrenaline and noradrenaline) [67]. Isoprenaline and dobutamine have similar effects in both transplanted and normal heart. Because atropine has no effect on a transplanted heart, isoprenaline and adrenaline should be readily available to manage bradycardia and hypotensive emergencies. In recent years, milrinone and levosimendan, inotropic vasodilators, have been included in the pharmacological arsenal. These drugs increase myocardial contractility without myocardial oxygen consumption (unlike catecholamines). In addition, they lead to arterial and venous vasodilatation and afterload decrease [68, 69]. **Table 6** summarizes the hemodynamic response of some commonly used drugs for resuscitation.

Heart transplant recipients may present with ongoing rejection with myocardial dysfunction, accelerated coronary atherosclerosis, or severe dysrhythmias, all of which must be diagnosed before surgery. Chronic allograft rejection usually presents as accelerated coronary artery disease. Therefore, heart transplant recipients may have significant myocardial ischemia without any clinical symptoms of pain and silent myocardial infarction on the ECG. Severe rejection can lead to significant systolic and diastolic dysfunction [70, 71].

General anesthesia is usually preferred, as there is a possibility of impaired response to hypotension after spinal or epidural anesthesia. A goal of anesthesia in this setting is the avoidance of significant vasodilation and acute decrease of the preload. Invasive hemodynamic monitoring is extremely useful during surgery that involves large volume shifts, due to the fact that these patients are preload-dependent and may be prone to myocardial dysfunction and/or

Drugs	SA node rate	AV conduction	SVR	BP	CO	Remark
Atropine	0	0	0	0	0	Cannot be used in bradycardia
Dopamine	↑	↑	0	E	↑	
Dobutamine	↑	↑	0	↑	↑	Effect on HR is more than normal heart
Adrenaline	↑	↑	0	↑	↑	
Noradrenaline	↑	↑	0	↑	E	
Isoprenaline	↑	↑	0	↓	↑	
Phenylephrine	0	0	0	↑	E	
Digoxin	0	↓				
Milrinone	0	0	↓	↑	↑	
Levosimendan	0	0	↓	↑	↑	

SA – sinoatrial; V – atrioventricular; SVR – systemic vascular resistance; BP – blood pressure; CO – cardiac output; HR – heart rate; 0 – no effect; and E – equivocal.

Table 6. Response of denervated heart to various cardiovascular drugs.

ischemia. Instead of invasive monitoring, intraoperative transesophageal echocardiography may be considered [72, 73]. All preoperative drug therapy should be continued during the perioperative period. If a pacemaker is in place, its proper function should be confirmed.

4.2. Lung transplant recipients

Denervation of the lungs after transplantation is associated with a lack of cough reflex below the tracheal anastomosis level and are unable to clear secretions unless they are awake. Therefore, they are prone to retention of secretions and silent aspiration [74]. These conditions may lead potential hazardous conditions especially in general anesthesia, such as bronchoconstriction and the increased risk of chest infection. In light of potential complications, it is preferable to perform a regional anesthesia whenever possible and if there is no contraindication [75].

Before elective surgery patients should undergo chest radiograph and spirometry to exclude chronic rejection and infection [76]. If allograft rejection or infection is suspected, elective surgery should be postponed and appropriate investigations should be performed.

Altered lymphatic drainage in the transplanted lung may cause interstitial fluid accumulation. It has been recommended that these patients be treated with diuretics and limited crystalloid infusion [77, 78]. Invasive hemodynamic monitoring is often required in heart-lung transplant recipients since there is a narrow line between the pulmonary edema occurrence and maintaining cardiac output with fluid load [79].

4.3. Kidney transplant recipients

Kidney transplant recipient have high incidence of cardiovascular diseases, especially elderly patients with diabetes and after years of dialysis procedures. Spectrum of disease can range from hypertension to severe coronary disease. It is wisely to approach them with caution. Cardiovascular complications are the leading cause of death in renal transplant recipients, accounting for 32% of all deaths [80].

After successful transplantation, renal function is restored, with no need for renal replacement therapy. Still, beware of prolonged drug action and excretion in kidney transplant recipients, due to the fact that their glomerular filtration rate and effective plasma flow can be significantly lower than in healthy subjects [81].

You should suspect at chronic graft rejection when azotemia, proteinuria, and hypertension are seen [82, 83]. One of the important parameters to consider in the prevention of graft failure is the maintenance of appropriate renal perfusion pressure. Perioperative fluid management must ensure restoration and maintenance of intravascular volume, in order to obtain good graft function. Diuretics should not be given without careful evaluation of the patient's volume status.

In anesthetic management, it is prudent to choose drugs that do not rely on the kidney for excretion. Nephrotoxic drugs should be avoided [84]. Cardiovascular instability can be present after a recipient has been recently hemodialysed due to hypovolemia and hypokalemia, causing arrhythmias and increased susceptibility to muscle relaxants [85].

4.4. Liver transplant recipients

Liver synthetic tests should normalize over time pointing out a good liver graft function. There is also gradual decrease of all liver enzyme levels, as graft function becomes normal. Recovery of drug metabolism capacity occurs immediately after reperfusion of the liver graft. Liver transplantation itself results in reversal of the hyperdynamic state that characterizes patients with end-stage liver disease and cardiac performance improves in the months after transplantation. Hypoxemia caused by ventilation/perfusion mismatch is reversed over the course of the first postoperative months. Patients with pre-existing true shunts may require more time to achieve reversal of hypoxemia, or hypoxemia may not resolve at all [86]. Hepatorenal syndrome gradually diminishes, renal function improves over time, and creatinine level may become normal. However, kidneys are still in danger of injury due to immunosuppression side effects [87].

The most severe complication of liver transplantation is hepatic artery thrombosis. It has often been associated with massive transfusion of blood products leading to hemoconcentration. Therefore, liver transplant recipients should have minimal blood viscosity (hematocrit approximately 28%) during the perioperative period [88].

No individual general anesthetic agents are contraindicated when hepatic and renal function is normal. If an epidural or spinal anesthesia is planned, clotting studies and platelet counts should be normal. Neither regional nor general anesthetic techniques were associated with deterioration of liver function assuming proper anesthetic and intensive care management [3, 25].

4.5. Pancreas transplant recipients

Pancreas transplantation provides the most effective method of glycemic and metabolic control. It can be done as a single organ transplant or simultaneously with kidney (predominantly in type 1 diabetes) (SPKT). SPKT is a treatment of choice for uremic diabetic patients when a living-related kidney donor is unavailable. After successful transplantation, pancreas transplant recipients do not require insulin to compensate for the stress response to surgery [89].

However, due to long-lasting diabetes effect, these patients are in high risk of developing cardiovascular diseases. It is prudent to manage these patients with the assumption that they have coronary artery disease [90]. Pancreas recipients still have persistent complications of diabetes such as gastropathy and neuropathy. Aspiration risk may be increased as a result of delayed gastric emptying. This population is also at increased risk for lymphoproliferative disorders secondary to immunosuppressant drugs and lymphoproliferative growth may compromise any part of the airway or mediastinum and cause life-threatening airway obstruction during sedation and anesthesia [91].

Amylase levels in serum and urine should be closely monitored. They can be our only window in the graft rejection recognition [92]. Glucose levels should also be monitored perioperatively. In normal functioning grafts, the suppression of endogenous insulin secretion during hypoglycemia is sufficient to enable a normal glucagon response from the transplanted pancreas, even in surgical stress [93]. In patients with failed pancreatic grafts, perioperative management of glucose levels and acid-base status is the same as that for any diabetic patient.

4.6. Intestine transplant recipients

There are three types of intestine transplantation: isolated intestinal transplantation, transplantation of combined intestine, and liver graft or multivisceral transplantation. The biggest problem in intestinal transplantation is graft rejection, and it is the main reason for morbidity and mortality. The diagnosis of rejection is confirmed by clinical symptoms, endoscopic appearance, and pathological specimens taken by endoscopy [94].

Denervation and lymphatic dysfunction of the intestine affect intestinal permeability and absorption. If the intestinal mucosa barrier is damaged by ischemia, rejection, or enteritis, bacteria translocate into the bloodstream and infections are often observed [95]. Some of these patients develop diarrhea and lose weight in the early post-transplantation period. Any imbalance in the electrolyte and acid-base status should be timely corrected. Fluid administration should be closely monitored to assure sufficient splanchnic perfusion. Venous access is of major consideration for the anesthesiologist due to chronic use of total parenteral nutrition and its thrombotic complications [96].

5. Special cases

5.1. Trauma

It is generally assumed that immunosuppressed patients are more susceptible to the effects of soft tissue damage and poor bone healing. Bone loss associated with chronic immunosuppressive therapy is a serious problem for most transplant recipients. These patients are prone to fractures (i.e. hip or compressive vertebral fracture) [97].

Only a few studies of traumatized transplant recipients have been reported. This is likely because of the infrequent presentation of these patients to trauma centers. The most common causes of trauma are car accidents and falls. The latest study by Scalea *et al.* determined that outcomes for traumatic injury in patients with organ transplants are not worse than that for non-transplant patients, despite common presumptions among physicians [98]. Transplant recipients sustaining trauma should receive the same initial resuscitation as any trauma victim. Patients should be assessed by a transplant surgeon as soon as possible and graft function should be closely assessed by a transplant team during hospitalization and after discharge from the trauma center [3]. Acute organ rejection within 6 months of admission for trauma is reported among 17% of solid organ recipients [99].

Transplant recipients, whose immune systems are already suppressed to prevent organ rejection, are presumed to be at greater risk of infection from traumatic injury. However, this was not observed in two latest studies [100]. Therefore, similar protocols of antimicrobial therapy should apply to both transplanted and non-transplanted patients to avoid the overuse of antimicrobial agents and ensure maintenance of the susceptibility patterns of pathogens.

Studies also show that transplanted organs are rarely injured in traumatic events. This is most likely related to careful selection of transplant recipients who are committed to self-care and continue to pursue healthy life style after transplantation.

5.2. Pregnancy

With the advances in transplantation medicine, female organ transplant recipients are able to conceive and carry pregnancies successfully to term. This state presents a unique challenge to attending physician, obstetrician, and anesthesiologist. These women are at an increased risk of comorbidities and obstetric complications. Therefore, all post-transplant pregnancies should be considered as high risk, and close monitoring is mandatory. Anesthesiologists are involved in the care of these patients for both labor analgesia and operative procedure. Anesthetic considerations include the effects of the physiologic changes of pregnancy on the transplanted organ, graft function in the peripartum period, and the maternal side effects and drug interactions of immunosuppressive agents. Anesthetic management should consider the important task of protecting graft function [101, 102].

Data are lacking regarding the optimal transplant-conception interval. The 2005 American Society of Transplantation Consensus Conference suggested that pregnancy 1 year after transplant is safe as long as the patient has stable graft function. This means: no episodes of rejection in the past year, a low risk for opportunistic infections, stable renal function (including in those receiving organs other than a kidney), and a low stable dose of maintenance immunosuppression [103].

Pregnancy does not appear to cause excessive or irreversible problems with graft dysfunction if the function of the transplanted organ was stable prior to pregnancy [104]. Maternal side effects of immunosuppression therapy include nephrotoxicity, hepatotoxicity, diabetes, and arterial hypertension, which could lead to possible dangerous complications. In kidney, heart, or heart-lung transplant recipients, the rate of complications, such as preeclampsia, premature labor, and risk of acute allograft rejection postpartum, is higher than that in the non-transplant population [105].

Current immunosuppressant drugs are not thought to be teratogenic and their use cannot be discontinued during pregnancy. All immunosuppressants cross the placenta. They are not strongly associated with the increased risk of congenital anomalies in the first trimester. However, they affect the immune system of fetus during the second and third trimesters and may result in premature delivery and low birth weight in newborn [106].

The anesthetic technique for cesarean section depends on indication, functional status of transplanted organ, and cardiovascular and hematological status. Central neuraxial blocks are not contraindicated if coagulation status is normal. However, documentation of paresthesia is important if regional anesthesia is planned. In the case of general anesthesia, all intravenous anesthetics and inhalational agents are safe. Neuromuscular function should be monitored particularly if the patient is receiving magnesium. Postoperative pain relief is provided with narcotics by epidural or spinal route if regional anesthesia is used or by parenteral opioids. Non-steroidal anti-inflammatory drugs should be avoided. Thromboprophylaxis should be administered because of the high risk of thromboembolic complications in these patients, especially after cesarean delivery. The threshold for admission to an intensive care or high-dependency unit should be low [107].

5.3. Laparoscopic surgery

Laparoscopic surgery is currently a widely accepted approach to several surgical fields because of its advantages in terms of postoperative pain reduction and easy patient recovery. The number of minimally invasive surgical procedures performed in transplant recipients is constantly increasing [108].

Lymphoceles can be successfully treated surgically after kidney transplantation by laparoscopy under general anesthesia [109, 110]. There are also reports of successful laparoscopic bariatric surgery after simultaneous pancreas and kidney transplantation [111]. Laparoscopic cholecystectomy is considered to be safe procedure in the transplant population. It has advantage of short hospital stay, low morbidity, maintenance of oral immunosuppression, and early return to preoperative routines. There is however a slightly higher rate of conversion to an open cholecystectomy among transplant patients compared to general population (27% vs. 11%, respectively) [112, 113]. Generally, laparoscopic approach may be useful even in solid-organ transplantation surgery as a diagnostic or treatment procedure in some surgical complications.

5.4. Outpatient and esthetic surgery

With shorter medical procedure duration and fewer complications, there is growth in popularity of outpatient or ambulatory surgery. Procedures performed are broad in scope: knee, shoulder, spine and eye surgery (cataract, laser surgery), plastic surgery, some types of esthetic surgery, and upper gastrointestinal endoscopy and colonoscopy [114].

Improved immunosuppression and lifespans have afforded solid organ transplant recipients the opportunity to seek outpatient and esthetic surgery. Most commonly performed procedures are soft tissue excisions with local flap coverage, facelifts, breast augmentation, and abdominoplasty. Among solid organ transplant recipients, kidney transplant recipients most often underwent plastic surgery, accounting for over 68% [115]. The complication rate is very low and ranges from 4 to 8% [116]. Delayed wound healing or wound disruption is reported as the most common complication and is associated with immunosuppression therapy, such as steroids [117].

It is extraordinarily important to manage these patients with a multidisciplinary approach. They should obtain clearance from the transplant surgeon and from the organ-specific specialist. The anesthesiologist should be familiar with the organ-specific needs in the perioperative period (i.e. maintaining preload for heart transplant patients, judicious fluid management in the renal patient, and avoidance of volatile anesthetics in liver transplants) to avert unintended consequences. It is more reasonable to use of general anesthesia over regional in the heart transplant patients. Perioperative antibiotic prophylaxis and stress-dose steroids should be administered prior to surgery. NSAIDs should be avoided in postoperative pain regimen [118].

Elective esthetic surgery can be performed safely in patients with a history of solid organ transplantation after a careful patient selection and multidisciplinary approach. These patients can potentially experience significant improvements in their quality of life with low morbidity.

6. Conclusion

The increasing prevalence of previously transplanted patients makes it likely that every anesthesiologist will care for patients with end-organ failure or a transplanted organ, either for accidental or transplant-related surgery in the future. Local, regional, or general anesthesia can be safely delivered to transplant recipients and a successful anesthetic and perioperative management can be provided. However, for the safe management of solid organ recipients, it is essential to have an appropriate knowledge of the physiology of the transplanted organ, the pharmacology of the immunosuppressive drugs, and the presence of associated organ dysfunction.

Many of the perioperative problems in the transplant population have not been specifically studied, and there are no formal recommendations for their management. Additional research should be performed in order to identify perioperative issues and facilitate the formulation of guidelines for anesthesia in this particular transplanted population.

Author details

Katarina Tomulić Brusich[1]* and Ivana Acan[2]

*Address all correspondence to: ktomulic@mail.com

1 Department of Anesthesiology and Intensive Care, The Magdalena Special Hospital for Cardiovascular Surgery and Cardiology, Croatia

2 Department of Anesthesiology and Intensive Care, University Hospital Merkur, Zagreb, Croatia

References

[1] Kostopanagiotou G, Smyrniotis V, Arkadopoulos N, Theodoraki K, Papadimitriou L, Papadimitriou J. Anesthetic and perioperative management of adult transplant recipients in nontransplant surgery. Anesthesia and Analgesia. 1999;**89**(3):613-622. PMID: 10475290

[2] Ashary N, Kaye AD, Hegazi AR, M'Frost EA. Anesthetic considerations in the patient with a heart transplant. Heart Disease 2002;**4**(3):191-198. PMID: 12028605

[3] Zeyneloglu P, Pirat A, Sulemanji D, Torgay A, Karakayali H, Arslan G. Perioperative anesthetic management for recipients of orthotopic liver transplant undergoing nontransplant surgery. Experimental and Clinical Transplantation 2007;**5**(2):690-692. PMID: 18194123

[4] Keegan MT, Plevak DJ. The transplant recipient for nontransplant surgery. Anesthesiology Clinics of North America. 2004;**22**(4):827-861. PMID: 15541938. DOI: 10.1016/j.atc.2004.05.006

[5] Shapiro R, Young JB, Milford EL, Trotter JF, Bustami RT, Leichtman AB. Immunosuppression: Evolution in practice and trends, 1993-2003. American Journal of Transplantation. 2005;**5**(4 Pt 2):874-886. PMID: 15760415. DOI: 10.1111/j.1600-6135.2005.00833.x

[6] Dickinson DM, Dykstra DM, Levine GN, Li S, Welch JC, Webb RL. Transplant data: Sources, collection and research considerations, 2004. American Journal of Transplantation. 2005;**5**(4 Pt 2):850-861. PMID: 15760413. DOI: 10.1111/j.1600-6135.2005.00840.x

[7] Reding R, Gras J, Sokal E, Otte JB, Davies HF. Steroid-free liver transplantation in children. Lancet. Dec 20, 2003;**362**(9401):2068-2070. PMID: 14697809. DOI: 10.1016/S0140-6736(03)15104-5

[8] Greig P, Lilly L, Scudamore C, Erb S, Yoshida E, Kneteman N, Bain V, Ghent C, Marotta P, Grant D, Wall W, Tchervenkov J, Barkun J, Roy A, Marleau D, McAlister V, Peltekian K. Early steroid withdrawal after liver transplantation: The Canadian tacrolimus versus microemulsion cyclosporin A trial: 1-year follow-up. Liver Transplantation. 2003;**9**(6):587-595. PMID: 12783400. DOI: 10.1053/jlts.2003.50102

[9] Ozbilgin M, Egeli T, Unek T, Ozkardesler S, Avkan-Oguz V, Sagol O, Ozbilgin S, Bacakoglu A, Astarcıoglu I. Incidence of late acute rejection in living donor liver transplant patients, risk factors, and the role of immunosuppressive drugs. Transplantation Proceedings. 2015;**47**(5):1474-1477. DOI: 10.1016/j.transproceed.2015.04.076

[10] Papalois VE, Hakim NS. New immunosuppressive drugs in organ transplantation. In: Hakim NS, editor. Introduction to Organ Transplantation. London: Imperial College Press; 1997. pp. 225-236

[11] Eide TR, Belenker S. Effect of cardiopulmonary bypass on plasma cyclosporin A levels in a renal transplant patient. Anesthesia and Analgesia. 1992;**74**:288-290. PMID: 1731551

[12] Campana C, Regazzi MB, Buggia I, Molinaro M. Clinically significant drug interactions with cyclosporin. An update. Clinical Pharmacokinetics 1996;**30**:141-179. PMID: 8906896

[13] Rancic N, Vavic NN, Kovacevic AM, Mikov MM, Drgojevic-Simic VM. Drug-drug interactions of tacrolimus. Hospital Pharmacology. 2015;**2**:291-296

[14] Aliabadi AZ, Zuckermann AO, Grimm M. Immunosuppressive therapy in older cardiac transplant patients. Drugs & Aging. 2007;**24**:913-932. PMID: 17953459

[15] Lill J, Bauer LA, Horn JR, Hansten PD. Cyclosporine-drug interactions and the influence of patient age. American Journal of Health-System Pharmacy. 2000;**57**(17):1579-1584. PMID: 10984808

[16] Gelb AW, Freeman D, Robertson KM, Zhang C. Isoflurane alters the kinetics of oral cyclosporine. Anesthesia and Analgesia. 1991;**72**(6):801-804. PMID: 2035864

[17] Freeman DJ, Sharpe MD, Gelb AW. Effects of nitrous oxide/oxygen/isoflurane anesthesia on blood cyclosporine concentrations in the rabbit. Transplantation. 1994;**58**:640-642. PMID: 8091495

[18] Pertek JP, Chaoui K, Junke E, Artis M, Coissard A, Frisoni A, Meistelman C. Effects of propofol on blood concentration of cyclosporine. Annales Françaises d'Anesthèsie et de Rèanimation. 1996;**15**(5):589-594. PMID: 9033752

[19] Cirella VN, Pantuck CB, Lee YJ, Pantuck EJ. Effects of cyclosporine on anesthetic action. Anesthesia and Analgesia. 1987;**66**(8):703-706. PMID: 3605689

[20] Crosby E, Robblee JA. Cyclosporine-pancuronium interaction in a patient with a renal allograft. Canadian Journal of Anesthesia. 1988;**35**(3 Pt 1):300-302. PMID: 3289771

[21] Gramstad L. Atracurium, vecuronium, and pancuronium in end-stage renal failure. British Journal of Anaesthesia. 1987;**59**:995-1003. PMID: 2888477

[22] Sidi A, Kaplan RF, Davis RF. Prolonged neuromuscular blockade and ventilatory failure after renal transplantation and cyclosporine. Canadian Journal of Anaesthesia. 1990; **37**(5):543-548. PMID: 1973635. DOI: 10.1007/BF03006323

[23] Backman SB, Fox GS, Stein RD, Ralley FE. Neostigmine decreases heart rate in heart transplant patients. Canadian Journal of Anaesthesia. 1996;**43**:373-378. PMID: 8697553. DOI: 10.1007/BF03011717

[24] Herborn J, Parulkar S. Anesthetic considerations in transplant recipients for nontransplant surgery. Anesthesiology Clinics. 2017;**35**(3):539-553. DOI: 10.1016/j.anclin.2017.04.009

[25] Ersoy Z, Ayhan A, Ozdemirkan A, Polat GG, Zeyneloglu P, Arslan G, Haberal M. Anesthetic and perioperative management of nontransplant surgery in patients after liver transplant. Experimental and Clinical Transplantation. 2017;**15**(Suppl 1):42-45. PMID: 28260430. DOI: 10.6002/ect.mesot2016.O24

[26] Demetris AJ, Murase N, Lee RG, Randhawa P, Zeevi A, Pham S, Duquesnoy R, Fung JJ, Starzl TE. Chronic rejection. A general overview of histopathology and pathophysiology with emphasis on liver, heart and intestinal allografts. Annals of Transplantation.. 1997;**2**(2):27-44. PMID: 9869851. PMCID: PMC3235804

[27] Libby P, Pober JS. Chronic rejection. Immunity. 2001;**14**(4):387-397. PMID: 11336684

[28] Dunn DL. Problems related to immunosuppression. Infection and malignancy occurring after solid organ transplantation. Critical Care Clinics. 1990;**6**(4):955-977. PMID: 2265389

[29] Suzuki Y, Kenjo A, Togano T, Yamamoto N, Ohto H, Kume H. Infectious diseases in solid organ transplant recipients: Analysis of autopsied cases in Japan. Journal of Infection and Chemotherapy. 2017;**23**(8):531-537. DOI: 10.1016/j.jiac.2017.05.001

[30] Bratzler DW, Houck PM; Surgical infection prevention guideline writers workgroup. Antimicrobial prophylaxis for surgery: An advisory statement from the national surgical infection prevention project. American Journal of Surgery. 2005;**189**(4):395-404. PMID: 15820449. DOI: 10.1016/j.amjsurg.2005.01.015

[31] Augustine SM. Heart transplantation. Long-term management related to immunosuppression, complications, and psychosocial adjustments. Critical Care Nursing Clinics of North America. 2000;**12**:69-77. PMID: 11051920

[32] Courson AY, Lee JR, Aull MJ, Lee JH, Kapur S, McDermott JK. Routine prophylaxis with proton pump inhibitors and post-transplant complications in kidney transplant recipients undergoing early corticosteroid withdrawal. Clinical Transplantation. 2016;**30**(6):694-702. DOI: 10.1111/ctr.12736

[33] Abualhassan N, Aljiffry M, Thalib L, Coussa R, Metrakos P, Hassanain M. Post-transplant venous thromboembolic events and their effect on graft survival. Saudi Journal of Kidney Diseases and Transplantation. 2015;**26**(1):1-5. PMID: 25579708

[34] Abdel-Razeq H. Venous thromboembolism prophylaxis for hospitalized medical patients, current status and strategies to improve. Annals of Thoracic Medicine. 2010;**5**(4): 195-200. DOI: 10.4103/1817-1737.69104

[35] Samama CM, Afshari A. ESA VTE guidelines task force. European guidelines on perioperative venous thromboembolism prophylaxis. European Journal of Anaesthesiology. 2018;**35**(2):73-76. DOI: 10.1097/EJA.0000000000000702

[36] Fussner LA, Heimbach JK, Fan C, Dierkhising R, Coss E, Leise MD, Watt KD. Cardiovascular disease after liver transplantation: When, what, and who is at risk. Liver Transplantation. 2015;**21**(7):889-896. DOI: 10.1002/lt.24137

[37] Bromberg JS, Alfrey EJ, Barker CF, Chavin KD, Dafoe DC, Holland T, Naji A, Perloff LJ, Zellers LA, Grossman RA. Adrenal suppression and steroid supplementation in renal transplant recipients. Transplantation. 1991;**51**:385-390. PMID: 1847249

[38] Marchetti P. New-onset diabetes after transplantation. The Journal of Heart and Lung Transplantation. 2004;**23**(5 Suppl):S194-S201. PMID: 15093805. DOI: 10.1016/j.healun.2004.03.007

[39] Johnston TD, Katz SM. Special considerations in the transplant patient requiring other surgery. Surgical Clinics of North America. 1994;**74**:1211-1221. PMID: 7940070

[40] De Hert S, Imberger G, Carlisle J, Diemunsch P, Fritsch G, Moppett I, Solca M, Staender S, Wappler F, Smith A. Task force on preoperative evaluation of the adult noncardiac surgery patient of the European Society of Anaesthesiology. Preoperative evaluation of the adult patient undergoing non-cardiac surgery: Guidelines from the European Society of Anaesthesiology. European Journal of Anaesthesiology. 2011;**28**(10):684-722. DOI: 10.1097/EJA.0b013e3283499e3b

[41] Hammer GB, Cao S, Boltz MG, Messner A. Post-transplant lymphoproliferative disease may present with severe airway obstruction. Anesthesiology. 1998;**89**:263-265. PMID: 9667319

[42] Bach A, Boehrer H, Schmidt H, Geiss HK. Nosocomial sinusitis in ventilated patients. Nasotracheal versus orotracheal intubation. Anaesthesia. 1992;**47**(4):335-339. PMID: 1519688

[43] Fuehner T, Wiesner O, DeWall C, Dierich M, Simon AR, Hadem J, Ivanyi P, Welte T, Gottlieb J. Self-expanding metallic stent placement with laryngeal mask in lung transplant recipients. Transplantation Proceedings. 2010;**42**(10):4595-4599. DOI: 10.1016/j.transproceed.2010.10.016

[44] Ejtehadi F, Carter S, Evans L, Zia M, Bradpiece H. General anaesthesia and emergency surgery in heart transplant recipient. Case Reports in Surgery. 2015;**2015**:256465. DOI: 10.1155/2015/256465

[45] Brusich KT, Acan I, Filipčić NV. Ventilator-associated pneumonia: Comparing cadaveric liver transplant and non-transplant surgical patients. Acta Clinica Croatica. 2016;**55**(3): 360-369. PMID: 29045094

[46] Chidambaran V, Ngamprasertwong P, Vinks AA, Sadhasivam S. Pharmacogenetics and anesthetic drugs. Current Clinical Pharmacology. 2012;**7**(2):78-101. PMID: 22432844

[47] Sneyd JR, Rigby-Jones AE. New drugs and technologies, intravenous anaesthesia is on the move (again). British Journal of Anaesthesia. 2010;**105**(3):246-254. DOI: 10.1093/bja/aeq190

[48] Campagna JA, Miller KW, Forman SA. Mechanisms of actions of inhaled anesthetics. The New England Journal of Medicine. May 22, 2003;**348**(21):2110-2124. PMID: 12761368. DOI: 10.1056/NEJMra021261

[49] Seutin VM. Mechanisms of actions of inhaled anesthetics. The New England Journal of Medicine. Aug 28, 2003;**349**(9):909-910. Author reply 909-10

[50] Dean M. Opioids in renal failure and dialysis patients. Journal of Pain and Symptom Management. 2004;**28**(5):497-504. PMID: 15504625. DOI: 10.1016/j.jpainsymman.2004.02.021

[51] Niscola P, Scaramucci L, Vischini G, Giovannini M, Ferrannini M, Massa P, Tatangelo P, Galletti M, Palumbo R. The use of major analgesics in patients with renal dysfunction. Current Drug Targets. 2010;**11**(6):752-758. PMID: 20041843

[52] De Wolf AM, Freeman JA, Scott VL, Tullock W, Smith DA, Kisor DF, Kerls S, Cook DR. Pharmacokinetics and pharmacodynamics of cisatracurium in patients with end-stage liver disease undergoing liver transplantation. British Journal of Anaesthesia. 1996;**76**(5):624-628. PMID: 8688259

[53] Baxi V, Jain A, Dasgupta D. Anaesthesia for renal transplantation: An update. Indian Journal of Anaesthesia. 2009;**53**(2):139-147. PMID: 20640114. PMCID: PMC2900097

[54] Barbara DW, Christensen JM, Mauermann WJ, Dearani JA, Hyder JA. The safety of neuromuscular blockade reversal in patients with cardiac transplantation. Transplantation 2016;**100**(12):2723-2728. PMID: 26760570. DOI: 10.1097/TP.0000000000001060

[55] Carlos RV, Torres MLA, de Boer HD. Reversal of neuromuscular block with sugammadex in five heart transplant pediatric recipients. Revista Brasileira de Anestesiologia. 2018 Jan 6. pii: S0034-7094(17)30194-0. DOI: 10.1016/j.bjan.2017.10.008. [Article in Portuguese]

[56] Gupta PK Hopkins PM. Regional anaesthesia for all? British Journal of Anaesthesia. 2012;**109**:7-9. PMID: 22696553. DOI: 10.1093/bja/aes169

[57] Tomulić Brusich K, Acan I, Kovačić Vicić V, Filipčić V. Supraclavicular nerve block: Does kidney transplantation make a difference? Periodicum Biologorum. 2015;**117**(2):331

[58] Freir NM Murphy C Mugawar M Linnane A Cunningham AJ. Transversus abdominis plane block for analgesia in renal transplantation: A randomized controlled trial. Anesthesia & Analgesia. 2012;**115**:953-957. PMID: 22763899. DOI: 10.1213/ANE.0b013e3182642117

[59] Cook TM, Counsell D, Wildsmith JA. Major complications of central neuraxial block: Report on the Third National Audit Project of the Royal College of Anaesthetists. British Journal of Anaesthesia. 2009;**102**:179-190. DOI: 10.1093/bja/aen360

[60] Feng ZY, Zhang J, Zhu SM, Zheng SS. Is there any difference in anesthetic management of different post-OLT stage patients undergoing nontransplant organ surgery? Hepatobiliary & Pancreatic Diseases International. 2006;**5**(3):368-373. PMID: 16911933

[61] Ahlers SJ, Van Gulik L, Van Dongen EP, Bruins P, Tibboel D, Knibbe CA. Aminotransferase levels in relation to short-term use of acetaminophen four grams daily in postoperative cardiothoracic patients in the intensive care unit. Anaesthesia and Intensive Care. 2011;**39**:1056-1063 PMID: 22165358

[62] Harris KP, Jenkins D, Walls J. Nonsteroidal anti-inflammatory drugs and cyclosporine. Transplantation. 1988;**46**:598-599. PMID: 3176159

[63] Mueller EA, Kovarik JM, Koelle EU, Merdjan H, Johnston A, Hitzenberger G. Pharmacokinetics of cyclosporine and multiple dose diclofenac during co-administration. Journal of Clinical Pharmacology. 1993;**33**:936-943. PMID: 8227465

[64] Klintmalm GBG, Husberg BS, Starzl TE. The organ transplanted patient: Immunological concepts and immunosuppression. In: Makowka L, editor. The Handbook of Transplantation Management. Austin, TX: Landes; 1995. pp. 72-108

[65] Bristow MR. The surgically denervated, transplanted human heart. Circulation. 1990; **82**:658-660. PMID: 2372914

[66] Swami AC, Kumar A, Rupal S, Lata S. Anaesthesia for non-cardiac surgery in a cardiac transplant recipient. Indian Journal of Anaesthesia. 2011;**55**(4):405-407. DOI: 10.4103/0019-5049.84849

[67] Ejtehadi F, Carter S, Evans L, Zia M, Bradpiece H. General anaesthesia and emergency surgery in heart transplant recipient. Case Reports in Surgery. 2015;**2015**:256465. PMID: 26788397. PMCID: PMC4695654. DOI: 10.1155/2015/256465

[68] Chen EP, Bittner HB, Davis RD, Van Trigt P. Hemodynamic and inotropic effects of milrinone after heart transplantation in the setting of recipient pulmonary hypertension. The Journal of Heart and Lung Transplantation 1998;**17**(7):669-678. PMID: 9703231

[69] Pérez Vela JL, Corres Peiretti MA, Rubio Regidor M, Hernández Tejedor A, Renes Carreño E, Arribas López P, Gutiérrez Rodríguez J, Perales Rodríguez De Viguri N. Levosimendan for postoperative ventricular dysfunction following heart transplantation. Revista Española de Cardiología. 2008;**61**(5):534-539. PMID: 18462658

[70] Hsu DT, Spotnitz HM. Echocardiographic diagnosis of cardiac allograft rejection. Progress in Cardiovascular Diseases. 1990;**33**:149-160. PMID: 2236563

[71] Schroeder JS, Shao-Zhou G, Hunt SA, Stinson EB. Accelerated graft coronary artery disease: Diagnosis and prevention. The Journal of Heart and Lung Transplantation. 1992;**11**:258-266. PMID: 1515448

[72] Steib A, Freys G, Otteni JC. Anesthesia for non-specific surgery in a post-transplantation patient. Annales Françaises d'Anesthèsie et de Rèanimation. 1993;**12**:27-37. PMID: 8338262

[73] Berberich JJ. Anesthesia for heart and heart-lung transplantation. In: Fabian JA, editor. Anesthesia for Organ Transplantation. New York: JB Lippincott; 1992. pp. 1-19

[74] McCarthy PM. Immediate postoperative care after thoracic organ transplantation. In: Shumway SJ, Shumway NE, editors. Thoracic Transplantation. Oxford: Blackwell Science; 1995. pp. 205-218

[75] Glanville AR, Burke CM, Theodore J, Baldwin JC, Harvey J, Vankessel A, Robin ED. Bronchial hyper-responsiveness after cardiopulmonary transplantation. Clinical Science. 1987;**73**:299-303. PMID: 3308288

[76] Gelb AW, Sharpe MD. Organ transplantation: Anesthetic considerations for the previously transplanted patient. In: Benumof JL, editor. Anesthesiology Clinics of North America. Philadelphia: WB Saunders; 1994. pp. 827-843

[77] Wekerle T, Klepetko W, Wisser W, Senbaklavaci O, Artemiou O, Zuckermann A, Wolner E. Incidence and outcome of major non-pulmonary surgical procedures in lung transplant recipients. European Journal of Cardio-Thoracic Surgery. 1997;**12**:718-723. PMID: 9458142

[78] Haddow GR. Anaesthesia for patients after lung transplantation. Canadian Journal of Anaesthesia. 1997;**44**:182-197. PMID: 9043732. DOI: 10.1007/BF03013008

[79] Boscoe M. Anesthesia for patients with transplanted lungs and heart and lungs. International Anesthesiology Clinics. 1995;**33**:21-44. PMID: 7657379

[80] Ponticelli C, Villa M. Role of anaemia in cardiovascular mortality and morbidity in transplant patients. Nephrology, Dialysis, Transplantation. 2002;**17**(Suppl 1):41-46. PMID: 11812911

[81] Santos J, Martins LS. Estimating glomerular filtration rate in kidney transplantation: Still searching for the best marker. World Journal of Nephrology. Jul 6, 2015;**4**(3):345-353. DOI: 10.5527/wjn.v4.i3.345

[82] Focosi D, Vistoli F, Boggi U. Rejection of the kidney allograft. The New England Journal of Medicine. Feb 3, 2011;**364**(5):485-486. Author reply 486. DOI: 10.1056/NEJMc1012440#SA1

[83] Marcén R. Immunosuppression and renal transplant rejection: Review of current and emerging therapies. Journal of Clinical Investigation. 2011;**1**(6):859-877. DOI: 10.4155/CLI.11.49

[84] Schmid S, Jungwirth B. Anaesthesia for renal transplant surgery: An update. European Journal of Anaesthesiology. 2012;**29**:552-558. DOI: 10.1097/EJA.0b013e32835925fc

[85] Sarin Kapoor H, Kaur R, Kaur H. Anaesthesia for renal transplant surgery. Acta Anaesthesiologica Scandinavica. 2007;**51**:1354-1367. PMID: 17944639. DOI: 10.1111/j.1399-6576.2007.01447.x

[86] Eriksson JS, Soderman C, Ericzon B-G, Eleborg L, Wahren J, Hedenstierna G. Normalization of ventilation/perfusion relationships after liver transplantation in patients with decompensated cirrhosis: Evidence for a hepatopulmonary syndrome. Hepatology. 1990;**12**:1350-1357. PMID: 2258151

[87] Millikan Jr WJ, Henderson JM, Stewart MT, Warren WD, Marsh JW, Galloway JR, Jennings H, Kawasaki S, Dodson TF, Perlino CA. Change in hepatic function, hemodynamics, and morphology after liver transplant. Physiological effect of therapy. Annals of Surgery. 1989;**209**(5):513-525. PMID: 2650642. PMCID: PMC1494074

[88] Tisone G, Gunson BK, Buckels JA, McMaster P. Raised hematocrit: A contributing factor to hepatic artery thrombosis following liver transplantation. Transplantation. 1988; **46**:162-163. PMID: 3293279

[89] Larsen JL, Duckworth WC, Stratta RJ. Pancreas transplantation for type I diabetes mellitus. Postgraduate Medicine. 1994;**96**(3):105-111. DOI: 10.1080/00325481.1994.11945895

[90] Knoll GA, Nichol G. Dialysis, kidney transplantation, or pancreas transplantation for patients with diabetes mellitus and renal failure: A decision analysis of treatment options. Journal of the American Society of Nephrology. 2003;**14**(2):500-515. PMID: 12538753

[91] Hammel L, Sebranek J, Hevesi Z. The anesthetic management of adult patients with organ transplants undergoing nontransplant surgery. Advances in Anesthesia. 2010;**28**(1):211-244. DOI: dx.doi.org/10.1016/j.aan.2010.09.001

[92] Pirson Y, Vandeleene B, Squifflet JP. Kidney and kidney-pancreas transplantation in diabetic recipients. Diabetes & Metabolism. 2000;**26**(Suppl 4):86-89. PMID: 10922978

[93] Rickels MR. Recovery of endocrine function after islet and pancreas transplantation. Current Diabetes Reports. 2012;**12**(5):587-596. DOI: 10.1007/s11892-012-0294-3

[94] Loo L, Vrakas G, Reddy S, Allan P. Intestinal transplantation: A review. Current Opinion in Gastroenterology. 2017;**33**(3):203-211. DOI: 10.1097/MOG.0000000000000358

[95] Girlanda R, Desai C, Matsumoto C, Fishbein T. Lymphatic leak after intestinal transplantation: Aspects of the donor technique. Progress in Transplantation. 2017;**27**(4):392-395. DOI: 10.1177/1526924817732943

[96] Nguyen-Buckley C, Wong M. Anesthesia for intestinal transplantation. Anesthesiology Clinics. 2017;**35**(3):509-521. DOI: 10.1016/j.anclin.2017.04.007

[97] Early C, Stuckey L, Tischer S. Osteoporosis in the adult solid organ transplant population: Underlying mechanisms and available treatment options. Osteoporosis International. 2016;**27**(4):1425-1440. DOI: 10.1007/s00198-015-3367-8

[98] Scalea JR, Menaker J, Meeks AK, Kramer ME, Kufera JA, Auman KM, Cooper M, Bartlett ST, Scalea TM. Trauma patients with a previous organ transplant: Outcomes are better than expected-a retrospective analysis. Journal of Trauma and Acute Care Surgery. 2013;**74**(6):1498-1503. DOI: 10.1097/TA.0b013e31828da918

[99] Barone GW, Sailors DM, Hudec WA, Ketel BL. Trauma management in solid organ transplant recipients. The Journal of Emergency Medicine. 1997;**15**(2):169-176. PMID: 9144057

[100] Tessier JM, Sirkin M, Wolfe LG, Duane TM. Trauma after transplant: Hold the antibiotics please. Surgical Infections (Larchmt). 2013;**14**(2):177-180. DOI: 10.1089/sur.2012.058

[101] Moaveni DM, Cohn JH, Hoctor KG, Longman RE, Ranasinghe JS. Anesthetic considerations for the parturient after solid organ transplantation. Anesthesia and Analgesia. 2016;**123**(2):402-410. DOI: 10.1213/ANE.0000000000001391

[102] Parikh BK, Shah VR, Bhosale G. Anesthesia for parturient with renal transplantation. Journal of Anaesthesiology Clinical Pharmacology. 2012;**28**(4):524-527. DOI: 10.4103/0970-9185.101948

[103] McKay DB, Josephson MA, Armenti VT, August P, Coscia LA, Davis CL, Davison JM, Easterling T, Friedman JE, Hou S, Karlix J, Lake KD, Lindheimer M, Matas AJ, Moritz MJ, Riely CA, Ross LF, Scott JR, Wagoner LE, Wrenshall L, Adams PL, Bumgardner GL, Fine RN, Goral S, Krams SM, Martinez OM, Tolkoff-Rubin N, Pavlakis M, Scantlebury V. Women's Health Committee of the American Society of transplantation. Reproduction and transplantation: Report on the AST consensus conference on reproductive issues and transplantation. American Journal of Transplantation. 2005;**5**:1592-1599. DOI: 10.1111/j.1600-6143.2005.00969.x

[104] Costantine MM. Physiologic and pharmacokinetic changes in pregnancy. Frontiers in Pharmacology. 2014;**5**:65. PMID: 24772083. PMCID: PMC3982119. DOI: 10.3389/fphar.2014.00065

[105] Casale JP, Doligalski CT. Pharmacologic considerations for solid organ transplant recipients who become pregnant. Pharmacotherapy. 2016;**36**(9):971-982. DOI: 10.1002/phar.1800

[106] Gerosa M, Meroni PL, Cimaz R. Safety considerations when prescribing immunosuppression medication to pregnant women. Expert Opinion on Drug Safety. 2014;**13**:1591-1599. PMID: 25189270. DOI: 10.1517/14740338.2014.951326

[107] Riley ET. Obstetric management of patients with transplants. International Anesthesiology Clinics. 1995;**33**:125-140. PMID: 7657378

[108] Merenda R, Gerunda GE, Neri D, Barbazza F, Di Marzio E, Meduri F, Valmasoni M, Faccioli AM. Laparoscopic surgery after orthotopic liver transplantation. Liver Transplantation. 2000;**6**(1):104-107. PMID: 10648587. DOI: 10.1002/lt.500060101

[109] Fuller TF, Kang SM, Hirose R, Feng S, Stock PG, Freise CE. Management of lymphoceles after renal transplantation: Laparoscopic versus open drainage. The Journal of Urology. 2003;**169**(6):2022-2025. PMID: 12771709. DOI: 10.1097/01.ju.0000063800.44792.61

[110] Lucewicz A, Wong G, Lam VW, Hawthorne WJ, Allen R, Craig JC, Pleass HC. Management of primary symptomatic lymphocele after kidney transplantation: A systematic review. Transplantation. Sep 27, 2011;**92**(6):663-673. DOI: 10.1097/TP.0b013e31822a40ef

[111] Zelones J, Biswas O, Mehran A. Laparoscopic sleeve gastrectomy after simultaneous pancreas-kidney transplant. The American Surgeon. 2012;**78**(5):613-614. PMID: 22546137

[112] Varga M, Kudla M, Vargova L, Fronek J. Cholecystectomy for acute cholecystitis after renal transplantation. Transplantation Proceedings. 2016;**48**(6):2072-2075. DOI: 10.1016/j.transproceed.2016.02.079

[113] Courcoulas AP, Kelly E, Harbrecht BG. Laparoscopic cholecystectomy in the transplant population. Surgical Endoscopy. 1996;**10**:516-519. PMID: 8658330

[114] Brownstein GM, Baker PA. Outpatient facility standards: What is necessary for satisfactory outcomes?. Clinics in Plastic Surgery. 2013;**40**(3):363-370. DOI: 10.1016/j.cps.2013.04.001

[115] MT V, F N. Is aesthetic surgery safe in the solid organ transplant patient? An international survey and review. Aesthetic Surgery Journal. 2016;**36**(8):954-958. DOI: 10.1093/asj/sjw044

[116] Sweis I, Tzvetanov I, Benedetti E. The new face of transplant surgery: A survey on cosmetic surgery in transplant recipients. Aesthetic Plastic Surgery. 2009;**33**(6):819-826. Discussion 827. DOI: 10.1007/s00266-009-9417-x

[117] Marik PE, Varon J. Requirement of perioperative stress doses of corticosteroids: A systematic review of the literature. Archives of Surgery. 2008;**14312**:1222-1226. PMID: 19075176. DOI: 10.1001/archsurg.143.12.1222

[118] Littlewood KE. The immunocompromised adult patient and surgery. Best Practice & Research. Clinical Anaesthesiology. 2008;**223**:585-609. PMID: 18831305

7

Immunosuppressive Minimization Strategies in Kidney Transplantation

Jorge Andrade-Sierra,
Pedro Alejandro Vazquez-Galvan,
Hernesto Hernandez-Reyes,
Lydia A. Mercado-Jáuregui,
Jonathan S. Chávez-Iñiguez,
Eduardo González-Espinoza,
Benjamin Gómez-Navarro and
José I. Cerrillos-Gutiérrez

Abstract

The long-term graft survival in renal transplantation results is still controversial, the toxicity and adverse reactions of the immunosuppressive drugs are implicated, as well as cellular and humoral antigen-specific immune mechanisms; therefore, different strategies for adapting immunosuppression are used to reduce the complications associated with the use of these drugs. Calcineurin inhibitors (CNI) require an adequate dose-dependent concentration leading to the appearance of drug-related adverse reactions. The variability in the required dose of CNI leads to minimization strategies that do not result in a higher acute rejection (AR) incidence when compared to other immunosuppressive agents. Early steroid withdrawal is another strategy, although with an increase in AR, but without an impact on the function and survival of the renal graft. The reduction of mycophenolate mofetil to 1.5 g/day seems to be a therapeutic option, decreasing the infectious, hematological and gastrointestinal adverse reactions. Finally, alemtuzumab, bortezomib, belatacept and cellular therapies are in the search for the new treatments, whose premise is the induction of donor-specific nonresponse in the context of operational tolerance or mixed chimerism. The use of adapted and adequate immunosuppression has led to variable results and some are very encouraging; however, they must be validated with experimental studies.

Keywords: renal transplantation, immunosuppressive minimization, acute rejection

1. Introduction

Renal transplantation (RT) is currently considered the best therapeutic option for renal replacement therapy in patients with end-stage renal disease (ESRD), with controversial results related to long-term graft survival [1–3]. Several factors can contribute to loss of the renal graft over time, which may be nonimmunological in nature, such as chronic nephrotoxicity due to drugs used for transplantation maintenance [particularly calcineurin inhibitors (CNI) tacrolimus (TAC) and cyclosporin] or for the side effects of immunosuppression when corticosteroids are involved, such as: infections, neoplasms, dyslipidemia, hypertension, cardiovascular disease, and new-onset diabetes mellitus (NODAT) that can lead to high mortality in patients with a functional graft [4–6]. Other conditions that induce long-term graft loss are the antigen-specific humoral and cellular immune mechanisms that contribute to an increase in the number and severity of episodes of acute rejection (AR), inducing chronic alloimmune damage [5–14]. These damage mechanisms raise the awareness that there must be a balance in posttransplantation immunosuppression; however, the new and powerful immunosuppressive drugs used today, and the alarming loss of kidney grafts, particularly due to the side effects of immunosuppression, have motivated transplant centers globally to try to minimize, suspend, or change the immunosuppressive maintenance drugs to try and further reduce the complications associated to them [15–39].

2. Minimizing immunosuppression with calcineurin inhibitors in kidney transplantation

The introduction of CNI has achieved exceptional short-term results in recent years in the field of allograft transplants, especially by reducing the rate of AR episodes, reaching, in the last 20 years, an overall graft survival of more than 90% in the first year [39]. However, the attention now focuses on the search for better long-term outcomes with strategies that sustain a low AR rate along with a decrease in the side effects of immunosuppression. The immunosuppressants have three effects: the therapeutic effect (rejection of suppression), unwanted consequences related to immunosuppression (infections, neoplasms, metabolic and hemodynamic disorders), and the nonimmune toxicity to tissues [40]. The nonimmune toxicity is immunosuppressive agent-specific and is related to the mechanism of action of the drug, since they target-specific molecules with certain functions in nonimmune tissues, conditioning progressive tissue damage, and gradual kidney graft failure. This, coupled with the death of the patient with a functional graft, encourages the new concept of focusing on nonimmune factors that intervene in the long term, evoking enthusiasm for strategies to minimize the side effects of CNIs.

3. Pharmacodynamics and nonimmune toxicity of the calcineurin inhibitors

In the classification of immunosuppressants, small molecules are included (from which the immunophilin-binding drugs are derived, such as CNIs, mechanism target of rapamycin (mTOR) inhibitor (imTOR), nucleotide blocking agents, and antimetabolites); the protein-depleting and nonlymphocyte-depleting agents (monoclonal and polyclonal antibodies), the intravenous immunoglobulin, and corticosteroids [40]. The effects of CNI are proportional to the serum concentration levels, since this depends on the saturation dose of its targets [40], which makes the dosage and the control of serum levels important in maintaining the balance between the desired immunosuppressant effect and the unwanted toxicity.

Cyclosporin A (CsA) is a fungal origin polypeptide (derived from *Tolypocladium inflatum),* composed of 11 amino acids, with a molecular weight of 1203 Da, which interacts by binding to its cytoplasmic receptor (cyclophilin); a protein from the family of immunophilins, forming a complex that binds to the calcineurin, inhibiting its normal phosphatase action on regulatory nuclear proteins (nuclear factor -KB and activator protein 1), preventing the cytokine production (IL-2), and eventually the T lymphocyte activation [41]. The adverse reactions to CsA, related to the serum concentration of the drug, include: nephrotoxicity, hypertension, hyperlipidemia, gingival hyperplasia, hirsutism, and tremor [42]; and, less frequently, hemolytic uremic syndrome, and NODAT [40].

In 2004, a longitudinal cohort where 888 renal biopsies were collected from 99 patients who were in immunosuppressive treatment with CsA for 10 years after renal transplantation, was evaluated; finding arteriolar hyalinosis as the most sensitive marker for nephrotoxicity due to CsA [43]. Another CNI introduced in the mid-1990s, that was initially called FK506 and is currently known as TAC, is a macrolide isolated from the fungi *Streptomyces tsukubaensis* that possesses suppressive effects similar to CsA (cell-mediated and humoral immune responses) [41]. The TAC binds to a protein called FKBP12 (binding protein of FK506–12) and a complex that inhibits the phosphatase activity of calcineurin, preventing the activation of the T cell, and selectively affecting the transcription of IL-2 and other cytokines. The adverse reactions are similar to those of CsA but with less incidence of hypertension, hyperlipidemia, hirsutism, and gingival hyperplasia; however, the incidence of NODAT and nephrotoxicity is higher [44].

The mechanism through which nephrotoxicity occurs is explained by the endothelial dysfunction associated with reduced production of local vasodilators (nitric oxide and prostaglandins) and increased production of vasoconstrictors (endothelin and thromboxane) [45].

The determination of the serum levels of the CNI is part of the management of immunosuppression in transplant recipients, due to the variability between patients (and the intra-patient variability). The inter-individual variability with TAC is explained by polymorphisms in genes that encode transporter proteins and enzymes that metabolize the drug. The TAC is metabolized in the intestine, liver, and kidney by cytochrome P450 (CYP) 3A4 and 3A5. Inter-individual differences in CYP3A activity are the most important determinants of variability in TAC metabolism. Polymorphisms in the CYP3A5 gene explain 40–50% of the variability in the TAC dose requirement to maintain adequate serum levels: the most studied one is the single nucleotide polymorphism CYP3A5*3. This allele causes a reduced enzymatic activity associating with the need to reduce the administered dose of TAC. On the other hand, when CYP3A5 is expressed, a dose of about 50% higher is required [46, 47]. To a lesser extent, the CYP3A4 genotype with impact on the determination of doses in transplant patients receiving TAC has also been identified. Individuals carrying the CYP3A4 * 1B allele reported up to a 35% dose reduction in order to achieve a therapeutic concentration. Similarly, it has been identified that the CYP3A4 * 22 variant reduces the enzymatic activity of CYP3A4, associated with a lower dose requirement. On the other hand, there are ethnic considerations that participate in allelic variability since Caucasian patients are commonly carriers of the CYP3A5 * 3 allele [46].

4. Minimization strategies of immunosuppression with calcineurin inhibitors

Given the nonimmunological toxic effects of CNI, two general strategies to reduce CNI are proposed: *de novo* minimization, where maintenance immunosuppression with CNI is sought immediately after transplantation at low doses subsequent to a powerful induction; and the second strategy, selective minimization, in which a class of immunosuppressants is avoided, showing a reduction of the undesired effects related to the drug. The Symphony study evaluated 1645 patients divided into four groups: (1) Standard dose of CsA, mycophenolate mofetil (MMF), and prednisone (PDN); (2) Low dose of CsA with induction therapy with daclizumab; (3) Low dose of TAC with induction with daclizumab; (4) Low dose of sirolimus (SRL) with induction with daclizumab. The primary aim was to reduce the nephrotoxicity using a low dose of CNI and SRL and to secondarily reduce the side effects, at the same time as maintaining the efficacy in terms of avoiding acute rejection, improving the overall survival of the patient and the graft. Their results at 1 and 3 years showed a better glomerular filtration rate (GFR) and graft survival in the group with low dose of TAC, as well as a low AR rate, compared with the SRL group [42, 48].

On the other hand, avoiding CNIs is the complete omission of these drugs from the maintenance immunosuppression regimen, while minimization schemes use reduced doses of CNI in order to avoid their nephrotoxicity [49]. Larso et al., compared regimens without CNI (SRL, MMF and PDN) and with CNI (TAC, MMF and PDN), in RT recipients, with similar results at 12 months in patient survival (98% SRL, 96% TAC, $p = 0.42$) and graft survival (94% SRL, 92% TAC, $p = 0.95$), as well as in the incidence of AR between both groups [50]. The regimens without CNI were also evaluated in the ORION51 study, which compared the efficacy of three schemes; (1) SRL + TAC with discontinuation of CNI at 13 weeks; (2) SRL + MMF; and (3) TAC + MMF. The SRL + MMF group presented more AR events (32.8%) compared to SRL + TAC (17.4%) and TAC + MMF (12.3%); however, the graft and patient survival were similar and there was the presence of hyperlipidemia in the group treated with SRL and NODAT in the group with TAC (**Table 1**) [51].

The BENEFIT study [52] compared two regimens (an intensive and a less intensive dose) with betalacept (selective T cell co-stimulation blocker) *versus* CsA in patients with living donor RT with standard criteria; finding better renal function with belatacept regimens (GFR of 65, 63, and 50 ml/min, respectively) but with a lower AR rate with CsA (22, 17 and 7%, respectively).

On the other hand, Weir et al. [53], who evaluated the efficacy and safety of the combination of MMF and SRL *versus* MMF and a CNI (TAC or CsA) at 24 months, found that the GFR was higher in the MMF/SRL regimen, with a similar AR rate in both groups.

Finally, a meta-analysis and systematic reviews related to these strategies have recently been published, with the aim of preventing nephrotoxicity and graft loss by a nonimmune character.

Immunosuppressor	Used dose in renal transplant	Adverse reactions	Minimization strategy
Tacrolimus	0.1–0.15 mg/kg/day divided in two doses	Nephrotoxicity, tremor, headache, dizziness, gingival hyperplasia, hypertension, carbohydrate intolerance, increased risk of infections and neoplasms.	Dose reduction; with lower nephrotoxicity without a higher acute rejection rate.
Cyclosporine	5–8 mg/kg/day divided in two doses	Nephrotoxicity, hypertension, hyperlipidemia, gingival hyperplasia, hirsutism, lymphoproliferative disorders associated to EBV, Kaposi sarcoma, TMA, HUS.	Dose reduction; improves the glomerular filtration rate and graft survival when compared to mTOR inhibitor.
Mycophenolate mofetil	2 g/day orally divided in two doses	Gastrointestinal: abdominal pain, nausea, vomits, diarrhea. Hematological: anemia, leukopenia, thrombocytopenia, increased risk of infections (especially viral), neoplasms.	Dose reduction not less than 1.5 g/day can decrease the gastrointestinal, hematological and infectious adverse reactions without an acute rejection rate increase.
Prednisone	0.5–1 mg/kg, orally divided in two doses with a taper of 5–10 mg/day indefinitely	Susceptibility to infections, obesity, osteonecrosis (avascular necrosis), hyperglycemia, hypertension, dyslipidemia, peptic ulcer, cushinoid features, long-term myopathy, osteoporosis, atherosclerosis, skin atrophy, cataracts.	Steroid withdrawal; better graft survival, lower risk of mortality, decrease in graft dysfunction with an improved metabolic and hemodynamic profile, although with contradictory results that may involve higher acute rejection rates proved by biopsy without affecting the long-term graft survival.
Alemtuzumab	30 mg/kg intravenously unique pre-transplant induction dose	Predisposition to severe infections (bacterial, viral, fungal) and increased risk of neoplasms.	Used as pre-transplant induction therapy allowing early steroid taper, CNI decrease or change to mTOR with a reduction in AR episodes in the first posttransplant year, without differences in graft survival in patients with low immunological risk and conventional therapy.
Bortezomib	1.3 mg/m^2 intravenously on day 1, 4, 8 and 11 for two cycles	Peripheral sensory neuropathies. Hematologic: anemia, leukopenia, thrombocytopenia Nausea, diarrhea, weakness.	Used as desensitization therapy, severe humoral rejection treatment, allowing an immunosuppression restart at an adjusted dose, being considered an immunosuppression minimization strategy.
Belatacept	10 mg/kg intravenously on posttransplant days 1, 5, 14 and then every 4 weeks indefinitely	Greater predisposition to lymphoproliferative disorders not associated to EBV, herpes virus and tuberculosis infections.	Adjuvant treatment with MMF and prednisone maintains a CNI-free immunosuppression with an increase in acute rejection in the first 6 months (posttransplant) but better long-term renal graft function compared with CsA.

Immunosuppressor	Used dose in renal transplant	Adverse reactions	Minimization strategy
Belimumab	Initial dose:120 mg intravenously, then 400 mg IV every 2 weeks indefinitely	Infusion related (bradycardia, myalgias, rash, urticarial, hypotension), depression, insomnia, nausea, diarrhea, bronchitis, pharyngitis, increased risk of viral infections.	Is in experimental phase, it can induce immunologic tolerance or mixed chimerism as an immunosuppression reduction strategy.

TMA, thrombotic microangiopathy; EBV, Epstein-Barr Virus; HUS, hemolytic uremic syndrome; mTOR, mechanistic target of rapamycin; CNI, calcineurin inhibitors; CsA, cyclosporine [50, 51, 53, 60, 61, 95, 97, 100, 101, 103].

Table 1. Immunosuppression in renal transplant, adverse reactions and minimization strategies.

Sawinski et al. [54], evaluated 88 clinical trials regarding CNI reduction strategies associated with MMF or imTOR in a meta-analysis (minimization of the CNI without suspending it, conversion to another immunosuppressant "imTOR," and withdrawal of the CNI in the post-transplant period or never used in the RT); finding the best results with the strategies in which the CNI was minimized, especially in the first 6 months without stopping it, with a lower incidence of AR (RR 0.80, 95% CI 0.68–0.95), graft loss (RR 0.71 95% CI 0.56–0.9), and better graft function and no differences in mortality (RR 0.87, 95% CI 0.66–1.15), compared to standard regimens with CNI. Nevertheless, it is important to mention that the majority of studies were based on CsA induction with basiliximab, thus more research is needed to determine the role with other immunosuppressants (TAC and thymoglobulin) and their doses, with the aforementioned strategies. Finally, a systematic review of 83 studies that included a total of 16,156 patients with a removing sample (RR 2.54; CI 95%: 1.56–4.12) or an avoiding sample (RR 2.16; CI 95%: 0.85–5.49) of CNI from the immunosuppression maintenance regimen, was associated to AR without a difference in graft loss (RR 0.96; CI 95%: 0.79–1.16), and with a lower incidence of hypertension in the CNI-abstained groups (RR 0.82, CI 95%: 0.71–0.95) [55].

5. Strategies for removing steroids from immunosuppression in kidney transplantation

Another tempting strategy for reduction of posttransplant immunosuppression is to withdraw or avoid the use of corticosteroids because of the numerous side effects, with the purpose of improving quality of life and reducing cardiovascular mortality.

This intervention has increased from 5 to 35% since the year 2000 until today, in RT recipients in the USA. Historically, the removal of steroids has been associated with the risk of precipitating AR [56, 57]; however, long-term safety in terms of patient and graft survival has been satisfactory with early steroid withdrawal (ESW); as Rizzaari shows [58] in a 10 year follow-up of 1241 RT recipients with graft survival, showing similar death in living donor RT recipients with maintained with steroids (79 *vs.* 73%) and with even an better survival in deceased donor RT (80 *vs.* 67%) with a report in their survival analyses free of AR, similar between the groups with and without corticosteroids. Lopez Soler et al. [59], similarly reported in a cohort undergoing ESW with a 10-year follow-up that showed better graft survival ($p = 0.023$), lower risk of mortality (0.23, $p \leq 0.011$), and less graft failure (0.57, $p = 0.026$).

Similar to minimization of the CNI, numerous meta-analyses have been published regarding a population undergoing ESW, both in the adult and pediatric populations, concluding, in some, a higher rate of AR, especially of mild characteristics, without greater impact in the function or graft survival, and with satisfactory results in the metabolic and hemodynamic profile, reducing cardiovascular morbidity and mortality (**Table 1**) [19, 20, 60, 61].

Knight et al. [19], evaluated a meta-analysis of 34 clinical trials with 5637 patients in regimens that included withdrawal or nonuse of steroids at any time of the transplantation, and found that the withdrawal of steroids was associated with a higher incidence of AR (RR 1.56; 95% CI 1.31–1.87), but with a lower incidence of hypertension (RR 0.64; 95% CI 0.50–0.83), diabetes (RR 0.90; 95% CI 0.85–0.94), and hypercholesterolemia (RR0.96; 95% CI 0.67–0.87); concluding that AR had no impact on function or survival of the grafts because it was considered mild.

Zhang et al. [60], in a meta-analysis of 13 clinical trials in 3520 patients with ESW after transplantation found a higher incidence of AR; but when the trials that used TAC were exclusively analyzed, the statistical significance was lost and only remained in those that used CsA. Studies that involve corticosteroid withdrawal associated with TAC in the immunosuppression regimen, document the development of borderline changes in AR, especially in the early stage of transplantation, without impact on function or survival of the graft [23, 62].

The current use of immunosuppression induction with anti-DC25 antibodies (basiliximab) or lymphocyte depletion (thymoglobulin) combined with MMF and TAC has favored that the minimization or elimination of the use of posttransplant steroids be safe with cell type AR rates comparable to those that maintain the use of the posttransplant steroid [16, 17, 20–27, 29–31, 58, 60, 63–67].

The good results from minimization or suspension of some immunosuppressants are encouraging because one of the main associated causes with poor long-term kidney graft survival is directly or indirectly related to the side effects of immunosuppressants that cause long-term complications and even a higher cardiovascular mortality [4, 11, 43, 68–71].

Experience with this intervention in our transplant center has shown satisfactory short-term (12 months) results with similar AR rates in immunosuppression with and without steroids, with lower glucose levels, lipids, and better blood pressure parameters, which leads to less use of antihypertensive and lipid-lowering drugs in the group without steroids [17, 23]. Nonetheless, despite the acceptable results found with these strategies the community dedicated to transplantation is concerned about what happens with these long-term immunosuppression strategies, especially since presently one of the main causes of graft loss is the chronic antibody-mediated rejection mainly associated to sub-immunosuppression.

Nonetheless, the sub-immunosuppression generated by minimization strategies or suspension of an immunosuppressant in the posttransplant context causes uncertainty regarding the formation of antihuman leukocyte antigen (HLA) antibodies [donor-specific antibodies

(DSA) or nondonor-specific antibodies (NDSA)] over time, with an increased risk of antibody-mediated AR and graft loss. Some studies show results in the incidence of DSA with immunosuppression regimens considered less potent, which could cause the appearance of humoral AR and long-term graft loss [33–37]. Kreijveld et al. [72] showed that the reduction or removal of TAC from immunosuppression in the posttransplant period does not generate antibodies and does not even predict the development of AR. As for steroids, the mechanism of suppression of antibodies by the B lymphocyte with the use of these drugs has created the idea that avoiding or removing steroids in the posttransplant period favors the appearance of antibodies against the major histocompatibility complex (MHC) and against other renal donor antigens. Even so, information related to the formation of DSA with the minimization or suspension of steroids posttransplantation is scarce [73–75].

6. Antihuman leukocyte antigen antibodies in kidney recipients with steroid withdrawal

One of the leading causes of long-term graft loss is interstitial fibrosis and tubular atrophy (IFTA) and the appearance of DSA posttransplant, which seems to play an important role in graft dysfunction.

The B lymphocyte antibody suppression combined with the use of steroids has created the idea that avoiding or removing these drugs in the posttransplant period may induce the appearance of antibodies. Unfortunately, there is not sufficient evidence to uphold that the withdrawal of steroids contributes to the increase in production of antibodies or if it is associated to a higher rejection rate and chronic graft dysfunction, that being with steroids in the immunosuppression regimen. Delgado et al. [73], in a retrospective study of 43 kidney recipients during posttransplant antibody monitoring, showed that patients with steroid withdrawal did not develop DSA compared to the steroid maintained group posttransplantation. Drugs such as MMF and thymoglobulin, in addition to interacting with T lymphocytes, inhibit the formation of B lymphocyte antibodies, so it is possible that the immunosuppression regimens that use these drugs provide greater safety even when steroids are avoided or suspended after the transplantation. Furthermore, the avoidance or withdrawal of steroids may enhance the myelosuppressive effect of MMF, since steroids induce greater activity of the hepatic enzyme uridine diphosphate-glucoronosyltransferase that degrades MMF [76]. In addition, steroids induce the cytochrome P450 isoenzyme 34ª responsible for the metabolism of TAC, and so avoiding these drugs would favor the increase of TAC serum levels, thereby increasing their immunosuppressive effect [77]. These possible mechanisms suggest that the appearance of DSA induced by the suspension of steroids after transplantation could be no different than in the immunosuppression schemes maintained by these drugs.

In a clinical trial recently performed at our center with living donor kidney transplant recipients who underwent protocolized biopsies every 3 months, it was found that the presence of AR was no different between patients who had an early steroid removal compared to those in which the drugs were sustained. However, the suspension of steroids has generated uncertainty about the risk of developing DSA posttransplant, over the course of time. Due to this concern, our team recently conducted a prospective cohort of 77 patients with low immunological risk (data not yet published) where findings revealed that the presence of cellular AR was a predictor for the formation of DSA against class II antigens, coinciding with the results of other authors [78]. There is currently little scientific evidence in which the absence of steroids in the posttransplant period may generate a greater presence of posttransplant DSA. Delgado et al. [73], observed that in a retrospective study of 43 kidney recipients during posttransplant antibody monitoring, patients with steroid suspension did not develop DSA compared to the group with maintained steroids. On the other hand, de Kort et al. [79] recently showed that in a population with steroids suspended using lymphocyte-depleting immunosuppressive induction (alentuzumab) and monotherapy with TAC, there was an increased risk for the development of DSA from an early posttransplant stage. Our study (data not yet published) also showed a higher incidence of DSA in patients with immunosuppression therapy without steroids appearing from a very early stage of the transplantation (<12 months). Unlike the study by de Kort et al. [79], 97% of our population undergoing steroid withdrawal used nonlymphocyte-depleting antibodies (basiliximab) with a double immunosuppression maintenance regimen based on MMF and TAC.

The immunoglobulin subclasses (IgG1/IgG3) capable of binding and activating the classical complement pathway (C1q) can predict the presence of antibody-mediated AR even with phenotypes of more severe damage (extensive microvascular inflammation and increased C4d deposition) and risk of kidney graft loss [80–83]. Undoubtedly, the measurement of antibody subclasses in patients subjected to a sub-immunosuppression state with minimization schemes or suspension of immunosuppression should be considered in order to discern whether the presence of these antibodies, according to the ability to fix complement, can generate chronic damage and lower the survival of the grafts. Finally, the benefits obtained from the nonsteroid schemes in the posttransplant stages in the lipid, metabolic, and blood pressure profiles, in our previously reported experience, should be considered for its possible risk of activating the immune system [17, 23].

7. Minimization strategies of mycophenolate mofetil in renal transplantation

Mycophenolate mofetil (MMF) has been established as the leading immunosuppressive regimen in most clinical trials and in almost 100% of the renal transplant centers in the world. With the initial use of CsA a daily dose of MMF was established at 2000 mg, while now, since the immunosuppressant regimen has changed to TAC significantly improving graft survival, the dose of MMF has not been established [84].

The MMF is an antiproliferative drug that requires de-esterification in gastrointestinal tissue for its absorption, thus releasing mycophenolic acid (MPA) that is freely absorbed and needs a $pH > 5.5$ to facilitate absorption in the small intestine. The most common use of MMF is still the prevention of AR in renal, pulmonary, cardiac, and hepatic organs, in adjunct with other immunosuppressive agents, which has shown to reduce AR by 20–40% in RT compared with azathioprine (AZA).

CsA and TAC have a different influence on enterohepatic circulation and the metabolism of MPA. The TAC increases serum levels of MMF and therefore exposure of the metabolite in the blood circulation in patients undergoing this immunosuppression regimen when compared to CsA, while the decrease in MMF dosage combined with TAC has not yet been well studied and no conclusive results have been established [85].

Clinical trials have tried to establish the MMF dosage. Doria et al. [86], included 901 patients with *de novo* RT, assigning three study groups with a MMF dose of <2000, =2000, and >2000 mg with thymoglobulin and an alemtuzumab-based induction, and no significant differences were found at 1 year follow-up regarding AR and graft loss; but they did find an increase, though not significant, in hematological complications related to leukopenia, anemia, and greater gastrointestinal disorders in patients with MMF doses of 2000 and >2000 mg.

These side effects have also motivated the establishment of adjusted dosing for certain populations. There are several controversies about whether reducing MMF dose modifies graft survival. Ji et al. [87], evaluated 128 patients with a low immunological risk at 12 months of follow-up, using immunological induction with basiliximab, methylprednisolone bolus (MPD) and TAC with a dosage of 0.1 mg/kg/day divided into two doses, PDN at 1 mg/kg/day at dose reduction, and MMF in different doses: = 500, <1500, and >1500 mg; finding, in the low dosage groups (=500 and <1500 mg), an increased number of cases of AR, renal graft dysfunction, and C4d deposition in follow-up biopsies, while the conventional dose group of MMF ≥ 1500 mg did not present any representative difference. Therefore, it is suggested that the dose should be individualized to the demographic characteristics of each population, under an integral evaluation of weight and height, and likewise that immunosuppression should not be reduced to doses less than 1 g of MMF per day nor suspension of the antimetabolite, since it jeopardizes the survival of the graft.

The side effects of MMF are divided into those due to gastrointestinal disease where diarrhea is the main manifestation with a frequency of up to 40–50% and in severe cases has been attributed as a cause of histologically inflammatory colitis type lesions similar to Crohn's disease.

Within the hematological side effects attributed to the drug there is leukopenia with or without neutropenia that can be potentiated by the use of other, concomitant drugs (Valganciclovir, trimethoprim with sulfamethoxazole, etc.) during the early period of RT. Other attributable side effects are hypogammaglobulinemia and severe anemia, especially in the first posttransplant months. The MMF has been associated with pneumonia due to pneumocystitis jirovecci, cytomegalovirus (CMV) disease, reactivation of Chagas disease, infection with Epstein-Barr virus (EBV), and risk of malignancy. On the other hand, patients with solid organ transplantation with hepatitis C seem to have better long-term outcomes with MMF therapy [88]. There is a strong association between the concentration of MPA, the pharmacological effects, and inter-individual variability between the MPA within the area under the curve (MPA AUC) estimated as the concentration of MMF after systemic elimination, enterohepatic recirculation, and the concentration before the dose (C 0) [89].

Two analysis tools have been used for the measurement of MPA plasma levels: high performance liquid chromatography (HPLC) and enzyme multiplied immunoassay technique (EMIT). The EMIT is less specific in the measurement of MPA than HPLC: the concentrations of MPA that are obtained by the EMIT method are typically higher than those of HPLC. The overestimation of the MPA concentration by the use of EMIT is approximately 24–35%. The degree of overestimation varies depending on the patients' characteristics, the time elapsed since the transplantation, and time of the blood sampling. However, in pediatric RT recipients the EMIT assay showed a diagnostic efficacy comparable to HPLC to assess the risk of AR, leaving EMIT as an acceptable monitoring tool for MPA. Therefore, either HPLC or EMIT can be used, although HPLC is a more specific analytical tool for the accurate assessment of MPA and metabolites [90, 91].

This clinical data supports the need for therapeutic monitoring of MPA. However, this could result in higher costs and time since the precise measurement of MPA AUC 0–12 h requires multiple blood samples during the dosing interval, which can be expensive and clinically impractical [91].

It is well established that in RT recipients, MMF reduces the risk of AR and improves graft survival; nonetheless, the side effects that include diarrhea in up to 37.3%, hematological alterations (leukopenia, anemia, thrombocytopenia), and an increase in the incidence of infections in 23–25% during the first year of transplantation, make it necessary to reduce the dose of MMF. Such side effects can be avoided by individualizing immunosuppression in patients, and other studies have demonstrated that the minimization strategies of immunosuppression must be adjusted according to the race, gender, and anthropometric characteristics at each transplant center [92].

8. New strategies for minimization of immunosuppressive therapy in kidney transplantation

8.1. Alemtuzumab

New strategies in the minimization of immunosuppression involve the use of alemtuzumab (humanized monoclonal antibody that targets CD52 on lymphocytes) used as a reduction strategy in doses of CNI and immunosuppression without steroids [93, 94].

Chan et al. [95], reported in 82 patients treated with alemtuzumab (TAC as monotherapy) *versus* 42 patients with daclizumab, TAC, and MMF; all with ESR, with results of a low AR incidence at 6 months posttransplant, and without differences in the survival of the graft or in its function, confirming the minimization of immunosuppression as a therapeutic strategy with this drug (**Table 1**).

In 3-year posttransplant follow-up studies, alemtuzumab combined with ESR has shown reduction in AR episodes in patients with low immunological risk compared to basiliximab-based induction, while the presentation of AR was similar in those patients with high immunological risk in whom immunosuppressive induction was compared with thymoglobulin. The main advantage of the use of alemtuzumab as a strategy to reduce immunosuppression is found in the availability to reduce the used dosage of CNI and the subsequent conversion to maintenance immunosuppression based on imTOR, whose main objective is to avoid chronic nephrotoxicity and improve graft survival and long-term function (**Table 1**) [96, 97].

The therapeutic effect of alemtuzumab is not different from the immunological induction with thymoglobulin in the areas of AR incidence, delayed graft function, CMV infection, development of NODAT, and use of granulocyte colony stimulant [98].

8.2. Proteasome inhibitors

Proteasome nonselective inhibitors prevent the antibody-mediated AR of the graft. However, adverse effects outweigh the benefits by limiting their application in clinical practice. Up till now, the inhibition of immunoproteasomes is effective in experimental models in the context of autoimmune diseases being used for several weeks of treatment, without significant side effects. The ONX 0914, a selective proteasome inhibitor (B5i) of the LMP7 subunit, prevents chronic rejection in allogenic kidneys transplanted in rodents. The selective inhibition of immunoproteasomes by ONX 0914 and bortezomib reduces the number of plasma cells and B lymphocytes, and suppresses the formation of donor-specific antibodies in transplanted organs.

In renal grafts, T lymphocyte, B lymphocyte, and macrophage infiltration is reduced, as well as the complement deposit, interferon-γ, interleukin-17, and IgG [99].

Several series of cases have shown the efficacy of bortezomib in reversing the severe antibody-mediated rejection, establishing the maintenance therapy in posttransplant patients, and has even been used as a desensitization treatment in recipients with a positive cross test considered highly sensitized with satisfactory results; formulating guidelines to establish strategies for adjusting immunosuppression in long-term RT recipients. However, there are contradictory results. The BORTEJECT study [100] used bortezomib as a treatment for late antibody-mediated AR in 44 patients, with a follow- up of 3 years, with immunosuppression based on imTOR or CNI, with MMF 1–2 g/day and PDN, without finding a significant difference in the incidence of AR and renal function compared with placebo. Therefore, studies that evaluate the use of the drug in the induction and maintenance of immunosuppression are necessary to allow the minimization or optimization of the therapy used in selected cases (**Table 1**).

8.3. Belatacept

Belatacept (CTLA-4 Ig fusion protein) is a new drug with a mechanism of action that allows CNI-free maintained immunosuppression. Clinical studies show a higher incidence of T cell-mediated AR in the first 6 months after transplantation, but show better long-term renal graft function. Likewise, the use of belatacept shows a lower incidence of DSA formation and less graft damage compared to the use of CsA. The most relevant adverse reactions include: herpes virus infections, tuberculosis, and a higher frequency of posttransplant lymphoproliferative disorders.

Belatacept has not yet been compared to a TAC/MMF-based regimen, considered the immunosuppression maintenance standard in RT.

The current immunosuppressive treatment, far from being perfect, has contributed to the overall improvement of the renal graft and patient survival, which contributes to overcoming the barrier for the development of new therapeutic agents. Consequently, most of the new drugs have failed in the course of transplantation, including janus kinase inhibitors (tofacitinib), sphingosine-1-phosphate receptor modulator (FTY720, fingolimod), protein kinase C inhibitor (sotrastaurin, AEB), inhibitors of adhesion anti-LFA-1 molecules (efalizumab), anti-ICAM-1, and the first generation of anti-CD40-ligand. Most of the current treatments, still in research and focused on the immunology of the transplant, are biological or cell-based treatments. The blocking of co-stimulation with the purpose to prevent T cell activation remains a point of interest. The ASKP1240, an anti-CD40 monoclonal antibody, has recently been tested in immunosuppression minimization regimens based on CNI dose reduction or suspension, compared to a control group based on standard dose TAC, finding higher AR and infection rates in the group treated with anti-CD40, so the future of this drug remains uncertain. More recently, CFZ533, a fully humanized monoclonal antibody has shown efficacy in primates, and clinical research is being initiated in humans (**Table 1**) [101].

8.4. Belimumab

Belimumab (human monoclonal antibody that inhibits B cell activating factor), approved for treatment in systemic lupus erythematosus (SLE), is in use in early-stage clinical studies for the prevention of antibody-mediated RA, as well as in patients sensitized with low titers of anti-donor-specific antibodies.

Cellular therapies represent an innovative therapeutic objective for the maintenance of long-term renal graft, and thus avoidance of adverse reactions related to the maintenance of immunosuppression. The premise of cell therapy is the induction of donor-specific nonresponse in the context of operational tolerance or mixed chimerism (**Table 1**) [100].

A single center study evaluated the autologous use of mesenchymal progenitor cells instead of the antibody-based induction with schemes based on low and high doses of CNI, comparing induction with basiliximab and standard maintenance with MMF-CNI. The induction of autologous mesenchymal progenitor cells resulted in a lower AR rate, a decrease in opportunistic infections, and better renal graft function 1 year after transplantation, concluding with conventional immunosuppressive maintenance [102].

Another study was carried out in hematopoietic progenitor cells transplant with HLA concordant kidney donors in adjunct with total lymphoid radiation and thymoglobulin, which resulted in persistent mixed chimerism with stable renal graft function and removal of all immunosuppressants in 50% of the patients (**Table 1**) [103].

The most recently used strategies include the use of a product based on hematopoietic stem cells "facilitating cells" co-administered with nonmyeloablative reconditioning in living donor kidney graft recipients, reaching, in five out of eight patients, a satisfactory donor-chimerism with successful immunosuppression maintenance withdrawal without evidence of AR or graft-versus-host disease [104].

The results of the previous studies, although very encouraging, should be validated in larger multi-centric controlled and randomized studies, from the safety-efficacy and cost–benefit points of view, compared with conventional immunosuppression therapy.

Author details

Jorge Andrade-Sierra[1,2,3*], Pedro Alejandro Vazquez-Galvan[2], Hernesto Hernandez-Reyes[2], Lydia A. Mercado-Jáuregui[3], Jonathan S. Chávez-Iñiguez[4], Eduardo González-Espinoza[2], Benjamin Gómez-Navarro[2] and José I. Cerrillos-Gutiérrez[2]

*Address all correspondence to: jorg_andrade@hotmail.com

1 Department of Physiology, University Health Sciences Center, University of Guadalajara, Guadalajara, Jalisco, Mexico

2 Department of Nephrology and Organ Transplant Unit, Specialties Hospital, National Occidental Medical Centre, Mexican Social Security Institute (CMNO IMSS), Guadalajara, Jalisco, Mexico

3 Department of Internal Medicine, Civil Hospital of Guadalajara Dr. Juan I. Menchaca, Guadalajara, Jalisco, Mexico

4 Department of Nephrology, Civil Hospital of Guadalajara "Fray Antonio Alcalde", Guadalajara, Jalisco, Mexico

References

[1] Meier-Kriesche HU, Schold JD, Srinivas TR, Kaplan B. Lack of improvement in renal allograft survival despite a marked decrease in acute rejection rates over the most recent era. American Journal of Transplantation. 2004;**4**(3):378-383

[2] Lamb KE, Lodhi S, Meier-Kriesche HU. Long-term renal allograft survival in the United States: A critical reappraisal. American Journal of Transplantation. 2011;**11**(3):450-462

[3] Meier-Kriesche HU, Schold JD, Kaplan B. Long-term renal allograft survival: Have we made significant progress or is it time to rethink our analytic and therapeutic strategies? American Journal of Transplantation. 2004;**4**(8):1289-1295

[4] Ojo AO, Hanson JA, Wolfe RA, Leichtman AB, Agodoa LY, Port FK. Long-term survival in renal transplant recipients with graft function. Kidney International. 2000;**57**(1):307-313

[5] Matas AJ, Humar A, Gillingham KJ, et al. Five preventable causes of kidney graft loss in the 1990s: A single-center analysis. Kidney International. 2002;**62**(2):704-714

[6] Nankivell BJ, Borrows RJ, Fung CL, O'Connell PJ, Allen RD, Chapman JR. The natural history of chronic allograft nephropathy. The New England Journal of Medicine. 2003; **349**(24):2326-2333

[7] Terasaki PI. Humoral theory of transplantation. American Journal of Transplantation. 2003;**3**(6):665-673

[8] Terasaki PI. A personal perspective: 100-year history of the humoral theory of transplantation. Transplantation. 2012;**93**(8):751-756

[9] Terasaki PI, Cai J. Humoral theory of transplantation: Further evidence. Current Opinion in Immunology. 2005;**17**(5):541-545

[10] Colvin RB, Smith RN. Antibody-mediated organ-allograft rejection. Nature Reviews Immunology. 2005;**5**(10):807-817

[11] Wiebe C, Gibson IW, Blydt-Hansen TD, et al. Rates and determinants of progression to graft failure in kidney allograft recipients with de novo donor-specific antibody. American Journal of Transplantation. 2015;**15**(11):2921-2930

[12] Sellares J, de Freitas DG, Mengel M, et al. Understanding the causes of kidney transplant failure: The dominant role of antibody-mediated rejection and nonadherence. American Journal of Transplantation 2012;**12**(2):388-399

[13] Nankivell BJ, Kuypers DR. Diagnosis and prevention of chronic kidney allograft loss. Lancet. 2011;**378**(9800):1428-1437

[14] Gaston RS, Cecka JM, Kasiske BL, et al. Evidence for antibody-mediated injury as a major determinant of late kidney allograft failure. Transplantation. 2010;**90**(1):68-74

[15] Cantarovich D, Hodemon-Corne B, Trebern-Launay K, Giral M, Foucher Y, Dantan E. Early steroid withdrawal compared with steroid avoidance correlates with graft failure among kidney transplant recipients with an history of diabetes. Transplantation Proceedings. 2013;**45**(4):1497-1502

[16] Woodle ES, Peddi VR, Tomlanovich S, Mulgaonkar S, Kuo PC, Investigators TS. A prospective, randomized, multicenter study evaluating early corticosteroid withdrawal with thymoglobulin in living-donor kidney transplantation. Clinical Transplantation. 2010;**24**(1): 73-83

[17] Andrade-Sierra J, Rojas-Campos E, Cardona-Munoz E, et al. Early steroid withdrawal in a renal transplant cohort treated with tacrolimus, mycophenolate mofetil and basiliximab. Nefrologia: Publicacion Oficial de la Sociedad Espanola Nefrologia. 2014;**34**(2):216-222

[18] Rike AH, Mogilishetty G, Alloway RR, et al. Cardiovascular risk, cardiovascular events, and metabolic syndrome in renal transplantation: Comparison of early steroid withdrawal and chronic steroids. Clinical Transplantation. 2008;**22**(2):229-235

[19] Knight SR, Morris PJ. Steroid avoidance or withdrawal after renal transplantation increases the risk of acute rejection but decreases cardiovascular risk: A meta-analysis. Transplantation. 2010;**89**(1):1-14

[20] Pascual J, Quereda C, Zamora J, Hernandez D, Spanish Group for Evidence-Based Medicine in Renal T. Updated metaanalysis of steroid withdrawal in renal transplant patients on calcineurin inhibitor and mycophenolate mofetil. Transplantation Proceedings. 2005;**37**(9):3746-3748

[21] Gonzalez-Molina M, Gentil MA, Burgos D, et al. Effect of long-term steroid withdrawal in renal transplant recipients: A retrospective cohort study. NDT Plus. 2010; **3**(Suppl_2):ii32-ii36

[22] Afaneh C, Cheng E, Aull MJ, et al. Renal allograft outcomes following early corticosteroid withdrawal in Hispanic transplant recipients. Clinical Transplantation. 2013; **27**(6):E611-E618

[23] Andrade-Sierra J, Rojas-Campos E, Cardona-Munoz E, et al. Early steroid withdrawal in recipients of a kidney transplant from a living donor: Experience of a single Mexican center. Transplantation Proceedings. 2016;**48**(1):42-49

[24] Iwamoto H, Hama K, Konno O, et al. Early steroid withdrawal in adult kidney transplantation at a single center. Transplantation Proceedings. 2012;**44**(1):179-181

[25] Lee YJ, Kim B, Lee JE, et al. Randomized trial of cyclosporine and tacrolimus therapy with steroid withdrawal in living-donor renal transplantation: 5-year follow-up. Transplant International. 2010;**23**(2):147-154

[26] Woodle ES, Alloway RR, Hanaway MJ, et al. Early corticosteroid withdrawal under modern immunosuppression in renal transplantation: Multivariate analysis of risk factors for acute rejection. Transplantation Proceedings. 2005;**37**(2):798-799

[27] Cantarovich D, Rostaing L, Kamar N, et al. Early corticosteroid avoidance in kidney transplant recipients receiving ATG-F induction: 5-year actual results of a prospective and randomized study. American Journal of Transplantation. 2014;**14**(11):2556-2564

[28] Nehus E, Liu C, Hooper DK, Macaluso M, Kim MO. Clinical practice of steroid avoidance in pediatric kidney transplantation. American Journal of Transplantation. 2015; **15**(8):2203-2210

[29] Woodle ES, Fujisawa Corticosteroid Withdrawal Study G. A prospective, randomized, multicenter, double-blind study of early corticosteroid cessation versus long-term maintenance of corticosteroid therapy with tacrolimus and mycophenolate mofetil in primary renal transplant recipients: One year report. Transplantation Proceedings 2005; **37**(2):804-808

[30] Teraoka S, Sato S, Sekijima M, et al. Comparative study of clinical outcome in kidney transplantation between early steroid withdrawal protocol using basiliximab, calcineurin inhibitor, and mycophenolate mofetil and triple regimen consisting of calcineurin inhibitor, mycophenolate mofetil, and steroid. Transplantation Proceedings. 2005; **37**(2):791-794

[31] Nagib AM, Abbas MH, Abu-Elmagd MM, et al. Long-term study of steroid avoidance in renal transplant patients: A single-center experience. Transplantation Proceedings. 2015;**47**(4):1099-1104

[32] Novosel MK, Bistrup C. Discontinuation of steroids in ABO-incompatible renal transplantation. Transplant International. 2016;**29**(4):464-470

[33] Kamar N, Del Bello A, Congy-Jolivet N, et al. Incidence of donor-specific antibodies in kidney transplant patients following conversion to an everolimus-based calcineurin inhibitor-free regimen. Clinical Transplantation. 2013;**27**(3):455-462

[34] Thierry A, Le Meur Y, Ecotiere L, et al. Minimization of maintenance immunosuppressive therapy after renal transplantation comparing cyclosporine A/azathioprine or cyclosporine A/mycophenolate mofetil bitherapy to cyclosporine A monotherapy: A 10-year postrandomization follow-up study. Transplant International. 2016;**29**(1):23-33

[35] Liefeldt L, Brakemeier S, Glander P, et al. Donor-specific HLA antibodies in a cohort comparing everolimus with cyclosporine after kidney transplantation. American Journal of Transplantation. 2012;**12**(5):1192-1198

[36] Croze LE, Tetaz R, Roustit M, et al. Conversion to mammalian target of rapamycin inhibitors increases risk of de novo donor-specific antibodies. Transplant International. 2014;**27**(8):775-783

[37] de Sandes-Freitas TV, Felipe CR, Campos EF, et al. Subclinical lesions and donor-specific antibodies in kidney transplant recipients receiving tacrolimus-based immunosuppressive regimen followed by early conversion to sirolimus. Transplantation. 2015; **99**(11):2372-2381

[38] Augustine JJ, Hricik DE. Minimization of immunosuppression in kidney transplantation. Current Opinion in Nephrology and Hypertension. 2007;**16**(6):535-541

[39] Golshayan D, Pascual M. Minimization of calcineurin inhibitors to improve long-term outcomes in kidney transplantation. Transplant Immunology. 2008;**20**(1-2):21-28

[40] Halloran PF. Immunosuppressive drugs for kidney transplantation. The New England journal of medicine. 2004;**351**(26):2715-2729

[41] Danovich GM. Handbook of Kidney Transplatation. 5th ed. Philadelphia, PA: Lippincott Williams & Wilkins; 2010. pp. 77-100

[42] Ekberg H, Tedesco-Silva H, Demirbas A, et al. Reduced exposure to calcineurin inhibitors in renal transplantation. The New England Journal of Medicine. 2007;**357**(25):2562-2575

[43] Nankivell BJ, Borrows RJ, Fung CL, O'Connell PJ, Chapman JR, Allen RD. Calcineurin inhibitor nephrotoxicity: Longitudinal assessment by protocol histology. Transplantation. 2004;**78**(4):557-565

[44] Srinivas TR, Meier-Kriesche HU. Minimizing immunosuppression, an alternative approach to reducing side effects: Objectives and interim result. Clinical Journal of the American Society of Nephrology. 2008;**3**(Suppl 2):S101-S116

[45] Haroon N, Singh A, Bhat ZY. Tacrolimus toxicity with minimal clinical manifestations: A case report and literature review. American Journal of Therapeutics. 2016;**23**(2):e631-e634

[46] Tang JT, Andrews LM, van Gelder T, et al. Pharmacogenetic aspects of the use of tacrolimus in renal transplantation: Recent developments and ethnic considerations. Expert Opinion on Drug Metabolism and Toxicology. 2016;**12**(5):555-565

[47] Thervet E, Loriot MA, Barbier S, et al. Optimization of initial tacrolimus dose using pharmacogenetic testing. Clinical Pharmacology and Therapeutics. 2010;**87**(6):721-726

[48] Ekberg H, Bernasconi C, Tedesco-Silva H, et al. Calcineurin inhibitor minimization in the symphony study: Observational results 3 years after transplantation. American Journal of Transplantation. 2009;**9**(8):1876-1885

[49] Issa N, Kukla A, Ibrahim HN. Calcineurin inhibitor nephrotoxicity: A review and perspective of the evidence. American Journal of Nephrology. 2013;**37**(6):602-612

[50] Larson TS, Dean PG, Stegall MD, et al. Complete avoidance of calcineurin inhibitors in renal transplantation: A randomized trial comparing sirolimus and tacrolimus. American Journal of Transplantation. 2006;**6**(3):514-522

[51] Flechner SM, Glyda M, Cockfield S, et al. The ORION study: Comparison of two sirolimus-based regimens versus tacrolimus and mycophenolate mofetil in renal allograft recipients. American Journal of Transplantation. 2011;**11**(8):1633-1644

[52] Vincenti F, Charpentier B, Vanrenterghem Y, et al. A phase III study of belatacept-based immunosuppression regimens versus cyclosporine in renal transplant recipients (BENEFIT study). American Journal of Transplantation. 2010;**10**(3):535-546

[53] Weir MR, Mulgaonkar S, Chan L, et al. Mycophenolate mofetil-based immunosuppression with sirolimus in renal transplantation: A randomized, controlled spare-the-nephron trial. Kidney International. 2011;**79**(8):897-907

[54] Sawinski D, Trofe-Clark J, Leas B, et al. Calcineurin inhibitor minimization, conversion, withdrawal, and avoidance strategies in renal transplantation: A systematic review and meta-analysis. American Journal of Transplantation. 2016;**16**(7):2117-2138

[55] Karpe KM, Talaulikar GS, Walters GD. Calcineurin inhibitor withdrawal or tapering for kidney transplant recipients. Cochrane Database of Systematic Reviews. 2017;**7**:CD006750

[56] Matas AJ. Minimization of steroids in kidney transplantation. Transplant International. 2009;**22**(1):38-48

[57] Vincenti F. Immunosuppression minimization: Current and future trends in transplant immunosuppression. The Journal of the American Society of Nephrology. 2003; **14**(7):1940-1948

[58] Rizzari MD, Suszynski TM, Gillingham KJ, et al. Ten-year outcome after rapid discontinuation of prednisone in adult primary kidney transplantation. Clinical Journal of the American Society of Nephrology. 2012;**7**(3):494-503

[59] Lopez-Soler RI, Chan R, Martinolich J, et al. Early steroid withdrawal results in improved patient and graft survival and lower risk of post-transplant cardiovascular risk profiles: A single-center 10-year experience. Clinical Transplantation. 2017;**31**(2):e12878

[60] Zhang X, Huang H, Han S, Fu S, Wang L. Is it safe to withdraw steroids within seven days of renal transplantation? Clinical Transplantation. 2013;**27**(1):1-8

[61] Pascual J, Quereda C, Zamora J, Hernandez D, Spanish Group for Evidence-Based Medicine in Renal T. Steroid withdrawal in renal transplant patients on triple therapy with a calcineurin inhibitor and mycophenolate mofetil: A meta-analysis of randomized, controlled trials. Transplantation. 2004;**78**(10):1548-1556

[62] Gaber AO, Moore LW, Alloway RR, et al. Acute rejection characteristics from a prospective, randomized, double-blind, placebo-controlled multicenter trial of early corticosteroid withdrawal. Transplantation. 2013;**95**(4):573-579

[63] ter Meulen CG, van Riemsdijk I, Hene RJ, et al. Steroid-withdrawal at 3 days after renal transplantation with anti-IL-2 receptor alpha therapy: A prospective, randomized, multicenter study. American Journal of Transplantation. 2004;**4**(5):803-810

[64] Rostaing L, Cantarovich D, Mourad G, et al. Corticosteroid-free immunosuppression with tacrolimus, mycophenolate mofetil, and daclizumab induction in renal transplantation. Transplantation. 2005;**79**(7):807-814

[65] Laftavi MR, Stephan R, Stefanick B, et al. Randomized prospective trial of early steroid withdrawal compared with low-dose steroids in renal transplant recipients using serial protocol biopsies to assess efficacy and safety. Surgery. 2005;**137**(3):364-371

[66] Andrade-Sierra J. Effect of early steroid withdrawal (ESW) in a Mexican kidney transplants recipients (KTR) cohort, treated with tacrolimus (TAC) and mycophenolate mophetil (MMF). The Journal of the American Society of Nephrology. 2010;**21**(TH-PO988):337A

[67] Aull MJ, Dadhania D, Afaneh C, et al. Early corticosteroid withdrawal in recipients of renal allografts: A single-center report of ethnically diverse recipients and recipients of marginal deceased-donor kidneys. Transplantation. 2012;**94**(8):837-844

[68] Vlaminck H, Maes B, Evers G, et al. Prospective study on late consequences of subclinical non-compliance with immunosuppressive therapy in renal transplant patients. American Journal of Transplantation. 2004;**4**(9):1509-1513

[69] Butler JA, Roderick P, Mullee M, Mason JC, Peveler RC. Frequency and impact of nonadherence to immunosuppressants after renal transplantation: A systematic review. Transplantation. 2004;**77**(5):769-776

[70] Sharif A, Baboolal K. Complications associated with new-onset diabetes after kidney transplantation. Nature Reviews Nephrology. 2012;**8**(1):34-42

[71] Budde K, Matz M, Durr M, Glander P. Biomarkers of over-immunosuppression. Clinical Pharmacology and Therapeutics. 2011;**90**(2):316-322

[72] Kreijveld E, Hilbrands LB, van Berkel Y, Joosten I, Allebes W. The presence of donor-specific human leukocyte antigen antibodies does not preclude successful withdrawal of tacrolimus in stable renal transplant recipients. Transplantation. 2007;**84**(9):1092-1096

[73] Delgado JC, Fuller A, Ozawa M, et al. No occurrence of de novo HLA antibodies in patients with early corticosteroid withdrawal in a 5-year prospective randomized study. Transplantation. 2009;**87**(4):546-548

[74] Lachmann N, Terasaki PI, Schonemann C. Donor-specific HLA antibodies in chronic renal allograft rejection: A prospective trial with a four-year follow-up. Clinical Transplants. 2006;**13**(1):171-199

[75] Li L, Chaudhuri A, Chen A, et al. Efficacy and safety of thymoglobulin induction as an alternative approach for steroid-free maintenance immunosuppression in pediatric renal transplantation. Transplantation. 2010;**90**(12):1516-1520

[76] Schuetz EG, Hazelton GA, Hall J, Watkins PB, Klaassen CD, Guzelian PS. Induction of digitoxigenin monodigitoxoside UDP-glucuronosyltransferase activity by glucocorticoids and other inducers of cytochrome P-450p in primary monolayer cultures of adult rat hepatocytes and in human liver. The Journal of Biological Chemistry. 1986; **261**(18):8270-8275

[77] Hesselink DA, Ngyuen H, Wabbijn M, et al. Tacrolimus dose requirement in renal transplant recipients is significantly higher when used in combination with corticosteroids. British Journal of Clinical Pharmacology. 2003;**56**(3):327-330

[78] Wiebe C, Gibson IW, Blydt-Hansen TD, et al. Evolution and clinical pathologic correlations of de novo donor-specific HLA antibody post kidney transplant. American Journal of Transplantation. 2012;**12**(5):1157-1167

[79] de Kort H, Willicombe M, Brookes P, et al. Microcirculation inflammation associates with outcome in renal transplant patients with de novo donor-specific antibodies. American Journal of Transplantation. 2013;**13**(2):485-492

[80] Loupy A, Lefaucheur C, Vernerey D, et al. Complement-binding anti-HLA antibodies and kidney-allograft survival. The New England Journal of Medicine. 2013;**369**(13):1215-1226

[81] Arnold ML, Ntokou IS, Doxiadis II, Spriewald BM, Boletis JN, Iniotaki AG. Donor-specific HLA antibodies: Evaluating the risk for graft loss in renal transplant recipients with isotype switch from complement fixing IgG1/IgG3 to noncomplement fixing IgG2/IgG4 anti-HLA alloantibodies. Transplant International. 2014;**27**(3):253-261

[82] Filippone EJ, Farber JL. Humoral immunity in renal transplantation: Epitopes, Cw and DP, and complement-activating capability--an update. Clinical Transplantation. 2015;**29**(4):279-287

[83] Everly MJ, Rebellato LM, Haisch CE, et al. Impact of IgM and IgG3 anti-HLA alloantibodies in primary renal allograft recipients. Transplantation. 2014;**97**(5):494-501

[84] Meier-Kriesche HU, Li S, Gruessner RW, et al. Immunosuppression: Evolution in practice and trends, 1994-2004. American Journal of Transplantation. 2006;**6**(5 Pt 2):1111-1131

[85] Park JM, Lake KD, Cibrik DM. Impact of changing from cyclosporine to tacrolimus on pharmacokinetics of mycophenolic acid in renal transplant recipients with diabetes. Therapeutic Drug Monitoring. 2008;**30**(5):591-596

[86] Doria C, Greenstein S, Narayanan M, et al. Association of mycophenolic acid dose with efficacy and safety events in kidney transplant patients receiving tacrolimus: An analysis of the mycophenolic acid observational Renal transplant registry. Clinical Transplantation. 2012;**26**(6):E602-E611

[87] Ji SM, Xie KN, Chen JS, et al. Retrospective evaluation of the effect of mycophenolate mofetil dosage on survival of kidney grafts based on biopsy results. Transplantation Proceedings. 2014;**46**(10):3383-3389

[88] Staatz CE, Tett SE. Pharmacology and toxicology of mycophenolate in organ transplant recipients: An update. Archives of Toxicology. 2014;**88**(7):1351-1389

[89] Oellerich M, Shipkova M, Schutz E, et al. Pharmacokinetic and metabolic investigations of mycophenolic acid in pediatric patients after renal transplantation: Implications for therapeutic drug monitoring. German study group on mycophenolate mofetil therapy in pediatric renal transplant recipients. Therapeutic Drug Monitoring. 2000;**22**(1):20-26

[90] Pawinski T, Hale M, Korecka M, Fitzsimmons WE, Shaw LM. Limited sampling strategy for the estimation of mycophenolic acid area under the curve in adult renal transplant patients treated with concomitant tacrolimus. Clinical Chemistry. 2002;**48**(9):1497-1504

[91] Jeong H, Kaplan B. Therapeutic monitoring of mycophenolate mofetil. Clinical Journal of the American Society of Nephrology. 2007;**2**(1):184-191

[92] Tornatore KM, Meaney CJ, Wilding GE, et al. Influence of sex and race on mycophenolic acid pharmacokinetics in stable African American and Caucasian renal transplant recipients. Clinical Pharmacokinetics. 2015;**54**(4):423-434

[93] Hanaway MJ, Woodle ES, Mulgaonkar S, et al. Alemtuzumab induction in renal transplantation. The New England Journal of Medicine. 2011;**364**(20):1909-1919

[94] Zachariah M, Nader ND, Brar J, et al. Alemtuzumab and minimization immunotherapy in kidney transplantation: Long-term results of comparison with rabbit anti-thymocyte globulin and standard triple maintenance therapy. Transplantation Proceedings. 2014; **46**(1):94-100

[95] Chan K, Taube D, Roufosse C, et al. Kidney transplantation with minimized maintenance: Alemtuzumab induction with tacrolimus monotherapy: An open label, randomized trial. Transplantation. 2011;**92**(7):774-780

[96] Friend PJ. Alemtuzumab induction therapy in solid organ transplantation. Transplantation Research. 2013;**2**(Suppl 1):S5

[97] Haynes R, Baigent C, Harden P, et al. Campath, calcineurin inhibitor reduction and chronic allograft nephropathy (3C) study: Background, rationale, and study protocol. Transplantation Research. 2013;**2**(1):7

[98] Zheng J, Song W. Alemtuzumab versus antithymocyte globulin induction therapies in kidney transplantation patients: A systematic review and meta-analysis of randomized controlled trials. Medicine (Baltimore). 2017;**96**(28):e7151

[99] Li J, Basler M, Alvarez G, Brunner T, Kirk CJ, Groettrup M. Immunoproteasome inhibition prevents chronic antibody-mediated allograft rejection in renal transplantation. Kidney International. 2018;**93**(3):670-680

[100] Eskandary F, Regele H, Baumann L, et al. A randomized trial of Bortezomib in late antibody-mediated kidney transplant rejection. The Journal of the American Society of Nephrology. 2018;**29**(2):591-605

[101] Lim MA, Kohli J, Bloom RD. Immunosuppression for kidney transplantation: Where are we now and where are we going? Transplantation Reviews (Orlando, Fla.). 2017; **31**(1):10-17

[102] Tan J, Wu W, Xu X, et al. Induction therapy with autologous mesenchymal stem cells in living-related kidney transplants: A randomized controlled trial. Journal of the American Medical Association. 2012;**307**(11):1169-1177

[103] Scandling JD, Busque S, Dejbakhsh-Jones S, et al. Tolerance and withdrawal of immunosuppressive drugs in patients given kidney and hematopoietic cell transplants. American Journal of Transplantation. 2012;**12**(5):1133-1145

[104] Leventhal J, Abecassis M, Miller J, et al. Chimerism and tolerance without GVHD or engraftment syndrome in HLA-mismatched combined kidney and hematopoietic stem cell transplantation. Science Translational Medicine. 2012;**4**(124):124ra128

8

Intestinal Transplantation

Georgios Vrakas

Abstract

Intestinal transplantation (ITx) has evolved in the past few decades moving from an experimental procedure to a life-changing modality for patients suffering from intestinal failure (IF). It is particularly for those with complications as a consequence of parenteral nutrition and/or who have a high risk of dying due to their underlying disease. In addition to this, intestinal transplantation is also increasingly considered for the treatment of conventionally unresectable abdominal tumors. With advancements in immunosuppressive drugs, induction regimens, standardization of surgical techniques and improved postoperative care, survival is increasing. The ultimate goal for intestinal transplantation would be to become as good and safe as total parenteral nutrition (TPN) and as such, it could become a viable first-line option of intestinal failure.

Keywords: intestinal failure, parenteral nutrition, multivisceral, intestine, liver, immunosuppression, intestinal transplant

1. History

Lillehei was the first to report an experimental isolated intestinal canine model in 1959 and Starzl reported the first multivisceral experimental canine model in 1960 [1, 2]. The first attempt in humans has been attributed to Deterling in Boston in 1964 [unpublished], whereas the first official report of human intestinal transplant was made by Lillehei in 1967 [1]. It should be noted that the first successful series were reported in the 1990s, coinciding with the introduction of more effective immunosuppression. The first attempts of intestinal transplantation (ITx) in the 1970s were largely disappointing because of high incidence of rejection of small bowel allografts, sepsis and technical complications [3]. The introduction of tacrolimus [4] revolutionized interest in ITx. The superior clinical outcomes from tacrolimus across a variety of organ transplantation compared with cyclosporine set the momentum for ITx as a life-changing therapy for patients with irreversible intestinal failure (IF) [5, 6].

Over the past 30 years, there has been a gradual increase in ITx cases, with nearly 2900 ITx cases performed worldwide, although there has been a decline in recent years [7]. This change could be attributed to the formation of specialized IF units to prevent and manage intestinal failure-associated liver disease (IFALD) [8]. Other possible factors include: inadequate reimbursement rates below the cost of performing the transplant; the extensive infrastructure demands required to address the frequent social problems of IF patients; concern over the narrow risk-benefit ratio for ITx in an era of improving outcomes with long-term total parenteral nutrition (TPN) for selected diseases [9] and/or the limited availability of experienced personnel to fill key positions. Finally, some transplant centers may be more willing to judiciously offer isolated liver transplants to patients with the short bowel syndrome and IFALD who have the potential for further intestinal adaptation [10, 11].

2. Indications

IF is characterized by the inability to maintain protein energy, fluid, electrolyte or micronutrient balance due to gastrointestinal disease. If the patient does not receive parenteral nutrition or become a recipient of an intestinal transplant, IF ultimately leads to malnutrition and even death.

The leading causes of IF differ between pediatric and adult populations (**Table 1**).

TPN is the current standard of care for patients with IF. Nevertheless, as survival following ITx improves, it is anticipated that ITx will become a valid alternative to total parental nutrition. However, because of significant complications that can arise from surgery and long-term use of immunosuppressive therapy, strict eligibility criteria exist to ensure appropriate patient selection.

Paediatric	**Adult**
Intestinal atresia	Crohn's disease
Gastroschisis	Superior mesenteric artery thrombosis
Crohn's disease	Superior mesenteric vein thrombosis
Microvillus involution disease	Trauma
Necrotizing enterocolitis	Desmoid tumour
Midgut volvulus	Volvulus
Chronic intestinal pseudo-obstruction	Pseudo-obstruction
Massive resection secondary to tumour	Massive resection secondary to tumour
Hirschsprung disease	Radiation enteritis

Table 1. Leading causes for intestinal transplantation in paediatric and adult populations.

Short bowel syndrome caused by surgical removal is the leading cause of IF (68%). As an early alternative to transplantation or total parenteral nutrition (TPN) for patients with short bowel syndrome, surgical bowel lengthening without transplant may be attempted. This requires the serial transverse enteroplasty (STEP) or longitudinal intestinal lengthening and tailoring (LILT) procedures. STEP and LILT are particularly successful in patients with decreased transit times and dilated bowel. These procedures lengthen the small bowel while keeping the total surface area the same. Bowel is either split lengthwise or cut obliquely at multiple points. This will lengthen the bowel and shrink the luminal diameter [12]. If successful, this may reduce the amount of TPN required, or negate its use altogether. If patients are not acceptable candidates for STEP or LILT, sometimes a reversal of small bowel direction may effectively increase transit times. If none of these operations are successful, the standard of care is TPN.

Currently, ITx has been mainly performed in patients who developed life-threatening complications attributed to IF and/or long-term TPN. In 2000, Medicare defined failure of TPN as impending or overt liver failure (elevated serum bilirubin and/or liver enzymes, splenomegaly, thrombocytopenia, gastroesophageal varices, coagulopathy, stomal bleeding, hepatic fibrosis or cirrhosis), thrombosis of two or more central veins, frequent and severe central venous catheter (CVC)-related sepsis and frequent severe dehydration [13]. In addition, other conditions associated with early death despite optimal TPN, such as congenital mucosal disorders and ultra-short bowel syndrome, are also included as per American Society of Transplantation guidelines [14].

The European guidelines recommend TPN as primary treatment for patients with IF, with early referral to specialist centers for optimal rehabilitative therapy and timely assessment of suitability for ITx. It recommends assessment for candidacy for transplantation for the presence of one or more indications parallel to American guidelines (failure of TPN, high risk of death attributable to underlying disease and IF with high morbidity or low acceptance of TPN) resulting in rates of transplant of 62, 26 and 12%, respectively [15]. Because of a statistically significant increased risk of death on TPN from liver failure due to IFALD and invasive intra-abdominal desmoids, direct referral for ITx should be considered [16]. IFALD is partly caused by omega-6 fatty acids in TPN formulas, which can be synthesized into inflammatory molecules. IFALD can range from steatohepatitis, cholestasis or hepatic fibrosis to end-stage liver disease. Children are more likely to have cholestatic liver disease than steatohepatitis [17]. Severe liver injury has been reported in as many as 50% of patients with IF who receive TPN for longer than 5 years; this is typically fatal. If patients have life-threatening infections, IFALD, or lose their venous access, 1-year mortality is 70% without ITx [18]. Conversely, patients with CVC-related complications or ultra-short bowel syndrome did not have an increased risk of death on TPN and no patients considered to be an ITx candidate with poor quality of life (QoL) or chronic dehydration actually died while remaining on TPN. This notable finding forms the basis of non-indications in previous European guidelines [19]. Despite very limited evidence exploring the role of quality of life (QoL) as an indicator for ITx, this holistic aspect may also be factored in the decision-making process [20] (**Table 2**).

North America	Europe
Failure of TPN	Impending or overt liver failure due to IFALD-related liver failure
Impending or overt liver failure	
Central venous thrombosis of 2 central veins	
Frequent and severe central venous catheter-related sepsis	
Frequent episodes of severe dehydration despite intravenous fluids in addition to TPN	
High risk of death attributable to underlying disease	CVC-related multiple venous thrombosis (in appropriately selected patients)
Intra-abdominal invasive desmoids tumour	Intra-abdominal desmoids
Intestinal failure with high morbidity and low acceptance of TPN	Individual case by case decision for patients with IF with high morbidity or low acceptance of TPN
Congenital mucosal disorders	
Ultra-short bowel syndrome (<10 cm in infants, <20 cm in adults)	
Need for frequent hospitalization, narcotic addiction or inability to function	
Patient's unwillingness to accept long-term TPN	

Table 2. Intestinal transplantation guidelines.

3. Contraindications

The contraindications of intestinal transplantation are the same as for all other transplants and are frequently reassessed. These include:

1. significant comorbidities;
2. active uncontrolled infections or malignancies that are not totally resectable during the transplant process;
3. psychosocial factors (e.g. lack of post-operative support network);
4. anatomical challenges that can prove the operation high risk such as inferior vena cava (IVC) and portal vein (PV) thrombosis. Previous laparotomies can also complicate the operation significantly; and
5. opiate dependence is very common and rehabilitation should be considered early.

4. Types of intestinal transplant

The choice of transplant type depends on the underlying cause of IF, quality of native organs, state of liver disease (if present) and history of previous abdominal surgeries. The main types of ITx are:

1. Small bowel transplant only (SBTx) (**Figure 1**): recommended for people with IF who have not developed liver disease. The arterial supply to the allograft is secured with anastomosis between the donor's superior mesenteric artery (SMA) and the recipient's infrarenal aorta; venous drainage is either onto the IVC or the recipient's portal vein (PV) or superior mesenteric vein (SMV) at the root of the mesentery.

2. Liver and small bowel transplant (SBLTx) (**Figure 2**): recommended for people with IF who also have advanced liver disease and extensive portomesenteric venous thrombosis precluding liver transplantation alone. The inclusion of a liver graft in combined liver-small bowel transplant has been associated with improved survival rates [21].

3. Multivisceral transplant (MVTx) (**Figure 3**): recommended for people with multiple organ failure and involves transplanting the stomach, pancreaticoduodenal complex, liver and small bowel.

4. Modified multivisceral transplant (MMVTx) (**Figure 4**): recommended for people with multiple organ failure and involves transplanting the stomach, pancreaticoduodenal complex and small bowel. The difference with the previous type is the exclusion of the liver. It is usually performed in patients with preserved liver function and coexisting pancreatic insufficiency such as patients with chronic pancreatitis, type I diabetes mellitus or cystic fibrosis, patients with intestinal dysmotility with concomitant severe gastroparesis and in cases with tumor involvement of the mesentery or the duodenum (e.g. in Gardner's syndrome) [22].

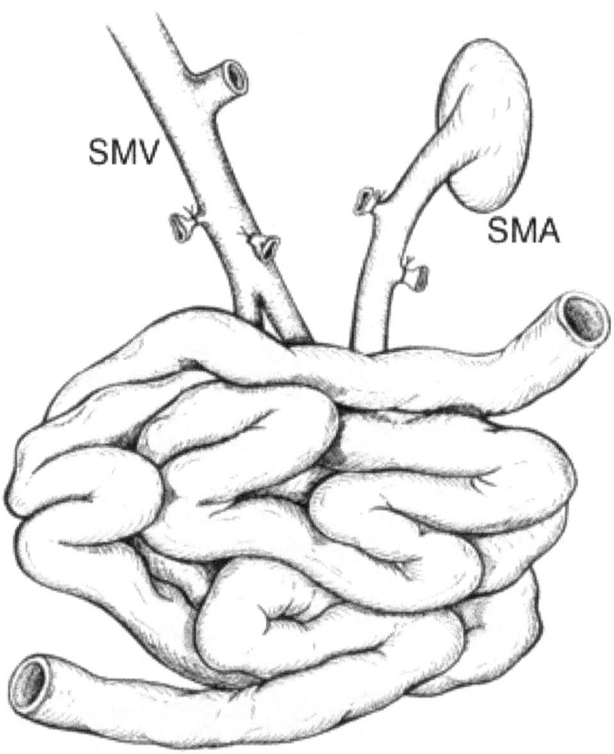

Figure 1. Small bowel transplant (SBTx).

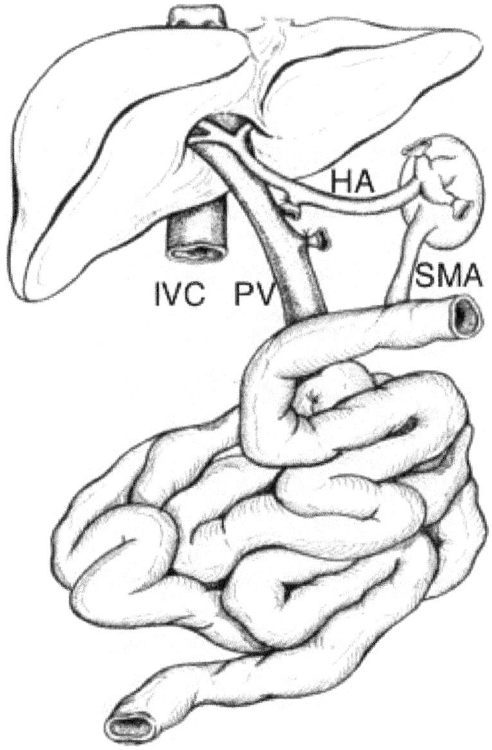

Figure 2. Liver and small bowel transplant (SBLTx).

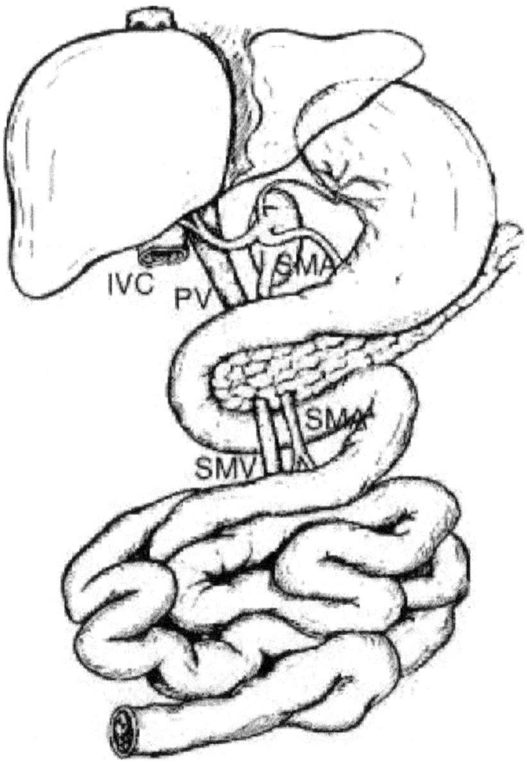

Figure 3. Multivisceral transplant (MVTx).

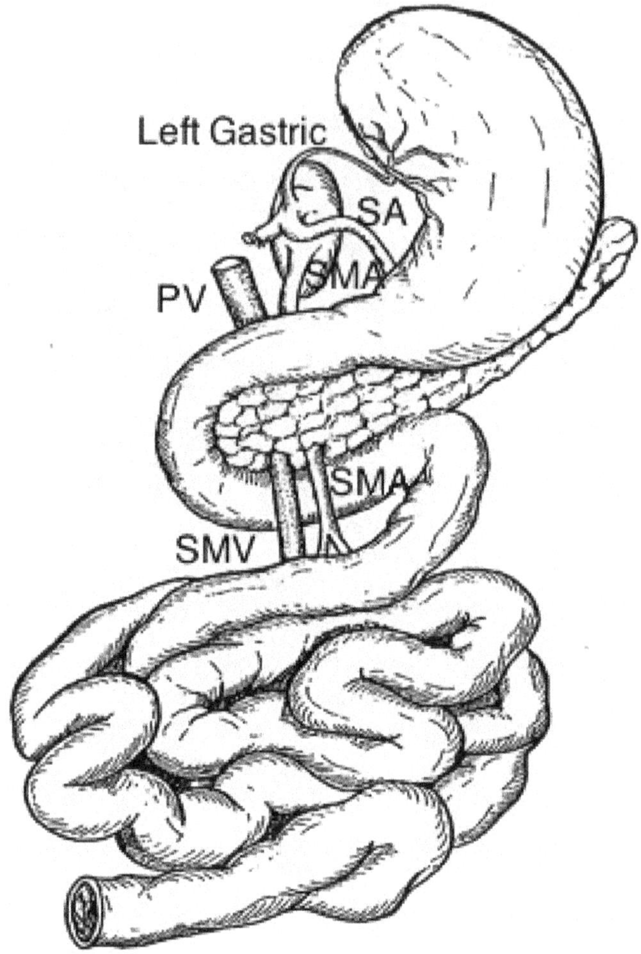

Figure 4. Modified multivisceral transplant (MMVTx).

In all the above ITx types, the right hemicolon can be included depending on the patient's native anatomy. Since 2000, there has been a sixfold increase in the inclusion of a colon segment resulting in a current inclusion rate of 30% [7]. The registry analysis has shown that inclusion of the colon did not adversely affect survival and recipients with a colon segment had a 5% higher rate of independence from supplemental parenteral nutrition (PN), as the retention of the ileocecal valve and the right colon enhance gut function through better fluid absorption and uptake of free fatty acids [23].

It's sometimes possible to carry out a small bowel transplant using a section of bowel donated by a living family member and the first standardized technique was reported by Gruessner and Sharp [24].

Because of previous surgery resulting in loss of abdominal wall domain and integrity, patients undergoing ITx face a problem with primary abdominal wall closure [25]. Surgical techniques such as reduction of the liver portion (left or right lobe) within the composite allograft [26], transplantation of composite abdominal wall tissue graft (**Figure 5**) [27, 28], the use of vascularized rectus sheath [29] and non-vascularized abdominal rectus fascia [30] have revolutionized abdominal wall reconstruction.

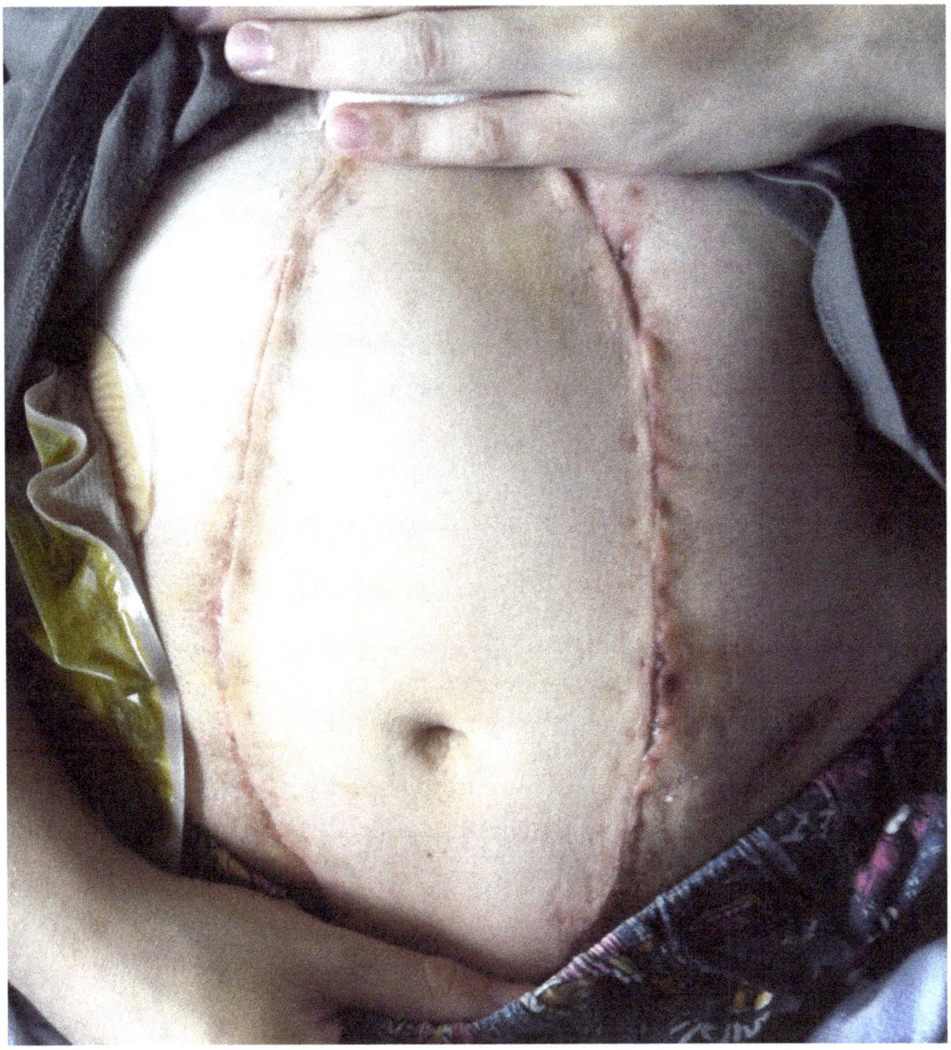

Figure 5. Abdominal wall transplant.

5. Recipient assessment

The assessment of a potential intestinal transplant recipient is robust and rigorous and needs to be done by a multidisciplinary team. This involves transplant surgery, gastroenterology, nutritional services, anesthesia, psychiatry and social work. However, due to the frequently pre-existing multiple comorbidities, consultation with other specialties may be required. Every assessment is 'tailor-made'.

Laboratory studies always include: full blood count (FBC), electrolytes and renal function, coagulation profile, ABO blood group, human leukocyte antigen (HLA) typing, panel-reactive antibody status, HIV and hepatitis B and C virus screening, cytomegalovirus (CMV) and Epstein-Barr virus (EBV) screening.

Liver biopsy is indicated, if liver disease is suspected. The native intestine should be assessed both by imaging and endoscopy.

Vascular access is of utmost importance and is assessed by magnetic resonance or computed tomography venogram. Securing upper-body vascular access is mandatory in cases where IVC occlusion is anticipated. Many patients will have central venous stenosis or obstruction and will mandate interventional radiology and/or vascular reconstruction before listing.

Manometry of the esophagus, stomach and rectum should be considered in patients with dysmotility disorders.

While on the waiting list, patients should be frequently reassessed, with specific attention given to any change in medical status, deterioration in liver function or vascular access.

6. Surgical technique

6.1. Intestinal retrieval

- Wide access to the abdominal cavity is needed and can be achieved via a midline incision from the suprasternal notch down to the symphysis pubis.
- The ascending colon and hepatic flexure are mobilized by using right-sided medial visceral rotation (Cattel-Braasch maneuver) that will expose the third and fourth portions of the duodenum.
- First, achieve control of the right common iliac artery or the distal abdominal aorta, which need to be mobilized for subsequent insertion of the infusion cannula.
- The structures of the hepatoduodenal ligament will have to be identified and slung for small bowel alone or modified multivisceral transplants.
- Depending on the type of transplant, sling the esophagus, the antrum or proximal jejunum.
- In case of MMVTx, the celiac axis has to be retrieved along with the left gastric and splenic arteries. This should be discussed with the liver implanting team in case of a left aberrant artery.
- Transect the gastrocolic ligament and, in case of large bowel retrieval, identify the middle colic vessels. Mark the transverse colon just distal to the vessels for the insertion of the gastrointestinal anastomosis (GIA) stapler. For small bowel, sling the ileum near the ileocecal valve.
- Expose the mesenteric root, abdominal aorta and infrahepatic IVC, including entry of the renal veins.
- If the pancreas is to be retrieved, the splenic flexure, spleen, and body and tail of pancreas are mobilized to allow adequate subsequent cooling of the pancreas.
- Perform proximal control for supraceliac cross-clamping, either above or below the diaphragm, depending on the presence of a cardiothoracic team.

- Cross-clamping of the supraceliac aorta is performed simultaneously with or immediately following venting of the IVC or atrium and cold perfusion is commenced.
- In situ cooling of abdominal organs, and exsanguination before removing the organs to the back table for preparation.
- University of Wisconsin (UW) Universal Organ Preservation solution for both in situ flushing and cold storage is most frequently used.
- Retrieve iliac, brachiocephalic and/or carotid arteries and veins as potential vascular grafts.

6.2. Back-table preparation of organs

Intestinal grafts require minimal back table; however, this depends on the retrieval technique and the extension of the allograft. Most commonly, back table involves to identify and tie the lymphatics. If the pancreas is retrieved along with a small bowel only graft, then it has to be removed/sacrificed on the back table.

6.3. Recipient operation

- Implantation begins commonly with adhesiolysis, as adhesions are usually abundant secondary to previous surgeries.
- Depending on the type of transplant, the aorta and IVC or SMA and SMV/PV are dissected and mobilized for the vascular anastomosis.
- The proximal and distal ends of the native digestive track are identified and dissected.
- Venous anastomosis to the graft is frequently performed to the recipient cava. However, when possible, venous anastomosis to the portal system is preferred.
- Arterial anastomosis is performed to the abdominal aorta via arterial jump graft.
- After reperfusion of the graft and careful hemostasis, the proximal and distal ends of the intestinal graft are anastomosed to the proximal and distal ends of the native digestive track. In some cases, the distal end is brought out as a permanent stoma.
- Most centers bring out a temporary stoma by utilizing various techniques (e.g. Bishop Koop), for post-operative endoscopic surveillance. This stoma is usually reversed in 6–12 months.
- Closure of the abdominal wall can be very challenging and should not be attempted under tension; if this is the case, keeping the abdominal wall open and planning for a sequential closing is preferable. Some centers are routinely performing abdominal wall transplantation from the same deceased donor in order to achieve closure.

7. Postoperative considerations

Patients are monitored in intensive therapy unit (ITU) post-operatively. It is common practice to administer broad-spectrum intravenous antibiotics and antifungals for 5–7 days post transplantation. Blood tests are sent daily and as well as arterial/venous blood gases to check bleeding and homeostasis.

Stoma output is monitored daily and will indicate the appropriate timing to resume enteral feeding via nasogastric tube or jejunostomy/gastrostomy. Some centers start elemental enteral feeding very early and gradually increase volumes depending on nasogastric tube aspirates. TPN is maintained for at least 2 weeks and can be discontinued once enteral nutrition is sufficient. Chyle leak can often be seen post-operatively due to the severed intestinal graft lymphatics. A no-fat or low-fat diet (<10 g/day) can be initiated as a first measure. Absorption of long-chain triglycerides, depends on lymphatic drainage, whereas medium-chain triglycerides are directly absorbed into the portal circulation.

Antiviral prophylaxis with intravenous ganciclovir (5 mg/kg OD) is common practice and regular CMV polymerase chain reaction (PCR) DNA tests are sent for monitoring. Oral valganciclovir is usually prescribed for 1-year post transplantation (900 mg OD). Epstein-Barr virus (EBV) is also monitored regularly by PCR. Trimethoprim-sulfamethoxazole is commonly used to prevent pneumocystis pneumonia for 1-year post operatively. Routine cultures are sent from all lines and most centers perform regular intestinal transplant endoscopies and biopsies via the stoma.

Oral medication is generally avoided in the early phase due to the unpredictable absorption and thus, bioavailability. Tacrolimus can be given sublingually and regular trough levels are sent for confirmation.

Plasma citrulline levels have emerged as a measure for overall for intestinal health as it is an indicator of enterocyte mass. However, compromised renal function is an important factor when considering plasma citrulline levels as a marker of intestinal failure as this potentially can increase circulating citrulline values [31]. Reduced citrulline levels can indicate the need for urgent investigations and also, commencement of TPN.

8. Immunosuppression

The intestine is the largest lymphoid organ in the body and hence, appropriate immunosuppression has been a real challenge. The lack of effective immunosuppressive agents hampered the first attempts of ITx in the 1960s. Over the years, advances in immunosuppression have transformed ITx with the intent of attenuating the intestinal allograft immunity and shifting it to a tolerogenic status [32].

Induction strategies to minimize rejection by reducing the recipient's T-cell load were implemented, initially with cyclophosphamide induction therapy, which was later replaced by daclizumab, an interleukin-2 receptor antagonist (IL2RA) [33]. Basiliximab, another IL2RA, in addition to tacrolimus and prednisone immunosuppression has also been utilized and shown to decrease the incidence of acute rejection [34, 35].

Alemtuzumab induction is becoming increasingly popular and Lauro et al. [36] reported significantly less early rejection episodes, with no sepsis implications. The use of Basiliximab monthly as part of maintenance immunosuppression has been associated with a decrease in acute rejection in liver-excluding transplants [37].

Immunosuppression regimen varies, with several protocols having been reported: Tacrolimus and steroids (35.8%) followed by tacrolimus, mycophenolate and steroids (18.7%), tacrolimus and mycophenolate without steroids in 15.4% of cases and tacrolimus alone in 13.8% of cases [38].

Target trough levels of tacrolimus vary between centers. Pittsburgh has reported target levels between 10 and 15 ng/ml in the first 3 months and thereafter 5–10 ng/ml [39]. Tacrolimus with low-dose steroids remains the most effective and durable long-term combination therapy [21] and is the most common maintenance immunosuppressive regimen [7].

Sirolimus, a rapamycin inhibitor, has been shown as a useful adjunct to tacrolimus in the presence of nephrotoxicity or rejection [40]. However, it carries the disadvantage of severe debilitating oromucosal ulceration. Azathioprine and mycophenolate mofetil have also been used as adjunctive immunosuppressive therapies [33]. Mycophenolate mofetil, however, causes symptomatic diarrhea (increased stoma output) and microscopically evident apoptosis in approximately 40% of solid organ transplant recipients, which could regrettably be mistaken for rejection [41].

9. Complications

Complications following ITx may result in graft failure and invariably death. Patients undergoing ITx have a higher incidence of life-threatening infectious complications than other transplant recipients. This is due to the high bacterial load of the transplanted graft [42]. Therefore, any breach to the intestinal transplant mucosal barrier can lead to bacterial translocation.

Graft loss would need TPN resuming and consideration of re-transplantation, which has a lower rate of success compared with the initial transplantation [43]. Common causes of graft loss include allograft rejection, infection, GVHD and post-transplant lymphoproliferative disorder (PTLD) [33].

9.1. Acute rejection

Allograft rejection has always been one of the most significant challenges to long-term graft and patient survival and can occur either as acute (commonly in the early phase, though can occur late) or chronic (typically taking months to years). Rejection can occur at any time but is most common in the first year, particularly the first 6 months. It affects 45% of ITx patients within the first post-transplant year, with implications on graft survival [7] and is mostly characterized by T-cell response to donor antigens.

Acute rejection should be suspected in all cases of bowel dysfunction (increased stoma output) and symptoms include fever, vomiting, abdominal pain and distension. Diagnosing acute rejection is always challenging and requires a combination of clinical, endoscopic and histopathological investigations. Intestinal allograft endoscopy and biopsies is the gold standard. However, diagnosis can be difficult to establish because of the patchy nature of rejection. Not to mention, that it is not always easy to differentiate between rejection and infection.

Most centers will endeavor to perform early, frequent endoscopies because of high prevalence of acute rejection in the early post transplantation phase [21] and then continue with regular endoscopies as part of their surveillance protocol [44].

The Oxford group, who is utilizing vascularized composite allograft (VCA) transplants from the same donor [45], is now mostly relying on the VCA as a surrogate marker for rejection and is not strictly adherent to early, intensive intestinal biopsy protocols [46]. They have reported that the VCA can provide lead time (about 7 days) before the onset of bowel dysfunction and this could be proven as a unique prognostic tool [45].

Rejection episodes are usually treated with pulses of methylprednisolone, and in resistant cases, thymoglobulin [32] or alemtuzumab [46].

A recent case series reported good outcomes in ITx of positive cross-match patients with only one patient developing acute rejection, with the use of intravenous immunoglobulin (IVIG) and rituximab [47]. Bortezomib, a proteasome inhibitor, has also been recently shown to be effective against donor-specific antibody (DSA)-related rejection [48]. Recently, Eculizumab, a monoclonal antibody that inhibits complement factor 5a, was shown to be effective in maintaining a 2-year rejection-free period in a highly sensitized patient [49]; however, high costs make this approach prohibitive for general use.

As mentioned before, biomarkers such as citrulline have gained interest in recent years. The prospective cohort study by Hibi et al. [50] reported excellent negative predictive value (range 93–99%) for citrulline levels as exclusionary marker for all types of acute rejection (cut-off point, 20 mmol/l) and moderate or severe acute cellular rejection (cut-off point, 10 mmol/l). Another study by the Bologna group [51] showed that citrulline sensitivity and specificity in detecting acute rejection, when adjusted for chronic renal failure, almost doubled the sensitivity of citrulline as a non-invasive marker of acute rejection in ITx. In general, citrulline can act as an exclusionary tool, as high levels are unlikely to be found in intestinal allograft rejection.

Recently, a large series evaluating video capsule endoscopy has shown to be potentially useful in the diagnostic management of patients with ITx [52]. Other non-invasive predictors of rejection include a recent retrospective study that revealed low insulin-like growth factor-1 and high calprotectin levels during malnutrition states post-ITx, and these findings should prompt the clinicians to investigate for acute rejection or infection [53]. Circulating apoptotic T cells following Caspase 3 activation may be a non-invasive marker for patients who are less likely to have rejection episodes than those who have lower levels [54].

9.2. Chronic rejection

Chronic rejection is diagnosed histologically with the identification of an obliterative arteriopathy in medium-sized vessels in the serosal layer with diffuse concentric intimal thickening [55]. This necessitates full-thickness biopsy and makes diagnosis challenging. Chronic rejection is clinically associated with diarrhea, ulceration, focal loss of mucosal folds, mural thickening and pruning of mesenteric artery arcades [55]. Surgery in such a hostile environment may lead to unwanted enterotomies and fistulae. Re-transplantation should therefore be considered. Evisceration is a potential life-saving option for ITx patients who developed severe rejection, and has similar survival rates with patients who underwent simultaneous enterectomy with re-transplantation; however, high sensitization may prevent re-transplantation [56].

9.3. Donor-specific antibodies

Preformed and de-novo DSAs have been associated with acute rejection and may be implicated in chronic rejection and graft loss [46, 57]. Five-year graft survival of less than 30% was noted in ITx patients who developed de-novo DSA, whereas survival rates of more than 80% were observed in recipients without DSA [44]. Yet, others have not found a statistically significant trend towards worsening outcomes [58] between those with or without de-novo DSA formation.

9.4. Infection

The use of immunosuppression in ITx poses a significant risk of infection and, historically, high levels of immunosuppressants have been utilized in ITx. Sepsis remains the most common cause of death and graft failure, accounting for over 50% of cases [7]. Bacterial infections are common in the early phase post-ITx and have a significant impact on patient survival. Invasive candidiasis has been reported as the commonest fungal infection [59].

Cytomegalovirus (CMV) and Epstein-Barr virus (EBV) viraemias are common and can be implicated in acute and chronic rejection as well as PTLD [60, 61]. CMV status is vital to anticipate the risk of developing de-novo infection in a non-infected recipient from the donor and through reactivation of a latent infection. CMV prophylaxis with oral valganciclovir is often continued for 1 year following ITx [62]. Most programs would not accept CMV-positive donors for CMV-negative recipients as this is high risk and should be avoided [63]. Last but not least, it has been demonstrated that isolated graft CMV disease without overt CMV viraemia can indeed occur [64].

9.5. Post-transplant lymphoproliferative disorder

In the updated 2016 WHO lymphoma classification, PTLD has been sub-classified as plasmacytic hyperplasia PTLD, infectious mononucleosis PTLD, florid follicular hyperplasia PTLD, polymorphic PTLD, monomorphic PTLD and classical Hodgkin lymphoma PTLD [65]. PTLD following SOT occurs in up to 20% with the highest incidence in intestinal and multi-organ transplants (5–20%), followed by lung and heart transplants (2–10%) and then by renal and liver transplants [66].

About 70% of cases of PTLD are associated with Epstein-Barr virus (EBV), especially in cases which occur early after transplantation. Pathogenesis of the disease is linked to EBV proliferation in the setting of chronic immunosuppression leading to an inhibition of T-cells immune function. However, in 30% of EBV-negative PTLD patients, pathogenesis is not clearly understood [67].

It is believed that in ITx, the lymphatic-rich intestinal allografts in combination with splenectomy and immunosuppression pose an increased risk for PTLD [68]. It has been reported that the presence of PTLD has significantly reduced patient survival within the first post-transplant year [69]. PTLD is treated with immunosuppression reduction and rituximab containing chemotherapy regimes in the presence of CD20 positive cases [70].

9.6. Graft versus host disease

The small intestine has abundant lymphoid cells that can mount an immunologic response to the host (i.e. a graft versus host disease [GVHD]) reaction. GVHD occurs in 5–7% of intestinal transplants, compared to 1% for solid organ transplants, and risk factors include younger age, MVTx recipients and intra-operative splenectomy [71]. It is more common in intestinal transplants due to the large volume of lymphatic tissue that is transplanted along with the graft. GVHD diagnosis is allegedly difficult to establish and patients usually present 1–8 weeks after transplantation with skin rash, ulceration of oral mucosa, diarrhea, lymphadenopathy or native liver dysfunction. Diagnosis is confirmed by skin or bowel biopsy.

Treatment strategies vary and most frequently involve tacrolimus, high-dose steroids or anti-thymocyte globulin (ATG) [71].

9.7. Renal dysfunction

Renal dysfunction is invariably seen post ITx due to a combination of high-dose tacrolimus therapy [72] and dehydration episodes, especially in the presence of stomas. The incidence of stage 4 or 5 CKD is 21.3% in patients with ITx [73] and approximately 9% of ITx patients will receive renal replacement therapy by a median of 7.4 years [74].

10. Graft and patient survival

Patient survival has been steadily improving because of improved first-year graft survival [7]. Graft survival has been reported for 1, 5 and 10 years at 74, 42 and 26%, respectively (SBTx); 70, 50 and 40% (MVTx); 61, 46 and 40% (SBLTx); overall patient survival was 76, 56 and 43%, respectively. Studies evaluating 1-year and 5-year patient survival rates at various transplant centers revealed comparable results [75, 76].

Patients on TPN have 1-year, 5-year, 10-year and 20-year survival of 91–93, 70–71, 55–59 and 28%, respectively, following IF commencement [77]. It should be noted, that 11–15% of deaths while on TPN were attributed to TPN complications (5–6% from sepsis or central-line sepsis and 6–9% from IFALD) [77]. A three-year prospective study reported 94 vs. 87% three-year survival in TPN non-transplant candidates vs. TPN transplant candidates who did not undergo transplantation. In addition, the three-year survival was 89 vs. 85 vs. 70% for those having first SBTx vs. transplant candidates with central venous catheter complications vs. candidates with parenteral nutrition-related liver failure [78].

11. Quality of life

Quality of life plays an important role in the decision-making for ITx candidates. ITx patients have reported better fatigue, gastrointestinal symptoms, stoma management/bowel movements, ability to holiday/travel and global health/QoL and probably better eating ability but worse sleeping patterns [79]. Others have found that ITx recipients have similar QoL to those who are stable on TPN, but both are better than those with complicated intestinal failure on TPN [80].

12. Future perspectives

ITx and its secrets have not been deciphered yet. The main issue remains the challenging balance between appropriate immunosuppression and over-immunosuppression. Therefore, ITx teams have been trying to develop markers that will provide adequate warning in case of rejection [45].

Multivisceral organ transplantation may solidify its role in the treatment of slow-growing abdominal cancers that are deemed "non-resectable" [81–83].

Another challenge will be to understand the physiology of the transplanted small bowel, such as its altered microflora and altered motility. New research has suggested that the flora composition within the graft may be a risk factor for acute rejection when more immunogenic species predominate [84].

Tolerance remains the 'Holy Grail' of transplantation and is characterized by increased allograft survival in the absence of immunosuppression and absent or reduced donor-specific response. Groups have used donor-specific blood transfusion in order to induce tolerance by upregulating graft protective memory Tregs [85]. Also, centers have introduced experimental models to induce microchimerism and tolerance by transplanting bone marrow along with the intestinal allograft [86]. These protocols could allow for sufficient immunosuppression with lower doses of immunosuppressants. This ongoing research may change the future of ITx.

13. Conclusion(s)

ITx continues to evolve and graft survival rates are nowadays more comparable with the results of other solid organ transplants. The main challenge is to develop immunosuppression protocols that can ensure long-term intestine graft function and less infectious complications. When this is accomplished ITx could potentially change from being a life-saving treatment to becoming a realistic first-line therapy for IF.

Author details

Georgios Vrakas

Address all correspondence to: georgiosvrakas@gmail.com

Oxford University Hospitals, Oxford, UK

References

[1] Lillehei RC, Goott B, Miller FA. The physiological response of the small bowel of the dog to ischemia including prolonged in-vitro preservation of the bowel with successful replacement and survival. Annals of Surgery. 1959;**150**:543-560

[2] Starzl TE, Kaupp HA Jr. Mass homo-transplantation of abdominal organs in dogs. Surgical Forum. 1960;**11**:28-30

[3] Kubal CA, Mangus RS, Tector AJ. Intestine and multivisceral transplantation: Current status and future directions. Current Gastroenterology Reports. 2015;**17**:427. DOI: 10.1007/s11894-014-0427-8

[4] Starzl TE, Todo S, Fung J, et al. FK 506 for liver, kidney, and pancreas transplantation. Lancet (London, England). 1989;**2**:1000-1004

[5] Todo S, Fung JJ, Starzl TE, et al. Liver, kidney, and thoracic organ transplantation under FK 506. Annals of Surgery. 1990;**212**:295-305

[6] Abu-Elmagd K, Reyes J, Todo S, et al. Clinical intestinal transplantation: New perspectives and immunologic considerations. Journal of the American College of Surgeons. 1998;**186**:512-527

[7] Grant D, Abu-Elmagd K, Mazariegos G, Vianna R, Langnas A, Mangus R, Farmer DG, Lacaille F, Iyer K, Fishbein T. Intestinal transplant registry & report: Global activity and trends. American Journal of Transplantation. 2015;**15**:210-219

[8] Pironi L, Joly F, Forbes A, et al. Long-term follow-up of patients on home parenteral nutrition in Europe: Implications for intestinal transplantation. Gut. 2011;**60**:17-25

[9] Zanfi C, Lauro A, Cescon M, et al. Comprehensive surgical intestinal rescue and transplantation program in adult patients: Bologna experience. Transplantation Proceedings. 2010;**42**:39-41

[10] Taha AM, Sharif K, Johnson T, Clarke S, Murphy MS, Gupte GL. Long-term outcomes of isolated liver transplantation for short bowel syndrome and intestinal failure-associated liver disease. Journal of Pediatric Gastroenterology and Nutrition. 2012;**54**:547-551

[11] Dell-Olio D, Beath SV, de Ville de Goyet J, et al. Isolated liver transplant in infants with short bowel syndrome: Insights into outcomes and prognostic factors. Journal of Pediatric Gastroenterology and Nutrition. 2009;**48**:334-340

[12] Iyer KR. Surgical management of short bowel syndrome. JPEN Journal of Parenteral and Enteral Nutrition. 2014;**38**(1 Suppl):53S-59S

[13] Buchman AL, Scolapio J, Fryer J. AGA technical review on short bowel syndrome and intestinal transplantation. Gastroenterology. 2003;**124**:1111-1134

[14] Kaufman SS, Atkinson JB, Bianchi A, et al. Indications for pediatric intestinal transplantation: A position paper of the American Society of Transplantation. Pediatric Transplantation. 2001;**5**:80-87

[15] Pironi L, Hebuterne X, Van Gossum A, et al. Candidates for intestinal transplantation: A multicenter survey in Europe. The American Journal of Gastroenterology. 2006;**101**:1633-1643

[16] Pironi L, Arends J, Bozzetti F, et al. ESPEN guidelines on chronic intestinal failure in adults. Clinical Nutrition. 2016;**35**:247-307

[17] Kumpf VJ. Parenteral nutrition-associated liver disease in adult and pediatric patients. Nutrition in Clinical Practice. 2006;**21**(3):279-290

[18] Reyes JD. Intestinal transplantation: An unexpected journey. Journal of Pediatric Surgery. 2014;**49**(1):13-18

[19] Staun M, Pironi L, Bozzetti F, et al. ESPEN guidelines on parenteral nutrition: Home parenteral nutrition (HPN) in adult patients. Clinical Nutrition. 2009;**28**:467-479

[20] Pither C, Wiles A, Butler A, et al. Quality of life in patients undergoing small intestinal transplantation. Gut. 2011;**60**(Suppl 1):A89-A189

[21] Fishbein TM. Intestinal transplantation. The New England Journal of Medicine. 2009;**361**:998-1008

[22] Cruz RJ Jr, Costa G, Bond GJ, et al. Modified multivisceral transplantation with spleen-preserving pancreaticoduodenectomy for patients with familial adenomatous polyposis "Gardner's syndrome". Transplantation. 2011;**91**:1417-1423

[23] Matsumoto CS, Kaufman SS, Fishbein TM. Inclusion of the colon in intestinal transplantation. Current Opinion in Organ Transplantation. 2011;**16**:312-315

[24] Gruessner RW, Sharp HL. Living-related intestinal transplantation: First report of a standardized surgical technique. Transplantation. 1997;**64**(11):1605-1607

[25] Loo L, Vrakas G, Reddy S, Allan P. Intestinal transplantation: A review. Current Opinion in Gastroenterology. 2017;**33**(3):203-211

[26] Reyes J, Fishbein T, Bueno J, et al. Reduced-size orthotopic composite liver-intestinal allograft. Transplantation. 1998;**66**:489-492

[27] Levi DM, Tzakis AG, Kato T, et al. Transplantation of the abdominal wall. Lancet. 2003;**361**:2173-2176

[28] Allin BSR, Ceresa CDL, Issa F, et al. A single center experience of abdominal wall graft rejection after combined intestinal and abdominal wall transplantation. American Journal of Transplantation. 2013;**13**:2211-2215

[29] Ravindra KV, Martin AE, Vikraman DS, et al. Use of vascularized posterior rectus sheath allograft in pediatric multivisceral transplantation-report of two cases. American Journal of Transplantation. 2012;**12**:2242-2246

[30] Gondolesi G, Selvaggi G, Tzakis A, et al. Use of the abdominal rectus fascia as a nonvascularized allograft for abdominal wall closure after liver, intestinal, and multivisceral transplantation. Transplantation. 2009;**87**:1884-1888

[31] Crenn P, Messing B, Cynober L. Citrulline as a biomarker of intestinal failure due to enterocyte mass reduction. Clinical Nutrition. 2008;**27**(3):328-339

[32] Rege A, Sudan D. Intestinal transplantation. Best Practice & Research. Clinical Gastroenterology. 2016;**30**:319-335

[33] Abu-Elmagd KM, Costa G, Bond GJ, et al. Five hundred intestinal and multivisceral transplantations at a single center: Major advances with new challenges. Annals of Surgery. 2009;**250**:567-581

[34] Sudan DL, Chinnakotla S, Horslen S, et al. Basiliximab decreases the incidence of acute rejection after intestinal transplantation. Transplantation Proceedings. 2002;**34**:940-941

[35] Farmer D, McDiarmid S, Edelstein S, et al. Induction therapy with interleukin-2 receptor antagonist after intestinal transplantation is associated with reduced acute cellular rejection and improved renal function. Transplantation Proceedings. 2004;**36**:331-332

[36] Lauro A, Zanfi C, Bagni A, Cescon M, Siniscalchi A, Pellegrini S, et al. Induction therapy in adult intestinal transplantation: Reduced incidence of rejection with "2-dose" alemtuzumab protocol. Clinical Transplantation. 2013;**27**(4):567-570

[37] Kubal CA, Mangus RS, Vianna RM, et al. Impact of positive flow cytometry crossmatch on outcomes of intestinal/multivisceral transplantation. Transplantation. 2013;**95**:1160-1166

[38] Smith JM, Skeans MA, Horslen SP, Edwards EB, Harper AM, Snyderf JJ, et al. OPTN/SRTR 2012 annual data report: Intestine. American Journal of Transplantation. 2014;**14**:97-111

[39] Reyes J, Mazariegos GV, Abu-Elmagd K, et al. Intestinal transplantation under tacrolimus monotherapy after perioperative lymphoid depletion with rabbit antithymocyte globulin. American Journal of Transplantation. 2005;**5**:1430-1436

[40] Lauro A, Dazzi A, Ercolani G, et al. Rejection episodes and 3-year graft survival under sirolimus and tacrolimus treatment after adult intestinal transplantation. Transplantation Proceedings. 2007;**39**:1629-1631

[41] Selbst MK, Ahrens WA, Robert ME, et al. Spectrum of histologic changes in colonic biopsies in patients treated with mycophenolate mofetil. Modern Pathology. 2009;**22**:737

[42] Akhter K, Timpone J, Matsumoto C, Fishbein T, Kaufman S, Kumar P. Six-month incidence of bloodstream infections in intestinal transplant patients. Transplant Infectious Disease. 2012 Jun;**14**(3):242-247

[43] Desai CS, Khan KM, Gruessner AC, et al. Intestinal retransplantation: Analysis of organ procurement and transplantation network database. Transplantation. 2012;**93**:120-125

[44] Abu-Elmagd KM, Wu G, Costa G, et al. Preformed and de novo donor specific antibodies in visceral transplantation: Long-term outcome with special reference to the liver. American Journal of Transplantation. 2012;**12**:3047-3060

[45] Gerlach UA, Vrakas G, Sawitzki B, et al. Abdominal Wall transplantation: Skin as a sentinel marker for rejection. American Journal of Transplantation. 2016;**c16**(6):1892-1900

[46] Weissenbacher A, Vrakas G, Chen M, Reddy S, Allan P, Giele H, Barnardo MCNM, Vaidya A, Friend PJ, Fuggle SV. De novo donor-specific HLA antibodies after combined intestinal and vascularized composite allotransplantation—A retrospective study. Transplant International. 2018 Apr;**31**(4):398-407

[47] Parekh R, Kazimi M, Skorupski S, et al. Intestine transplantation across a & positive crossmatch with preformed donor-specific antibodies. Transplantation Proceedings. 2016;**48**:489-491

[48] Fujiwara S, Wada M, Kudo H, et al. Effectiveness of bortezomib in a patient with acute rejection associated with an elevation of donor-specific HLA antibodies after small-bowel transplantation: Case report. Transplantation Proceedings. 2016;**48**:525-527

[49] Fan J, Tryphonopoulos P, Tekin A, et al. Eculizumab salvage therapy for antibody-mediated rejection in a desensitization-resistant intestinal re-trans-plant patient. American Journal of Transplantation. 2015;**15**:1995-2000

[50] Hibi T, Nishida S, Garcia J, et al. Citrulline level is a potent indicator of acute rejection in the long term following pediatric intestinal/multivisceral transplantation. American Journal of Transplantation. 2012;**12**(Suppl 4):S27-S32

[51] Pironi L, Guidetti M, Lauro A, et al. Plasma citrulline after small bowel transplantation: Effect of time from transplantation, acute cellular rejection and renal failure. Clinical Transplantation. 2015;**29**:1039-1046

[52] Varkey J, Oltean M, Pischel AB, et al. Initial experience of video capsule endoscopy after intestinal transplantation. Transplant Direct. 2016;**2**:e119

[53] Vrakas G, O'Connor M, Matsou A, et al. Markers of malnutrition after intestinal transplantation: The role of IGF-1 and calprotectin. Journal of Clinical Biochemistry and Nutrition. 2015;**56**:64-65

[54] Ashokkumar C, Sun Q, Ningappa M, et al. Antithymocyte globulin facilitates alloreactive T-cell apoptosis by means of caspase-3: Potential implications for monitoring rejection-free outcomes. Transplantation. 2015;**99**:164-170

[55] Demetris AJ, Murase N, Lee RG, et al. Chronic rejection. A general overview of histopathology and pathophysiology with emphasis on liver, heart and intestinal allografts. Annals of Transplantation. 1997;**2**:27-44

[56] Nagai S, Mangus RS, Anderson E, et al. Intestinal graft failure: Should we perform the allograft enterectomy before or with re-transplantation? Transplantation. 2017;**101**:411-420

[57] Cheng EY, Everly MJ, Kaneku H, Banuelos N, Wozniak LJ, Venick RS, Marcus EA, McDiarmid SV, Busuttil RW, Terasaki PI, Farmer DG. Prevalence and clinical impact of donor-specific alloantibody among intestinal transplant recipients. Transplantation. 2017;**101**(4):873-882

[58] Kubal C, Mangus R, Saxena R, et al. Prospective monitoring of donor-specific & anti-HLA antibodies after intestine/multivisceral transplantation. Transplantation. 2015;**99**:e49-e56

[59] Florescu DF, Sandkovsky U. Fungal infections in intestinal and multivisceral transplant recipients. Current Opinion in Organ Transplantation. 2015;**20**:295-302

[60] Timpone JG, Girlanda R, Rudolph L, Fishbein TM. Infections in intestinal and multivisceral transplant recipients. Infectious Disease Clinics of North America. 2013;**27**:359-377

[61] Timpone JG, Yimen M, Cox S, et al. Resistant cytomegalovirus in intestinal and multivisceral transplant recipients. Transplant Infectious Disease. 2016;**18**:202-209

[62] Allan PJ, Vaidya A, Lal S. Small bowel transplantation. In: Nutritional Management of Inflammatory Bowel Diseases. Cham: Springer International Publishing; 2016. pp. 215-230

[63] Ambrose T, Sharkey LM, Louis-Auguste J, et al. Cytomegalovirus infection and rates of antiviral resistance following intestinal and multivisceral transplantation. Transplantation Proceedings. 2016;**48**:492-496

[64] Avsar Y, Cicinnati VR, Kabar I, et al. Small bowel transplantation complicated by cytomegalovirus tissue invasive disease without viremia. Journal of Clinical Virology. 2014;**60**:177-180

[65] Swerdlow SH, Campo E, Pileri SA, et al. The 2016 revision of the World Health Organization classification of lymphoid neoplasms. Blood. 2016;**127**:2375-2390

[66] Petrara MR, Giunco S, Serraino D, et al. Post-transplant lymphoproliferative disorders: From epidemiology to pathogenesis-driven treatment. Cancer Letters. 2015;**369**:37-44

[67] Bishnoi R, Bajwa R, Franke AJ, Skelton WP 4th, Wang Y, Patel NM, Slayton WB, Zou F, Dang NH. Post-transplant lymphoproliferative disorder (PTLD): Single institutional experience of 141 patients. Experimental Hematology & Oncology. 2017;**6**:26

[68] Lauro A, Arpinati M, Pinna AD. Managing the challenge of PTLD in liver and bowel transplant recipients. British Journal of Haematology. 2015;**169**:157-172

[69] Abu-Elmagd KM, Mazariegos G, Costa G, et al. Lymphoproliferative disorders and de novo malignancies in intestinal and multivisceral recipients: Improved outcomes with new outlooks. Transplantation. 2009;**88**:926-934

[70] Trappe R, Oertel S, Leblond V, et al. Sequential treatment with rituximab followed by CHOP chemotherapy in adult B-cell post-transplant lymphoproliferative disorder

(PTLD): The prospective international multi-centre phase 2 PTLD-1 trial. The Lancet Oncology. 2012;**13**:196-206

[71] Mazariegos GV, Abu-Elmagd K, Jaffe R, Bond G, Sindhi R, Martin L, et al. Graft versus host disease in intestinal transplantation. American Journal of Transplantation. 2004;**4**(9):1459-1465

[72] Suzuki M, Mujtaba MA, Sharfuddin AA, et al. Risk factors for native kidney dysfunction in patients with abdominal multivisceral/small bowel transplantation. Clinical Transplantation. 2012;**26**:E351-E358

[73] Ojo AO, Held PJ, Port FK, et al. Chronic renal failure after transplantation of a nonrenal organ. The New England Journal of Medicine. 2003;**349**:931-940

[74] Abu-Elmagd KM, Kosmach-Park B, Costa G, et al. Long-term survival, nutritional autonomy, and quality of life after intestinal and multivisceral transplantation. Annals of Surgery. 2012;**256**:494-508

[75] Ceulemans LJ, Monbaliu D, De Roover A, et al. Belgian multicenter experience with intestinal transplantation. Transplant International. 2015;**28**:1362-1370

[76] Ramisch D, Rumbo C, Echevarria C, et al. Long-term outcomes of intestinal and multivisceral transplantation at a single center in Argentina. Transplantation Proceedings. 2016;**48**:457-462

[77] Dibb M, Soop M, Teubner A, et al. Survival and nutritional dependence on home parenteral nutrition: Three decades of experience from a single referral centre. Clinical Nutrition. 2017 Apr;**36**(2):570-576

[78] Pironi L, Forbes A, Joly F, et al. Survival of patients identified as candidates for intestinal transplantation: A 3-year prospective follow-up. Gastroenterology. 2008;**135**:61-71

[79] Pironi L, Baxter JP, Lauro A, et al. Assessment of quality of life on home parenteral nutrition and after intestinal transplantation using treatment-specific questionnaires. American Journal of Transplantation. 2012;**12**:S60-S66

[80] Cameron EAB, Binnie JAH, Jamieson NV, et al. Quality of life in adults following small bowel transplantation. Transplantation Proceedings. 2002;**34**:965-966

[81] Allan P, Reddy S, Moran B, Vrakas G, Giele H, Mohamad F, Gilbert J, Sinha S, Vaidya A, Cecil T, Friend P. Cytoreductive surgery and small bowel transplantation is a feasible option for patients with end-stage pseudomyxoma peritonei. Gut. 2016;**65**:A106-A107

[82] Chi Z, Mangus RS, Kubal CA, Chen S, Lin J. Multivisceral transplant is a viable treatment option for patients with non-resectable intra-abdominal fibromatosis. Clinical Transplantation. 2017 [Epub ahead of print]

[83] Frilling A, Giele H, Vrakas G, Reddy S, Macedo R, Al-Nahhas A, Wasan H, Clift AK, Gondolesi GE, Vianna RM, Friend P, Vaidya A. Modified liver-free multivisceral transplantation for a metastatic small bowel neuroendocrine tumor: A case report. Transplantation Proceedings. 2015 Apr;**47**(3):858-862

[84] Voswinkel J, Francois S, Gorin NC, Chapel A. Gastro-intestinal autoimmunity: Preclinical experiences and successful therapy of fistulizing bowel diseases and gut graft versus host disease by mesenchymal stromal cells. Immunologic Research. 2013 Jul;**56**(2-3):241-248

[85] Ceulemans LJ, Braza F, Monbaliu D, Jochmans I, De Hertogh G, Du Plessis J, Emonds MP, Kitade H, Kawai M, Li Y, Zhao X, Koshiba T, Sprangers B, Brouard S, Waer M, Pirenne J. The Leuven immunomodulatory protocol promotes T-regulatory cells and substantially prolongs survival after first intestinal transplantation. American Journal of Transplantation. 2016 Oct;**16**(10):2973-2985

[86] Sheng Sun D, Iwagaki H, Ozaki M, Ogino T, Kusaka S, Fujimoto Y, Murata H, Sadamori H, Matsukawa H, Tanaka N, Yagi T. Prolonged survival of donor-specific rat intestinal allograft by administration of bone-marrow-derived immature dendritic cells. Transplant Immunology. 2005 Mar;**14**(1):17-20

9

Organ Donation Course in Medical Education Program

Nilufer Yılmaz, Sibel Demiral and
Taylan Özgür Sezer

Abstract

The number of patients waiting for organ transplantation is increasing. Today, living donors and cadaveric donors comprise the donor pool. Although it varies from country to country, organ transplants are mostly based on living donors because the cadaveric donor pool is not enough. There are different alternatives to increase the cadaveric donor pool. One of them is to raise awareness of organ donation in undergraduate medical education. Unfortunately, its effectiveness is controversial. In this section, to increase the effectiveness of the organ donation course given in medical education programs, a method proposal is presented. Medical professionals' knowledge of and attitudes toward donation have an impact on donation rates. It is possible that these attitudes and knowledge are molded during pre-graduation. As such, educating medical students may be an important factor in increasing organ donation. Learners' participation in an educational program is one of the most important factors contributing to learning. Flipped classroom is a student-oriented education method based on the combination of in- and out-of-class activities. With the use of the flipped classroom method in organ donation courses offered in medical education programs, students' knowledge and skills that enable them to discuss the topic of donation with patients can be improved.

Keywords: organ donation, medical education, flipped classroom

1. Introduction

The number of patients waiting for organ transplantation is increasing. Today, living donors and cadaveric donors comprise the donor pool. Although it varies from country to country, organ transplants are mostly based on living donors because the cadaveric donor pool is not enough. There are different alternatives to increase the cadaveric donor pool.

One of them is to raise awareness of organ donation in undergraduate medical education. Unfortunately, its effectiveness is controversial. In this section, to increase the effectiveness of the organ donation course given in medical education programs, a method proposal is presented.

Medical professionals' knowledge of and attitudes toward donation have an impact on donation rates. It is possible that these attitudes and knowledge are molded during pre-graduation. As such, educating medical students may be an important factor in increasing organ donation [1, 2]. Learners' participation in an educational program is one of the most important factors contributing to learning. Today's learner has a good command of digital technology, accesses information easily, and can easily adapt to changing learning styles and needs, and thus they have distinct differences from previous generations in thinking, and processing of information, which necessitates the use of alternative education methods. Flipped classroom (FC) is a student-oriented education method based on the combination of in- and out-of-class activities. With the use of the flipped classroom education method in organ donation courses offered in medical education programs, students' knowledge and skills that enable them to discuss the topic of donation with patients can be improved.

2. What is the flipped class model?

Flipped class model is a model which emerged following transformation of the blended learning as a result of the changes that have taken place in both technology and the notion of education [3]. The flipped learning approach describes a learning process, which progresses counter-wise the teacher-centered and traditional approach that is confined to within the four walls. In the traditional teaching approach, conveyance of a topic is realized through a teacher-centered approach in a classroom setting, while digestion of the topic takes place out of the classroom by the learner and through homework-like practices. Flipped learning approach, on the other hand, is a model of learning that proceeds in the opposite direction of the traditional teaching process, in which the learners watch pre-prepared video lessons before the actual class usually at home, and digest the topic in the classroom through several activities [4]. As an educational technique, the flipped class model is not a novel idea but has gained a reputation with the recent technological advances and the increasing access to computers and mobile devices regardless of time and space.

Flipped class model is defined as "a blended learning model that combines the traditional face-to-face teaching and online components." The learning models blended by Staker and Horn [5] are divided into four groups as the rotation model, flex model, self-blend model, and enriched virtual model. Within this classification, flipped class model falls under the rotation model category. The taxonomy developed by Staker and Horn [5] is presented in **Figure 1** [5].

Flipped class model can be described as an innovative model facilitated by the advances in technology. The objective of this model is to offer learning opportunities independently from time, space, and means and to create settings of active learning where interaction is prioritized. Flipped class model encompasses utilization of all sorts of Internet technologies to enforce

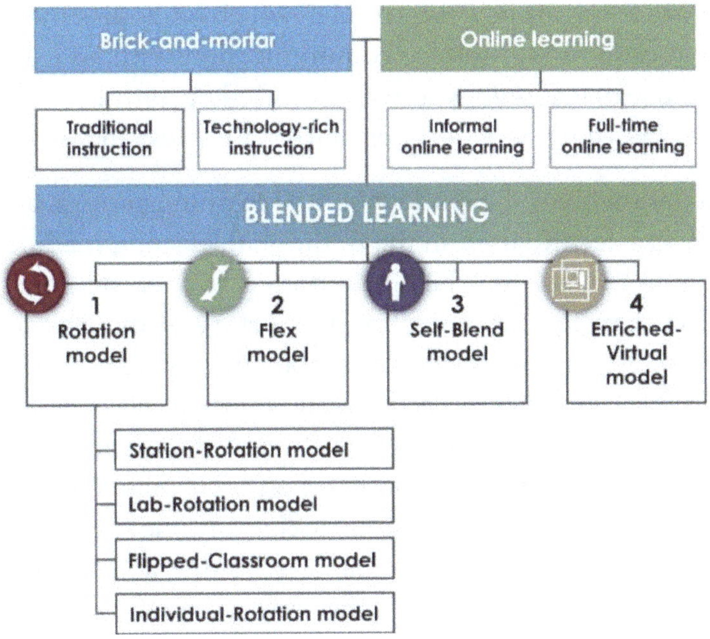

Figure 1. Blended learning taxonomy. Source: Staker and Horn [5].

in-class learnings, and thus the educator spares more time to interact with the student rather than delivering the lecture. In traditional educational settings, students devote their class time to listening to the lecture and, if time remains, practices about the information they have just learned [4, 6, 7]. In this model, on the other hand, the traditional classroom paradigm is reversed to enable students to learn the concepts of the lecture outside the classroom through online educational tools such as video, film, and audio materials. Thus, in-class time is devoted to discussions, problem-solving, and practical training [3, 4, 8, 9].

The activities covered in and out of the classroom for students and instructors in traditional education and flipped class models are presented in **Figure 2** [10].

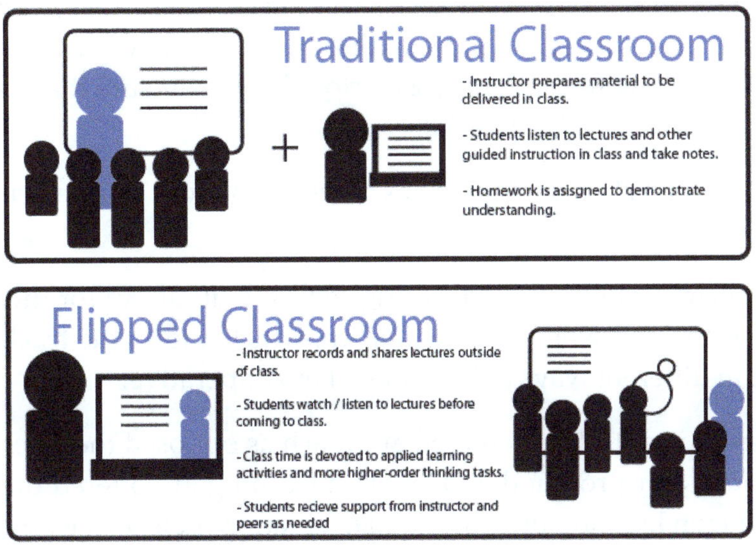

Figure 2. Features of traditional education and flipped classroom. Source: Saint Louis University [10].

As can be seen in **Figure 2**, the flipped class model, which embodies the combination of active education models that require face-to-face communication with educator-centered methods that make less limited use of technology as well as varied opportunities offered through activities in and out of the classroom, will perhaps help us to access today's learners more easily.

The flipped class model involves the students in the learning process and combines the benefits of direct delivery of a lecture used in the traditional learning method with those of active learning. Hence, flipping the classes is being supported as a teaching method that will enable usage of the time to be devoted for delivering the lecture in the classroom much more efficiently through the use of currently available technologies which facilitate access to information. Thus, active learning methods that can be used within the classroom offer the opportunity for teachers to act as a guide while assisting the students to advance their skills such as peer communication, collaborative learning, and taking on their own learning responsibility, thus improving active learning activity. The skill of taking on one's own learning responsibility is reinforced by coming to the class prepared and assuming active roles in in-class activities [11–13]. This method offers advantages to the instructor as well, particularly enabling them to understand and correct the thinking/reasoning errors of the learner and achieve the learning goals with more interactive methods instead of delivering a lesson in the classroom [11, 14]. Besides, although it takes time to prepare, the flipped class model allows the teachers to actualize transformative experiences for their students, build flexible teaching strategies, and make the lessons appealing [15].

The underlying idea of the flipped class model is to devote in-class time to active learning. This is a model that encourages the use of technology in the classroom as well as at home (e.g., video records) for active learning. With the flipped class model, most of the time spent in the classroom is used for communication in comparison to the traditional teaching [16]. This model is student centered. Each student has the responsibility to understand the material at a basic level before coming to the class, and this enables the student to take interest and participate in classroom discussions [17, 18]. Knowledge acquisition takes place at the own pace and guidance of the student; when and how the student will view the content is at their own control. The instructor provides guidance on the content, interactive practices, and creative thinking to facilitate learning, ensures deepening the information, and offers feedback. By offering materials of varying formats, the instructor also makes sure that learners with different learning styles are addressed to [18–20].

The features of the flipped class model are described as follows, emphasizing the word "flip" as an acronym [21]:

- Flexible Environment: It describes a learning setting that allows for the flexibility for students to choose when and where they will learn, which allows the teacher to organize the learning setting in different ways to be personal or cooperative.

- Learning Culture: It is a student-centered approach as opposed the teacher-centered traditional model. Means for profound and creative learning are offered during in-class time. Involved in their own learning processes and evaluating their own learnings, students participate actively to the structuring of information.

- Intentional Content: Educators focus on helping the students improve their conceptual understanding. Educators decide what they will teach and what materials the students will study themselves.
- Professional Educator: The role of educators is more important in the flipped class model. In this model, educators must continuously observe the students, offer instantaneous feedback, and assess the students. Although educators have a less visible role in the classroom in this model, they are the required element for the flipped class model to develop.

With the growing interest toward the flipped class model, Bergmann et al. describe that the model leads to misunderstandings by the practitioners of it. According to the authors, flipped class practices [22]

- are not synonymous with online videos. In this model, interactions emerging during face-to-face time and meaningful learnings are more important
- are not online lessons
- are not replacement of instructors and teaching by videos
- do not mean unplanned, non-programmed, and disorganized work by students
- do not mean that students will spend the whole lesson time looking at a computer screen
- do not mean that students will study alone

3. The advantages and disadvantages of the flipped class model

Flipped class model seems advantageous, in that it encourages single-handed learning, new ideas arise in platforms of discussion, individuals come prepared to the subject, allows flexibility in watching videos, helps understanding of the subject, contributes to pre-learning, motivates learning, and offers the opportunity for the individuals in accordance with their characteristics. Besides, the flipped class model increases student's commitment to the lesson, strengthens team skills, provides individualized student guidance, focuses on class discussions and offers freedom of teaching [23, 24].

On the other hand, the flipped class model appears disadvantageous because of problems with Internet access, students coming to the classroom without necessary pre-work, some students resisting to new applications, and lack of simultaneous feedback [25].

Besides, Bergmann and Sams [4] described two major problems that may be experienced in the flipped class model as the lack of means to check whether the students have watched the video and the vagueness of what the students who have not watched the video prior to the lesson will do in the classroom, and offered the following suggestions for the problems [4]:

- to verify whether the students have watched the video, having the students log in to the page with a username and password, or come to the classroom with questions on the video prepared beforehand.

- for the students who have not watched the video, having them watch it on a computer kept at the classroom. Thus, the students will understand the importance of participating in classroom activities.

4. Theoretical bases of the flipped classroom practice

The flipped class model regards education as a lifelong process. This model is a learning approach that is based on the pragmatist philosophy. Pragmatist approach appraises accuracy or reality only by looking at the consequences of the action and emphasizes benefit. All knowledge and theories are used to make life easier. In this sense, the value of a knowledge or thought is associated with its being beneficial. Therefore, outcomes, or in other words implementations rather than theory, stand out. The student is thus carried to the center of education. The reflection of pragmatism to education manifests as progressivism and reconstructivism advocating the concepts of change, experiences derived by the individual, and learning responsibility.

Progressivism, in reaction to the oppressive and conservative approach of traditional education, considers the essence of truth as change and freedom. In this understanding, training that is intertwined with the evolving life should naturally be progressive. Progressivism places students, who develop themselves and learn to learn through personal experiences, at the center of education. It advocates a teaching approach which preserves the core of change and aim at exhibiting democratic behavior [26, 27].

On the other hand, reconstructivism considers education as a means to achieve a more modern society. The society must renew and reshape constantly. Potential detrimental effects originating from changes would otherwise be unavoidable. Because change is inevitable. In this understanding, the role of actualizing change is entrusted to students who are described as social engineers. Schools should therefore raise social engineers who are able use the fundamental dynamics of change, that is, science and technology. Reconstructivists object to teaching traditional subjects at schools. Methods to solve ever-changing problems should be taught instead. Because only thus can it respond to the requirements of modern life. What is being tried to convey here with the modern life concept is, according to reconstructivists, is group life. From this perspective, school is a special social institution established to prepare students to group living [27].

Contemporary philosophical approaches developed later entrusted schools with the task to reach more modern societies. It was expected from the schools to perform this task to focus on developing problem-solving and learning to learn skills and be able to transform themselves into life settings that support cooperative learning so that the student may be more active in their lifelong learning processes. Also, an emphasis has emerged to use some models when performing this task. As the first of these models, the flipped class model was proposed and began to be used in these schools.

The main reason to use the flipped class model was to have the students at the center, to create a learning setting which involves activities that target research making, creativity, and problem-solving to transform classrooms into a laboratory or a studio to strip teachers out of their information-radiating roles and students out of their roles as actors who are merely takers of information and to convert them into individuals by processing and shaping them, shortly, to introduce a "constructivist" consciousness. The pedagogic foundations of the flipped classroom approach are based on the constructivist learning theory. According to this theory, students do not take the information as is during the learning process. On the contrary, students take information as active constructive participants throughout the learning process and the responsibility of learning is solely on the student. The process or restructuring information is accomplished through problem-based learning, simulation and pair-share-like active learning strategies. In a flipped classroom, out-of-classroom learning processes depend entirely on self-controlled learning. In-class learning activities comprise higher-order cognitive activities that utilize active learning techniques including decision-making and problem-solving, which students perform through interaction. Constructivist theory does not deny the role of instructor in the learning process. According to the constructivist theory, the instructor is not the wise man who knows everything on the scene but the person who take sides and collaborates with the student during the learning process. Also in a flipped classroom, the instructor does not deliver a lecture but assumes to role of facilitating the learning process in the classroom [28–33].

In summary, the flipped class model encompasses such concepts as constructivist approach, research-based method, active learning, and student-centered learning [13].

5. Flipped class model and Bloom's taxonomy

In 1956, Benjamin Bloom described the incrementally organized "Cognitive Domain" taxonomy. The main theme of this taxonomy was gradual and hierarchical listing of the things the educators want the students to know (learning targets). Bloom's taxonomy—which consists of remembering, understanding, applying, analyzing, evaluating, and creating stages—progresses from simple, concrete, and easy-to-learn behaviors representing the first step of learning to more complex, abstract, and harder-to-learn behaviors. It was also taken into consideration that each behavior is to be the prerequisite for the other, where they pertain to the same subject. In other words, the first behavior is the precondition of the behavior in the second step. Moreover, the first behavior is included in the behavior in the second step.

In the traditional classroom practice, the educator presents the new information by delivering a lecture. In this process, the students are considered to have reached the first two steps of Bloom's taxonomy, that is, remembering and understanding. After the class, students perform by themselves as homework the exercises of the more complicated higher steps. In the flipped classroom, on the other hand, students carry out the part that involves the relatively easier initial steps, that is listening to the lecture, at home by themselves. Practices for the difficult and complicated higher steps are accomplished through active learning methods accompanied by the educator. The students can thus advance up to higher-order cognitive skill stages in the taxonomy (**Figure 3**) [4, 33–35].

When viewed from the perspective of the reorganized Bloom's taxonomy, learnings at the level of the first to steps of understanding and remembering are accomplished by preparing

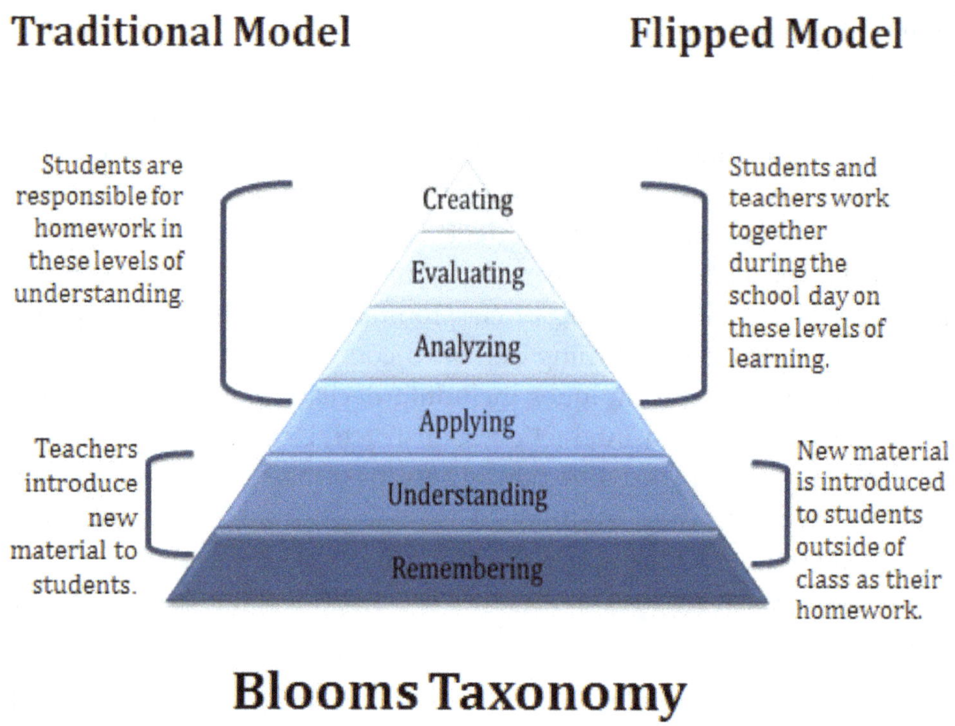

Figure 3. Bloom's taxonomy related to traditional and flipped learning. Source: Ouda and Ahmed [33].

materials at home, while learnings at the levels of applying, analysis, evaluation, and creating are achieved during the active learning processes including in-class practices, discussion, and problem-solving. An important advantage of the flipped class model is that it can incorporate the learning targets of each step in the Bloom's taxonomy.

6. Emergence of the flipped class concept

The conception of traditional teaching describes a process where the educator is deemed as the primary source of information and the action of learning is confined to within school walls and school time. However, the advancing education, technological opportunities, rapidly growing body of knowledge, and changing student profile force learning concepts to change and transform. With the changing educational paradigms, new learning approaches, models, and strategies to enhance the efficacy of learning in learning processes and encourage the learners in this respect are being sought [36–38].

Although referred by a different name, the foundations of the flipped class model were first laid in Miami University by the professors of departments that involve too much reading tasks including law, philosophy, sociology, and psychology because the duration of lectures was not enough to deliver the content [3]. With this model that was first being used in higher education, it was aimed to develop a system that will meet the learning requirements of students with varying styles of learning. Covering different educational resources and appealing to all learning styles, the system was named "Inverted Classroom". When planning the system, Lage et al. [3] first determined the subject and then recorded to videotapes while delivering the determined lecture during the class. The recorded lesson was copied and handed to

the students. Students who wished so found the opportunity to watch the lecture over and over again and could fill their gaps of the subject. Later, PowerPoint presentations used during the lecture were voiced over and uploaded to web together with complete lecture notes, making them available to students. Getting the printouts of the written resources uploaded to the web, students were able to take the necessary notes on these resources and found the opportunity to undertake a more comprehensive and planned work. Coming to subsequent classes after studying the ready lecture notes they have, students discussed the points they could not understand in the company of their teachers right at the beginning of the lesson and practiced in depth on the subject once the points that could not be understood were eliminated, and engaged in laboratory work where they put their learnings into practice. For all these, a website dedicated for the lecture to access all students and address every learning style was built. The built website was uploaded with materials such as previous exam questions, worksheets, lecture presentations and lecture video records, and were shared with students. Students' questions were answered online in chat rooms created during specific time frames. A virtual library was put together over the established website. This education model was even offered for the appreciation of students and lecturers and a questionnaire and an assessment scale including open-ended questions were applied. While the developed model was received very well by students and lecturers, this first detailed and elaborately planned implementation did not attract the anticipated attention.

The individuals who ensured that the flipped model survived up to the present time and found widespread use were Jonathan Bergmann and Aaron Sams who worked as chemistry teachers in the Woodland Park High School, USA (2007). Bergman and Sams observed that students who could not attend a lesson for various reasons (students taking part in sports games, miscellaneous activities) were unable to fill their learning gaps afterwards. To solve this problem, the duo initially developed a software that could voice over PowerPoint presentations and convert them into a video format and had the students who could not attend a lesson for various reasons watch these videos. The students who could not attend classes learned their missed lessons by these videos. This attracted the attention of other students, and the videos were made available for viewing for all students, regardless of their attendance to the class. By means of the videos, students who missed classes were able to learn the lesson, while those who attended the classes found the opportunity to rehearse and capture the notes they had missed during the lesson. Shortly, these videos were heard of by other schools, students, and teachers who also began to use the videos. With the videos gaining fame in a short span of time, Sams raised the idea of replanning the teaching process. Bergman and Sams [4] asked "When do students really need teachers?" and argued that students needed teachers when they were solving problems at home rather than when the lecture was delivered, and that the students could learn the subject by themselves through videos. Bergman and Sams uploaded other lessons to web in the same way and described students how they should watch videos and take notes before coming to the class. Because when the students arrived at the classroom, the bits that were not understood were now apparent, the parts of the content that were not apprehended were figured out rapidly, and more time was spared for problem-solving and laboratory activities for which students actually needed a teacher [4].

In short, the method of these two teachers has created a great deal of impression and, in 2012, the faculty staff of Northern Colorado University established a database by packing lecture contents to videos. Later on, Salman Khan, with the math videos he recorded without any commercial purpose, helped the model spread wider and be known as "Flipped Classroom" [39].

The title of the book released by Bergmann and Sams in 2012 was "Flip your classroom; reach every student in every class every day" [4]. As the title suggests, the main objective of the "flipped classroom" method is to make classroom lessons available using technology and to reach all students with different types of learning by making in-class activities more active.

7. Implementing the flipped classroom method

Flipped classrooms is a method in which the learner, viewing the learning topics by means of virtual technologies and videos prior to the classroom lecture and makes preparations and then comes to the classroom, engages in face-to-face interaction with the instructor and peers with the instructor assuming the role of a guide and facilitator. There are two distinct components of the flipped classroom exercise. These are out-of-class and in-class activities. Out-of-class activities is a platform involving technical equipment which aims to form a resource for learning where the learners will access the information they will acquire themselves. In-class activities are the part where interactive methods are used [4, 13, 40–42]. **Figure 4** demonstrates the planning of out-of-class and in-class activities in the flipped classroom exercise.

The cyclical steps in **Figure 5** can be used in structuring lectures in flipped classrooms [42].

Step 1. The content and learning outcomes should be prepared.

- Students should be informed of the flipped classroom method and should be clearly explained what are being expected of them.

Step 2–3. Technical hardware to be used out of and in the class should be prepared, choosing systems that all students can use easily and uninterruptedly (**Table 1**) [40].

- Out-of-class teaching materials suitable for the content and learning outcomes of the chosen lecture should be prepared (**Table 1**). When preparing teaching materials, various resources

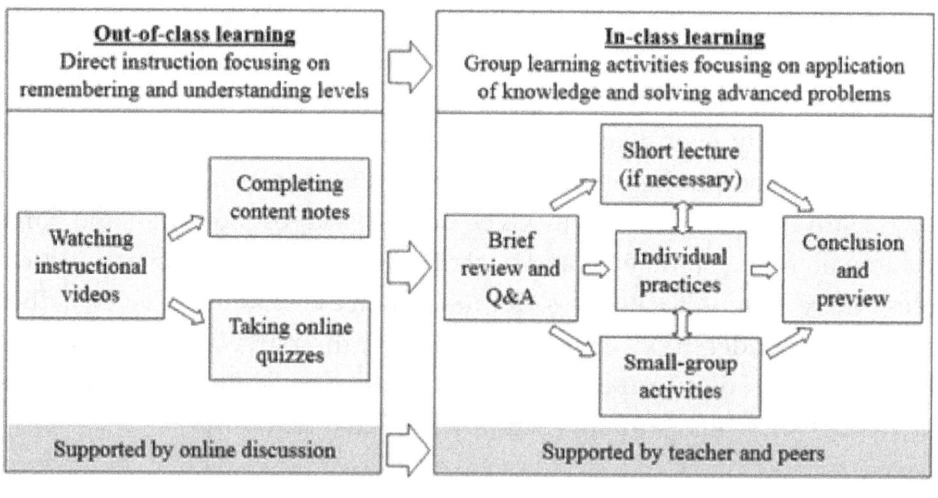

Figure 4. Out-of-class and in-class activities. Source: Lo and Hew [41].

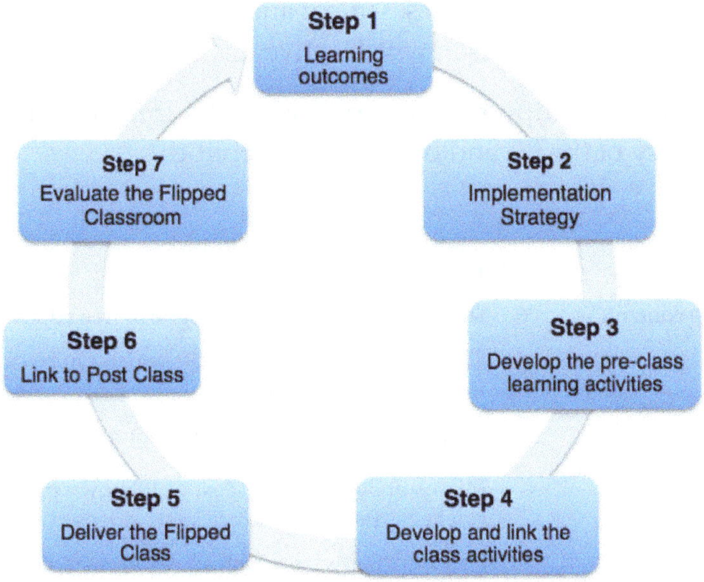

Figure 5. Structuring lectures in flipped classrooms. Source: Karanicolas and Snelling [42].

including lecture notes, research tasks, field work, papers, voiced-over PowerPoint presentations, reports, cases, websites, blog contents, educational games, videoconference recordings, demonstration, and lecture videos can be made use of [43–46].

- For suitable videos, web-sourced open resources may be used, but educators may also make their own videos. Bergmann and Sams [47] recommend that video lessons be prepared by the educator personally [47]. Video lessons prepared by the educator make it possible to initiate student-educator interaction during out-of-classroom activities, resulting in readier acceptance of the model among students [48]. The duration of video lessons is very important. Prolonged video lessons are hard to watch alone, which reduces the success of the exercise, and are also not welcomed by the students [45, 49, 50]. The recommendation is mini video lessons of 20–30 mın in duration [50, 51].

Step 4. In-class activities should be planned. Methods such as discussion sessions, group work, project development work, problem-solving, question-answer exercises, and case discussions can be used in in-class activities. The key is to prefer teaching methods in which knowledge can be used with the highest efficiency. The more in-class activities are supported by the educator, the higher cognitive learning, and reasoning skills will develop [11].

Step 5–6. Flipped class model should be delivered and information on how post-class link will be made should be provided.

Step 7. Assessment and evaluation method should be decided at the very beginning and should be appropriately structured.

- Flipped classrooms possess quite suitable conditions for both formative and summative evaluation [52]. Although studies do not indicate increased success versus the classical system in summative evaluation scales, there is compelling evidence that it improves analytical thinking skills of the learner [4, 6, 13, 32, 49, 50, 53–55]. The assessment and evaluation method should be changed when the model is not improving students' examination success [40]. Also according to the constructivist theory, assessment and evaluation methods should be changed accordingly after teaching processes in which active teaching strategies are extensively used.

- Formative evaluations are important in monitoring the improvement of the learner and checking the efficiency of the in- and out-of-class activities.

Resource	Features
Externally produced video content	iTunesU: Large online catalogue of free educational content
	TED-Ed: Free videos available which can be customized by educators for use with own students
	Vimeo: Video-sharing website, not restricted to educational content
Presentation software	Microsoft PowerPoint: Most well-known presentation software, slides can be narrated to produce short videos
	Powtoon: Software which allows users to develop colorful animated presentations
Screencasting software	Camtasia: Allows capture and personalization of videos, can be viewed from mobile devices
	ShowMe: Free iPad app that allows educators to create and share whiteboard-style lessons with students
Learning management systems	Moodle: Open source web platform for online learning activities
	Blackboard: Commercially available platform for online learning activities
Other content delivery applications	Edmodo: Virtual learning environment with online discussion and poll facilities
	DropBox: Web-based repository that allows educators and students to share documents and large attachments
	Educlipper: Online social platform that allows educators to collect, store, and share web resources with students
Social networking applications	Twitter: Online social networking platform where "hashtag" categories allow students to hold online, interactive discussions during class
	Wikispaces Classroom: Wiki application which allows students working in small groups to record and playback discussions, either to group or during plenary session
Video-calling and webcast software	Skype: Videoconferencing tool that allows outside speakers to be involved in classroom discussions from a different location
	GoToMeeting: Webcasting tool that allows educators to share screens and interact with an outside speaker
Audience response systems	TurningPoint: Commercially available "clicker"-operated system, allows real-time feedback and polling
Other polling applications	Poll Everywhere: Web-based alternative to clickers. Free for audience size up to 40 people

Source: Moffett [40]

Table 1. Learning resources that can be used in a flipped classroom [40].

8. What should be paid attention to in a flipped classroom?

It is possible to say that the flipped learning approach contributes to more active involvement of learners in the learning process and help them learn better by increasing their motivation. However, it also appears that very diligent and meticulous work is required in implementing it. There are many points to consider, especially by the educator, in implementing the flipped classroom concept. Foremost among these is the preparation of videos that are included in out-of-class activities. When preparing videos, having an extended video length causes students to get distracted and reduces the viewability of the video, decreasing the success of the practice. Therefore, the recommended duration for the videos was limited as 20–30 min [38, 50, 51]. It may also be useful to add motivating elements to the videos and to add worksheets or questions at the end of the videos to be able to understand whether students have watched the video [45, 47, 51]. Videos prepared by the educator will improve acceptance of the model by the students. This is because flipped classroom exercise should be adopted not only by the educators but also by the students [37]. The practice should be clearly explained to the students for them to adopt the model. Studies report that students find it difficult to internalize the practice when they are not open to change and sometimes because of cultural habits, especially in Asian countries [46, 56]. Students and educators who are equipped with knowledge about their duties and responsibilities surrounding this practice will contribute to successful implementation of it.

Another point to consider is to encourage students to come to the class prepared. For this, in- and out-of-classroom activities should be defined and planned very well and executed according to the plan. Effective use of time and material and the qualities of in- and out-of-classroom activities are the factors that directly affect learning [49, 50]. For example, out-of-classroom activities should be planned so as not to place excessive burden on the student and care should be taken to ensure that materials are comprehensible, especially for difficult subjects. In addition, out-of-classroom activities should be arranged to cover not more than 60 min a day. In in-class activities, on the other hand, approaches should be offered to learners, which allow them to ask questions to improve their deep learning skills, to make associations by following the flow of thoughts, and to make assessments and estimations. Learnings should be supported by proper feedback at proper times and opportunities should be offered for the learner to reflect so that they can comprehend their own learnings. This not only supports learning efficacy but may also be used to formatively evaluate student's knowledge [43–45]. Methods to be used in assessment and evaluation should also be structured to the content and targets of education. Quizzes measuring conventional knowledge should not be maintained when the classrooms are flipped.

9. The place of flipped classrooms in medical education

The future of medical education lies in technology. The cost and efficiency technology allows represent a paradigm shift in how we teach and utilize faculty, space, finances, and other resources [57]. Today's physicians who completed their education in the previous century are now face to face with new medical students with different ways of thinking and learning. Today's medical students' characteristics are their good command on digital technologies, easy access to information, and changing learning styles and needs, and they exhibit differences in thinking and processing information compared with the generations before them [4, 12]. This makes it imperative to develop alternative teaching-training methods in medical education.

Looking at the medical education literature, examples of implementing the flipped classroom model are seen in the medical faculties in the USA and Central Asian countries. The most radical declaration for the method took place in the Medical Faculty of Stanford University. A model for medical education before graduation based on the flipped classroom philosophy was described by faculty members, Prober and Khan [58]. The two faculty members declared that the current systems were not flexible and did not support individual learning, and that they intended to make the method more common and increase its utilization [56]. There are also attempts to implement the model in Hawaii, as the joint major project of the Accreditation Council for Graduate Medical Education (ACGME) and local medical faculties [59]. Gillous et al. [60] reported that this method was used in the first year of educational programs in medical faculties in France since 2006 [60]. Interestingly, favorable results of the studies performed with the flipped classroom approach in medicine, nursing, and pharmacy domains have been influential in regarding the flipped classroom concept as a pedagogical model.

It can also be seen in the literature that flipped classrooms is a method, which can be used in medical education. Attention of students with intensive course load particularly during the preclinical education period can be grabbed and their motivation can be increased. Also, this method seems to be an opportunity in learning basic mechanisms and integrated pathophysiologic information in the preclinical phase. And in clinical education, flipped classroom can be used in acquiring higher-order cognitive skills such as critical thinking and evidence-based reasoning and application of clinical knowledge including deep learning strategies (approaching patients, initial diagnosis, differential diagnosis, treatment, complementary approach, etc.).

Current evidence suggests that the flipped classroom approach in health professions' education overall yields a statistically significant improvement in learner performance compared with traditional teaching methods. In addition, the flipped classroom would be more effective when instructors use quizzes at the start of each in-class session [61].

In summary, flipped classrooms can be used in medical education in courses and applied training which require conveying the knowledge to a learning level of and above analysis in Bloom's taxonomy. This should therefore be taken into account when determining the content and targets of learning.

10. Using flipped classrooms in organ donation courses

Many organs should function in certain harmony for the human organism to work perfectly. Diseases occur when dysfunction appears in any of these organs. If the dysfunction is left untreated or becomes irreversible, this means that a threat to life has begun to shape, and life expectancy decreases as functional loss progresses. A person at this stage requires a new organ to sustain life. If that organ is the kidney, the person must be confined to dialysis machines for the rest of his/her life but if the organ with failure is the heart, lungs, or liver, death is inevitable. Unfortunately, all these patients could lose their lives if donation is not found in good time. One should bear in mind that organ transplantation is the only hope for these patients to survive. Excellent results can be achieved and lives can be saved with organ transplantation, but, unfortunately, people seem not to be sensitive enough regarding the topic of organ donation. When cadaveric organ donation falls short, the frequency of transplantations from living donors increases to prevent life losses. Under these circumstances, individuals with brain death are buried along with their organs, while healthy people are forced to give their organs to their significant other.

There is globally an increasing number of patients whose lives depend solely on organ or tissue transplantation. This increase also escalates the importance of organ and tissue transplantation. Many studies are being performed on this topic, particularly to raise awareness, but the effectiveness of these studies are disputable. People's awareness needs to be raised to increase cadaveric organ transplantations. The major role here belongs to physicians. Raising awareness is only possible by ensuring that physicians or candidate physicians understand the importance of topics such as cadaveric transplantation, donation, and brain death. By including organ donation as a topic in continuing professional development and undergraduation, medical education programs may emphasize the importance of the subject for physicians or candidate physicians. However, the effectiveness of these activities will still be disputable as long as they remain as didactic courses.

The flipped classroom model, which is an active teaching method, can be used in organ donation courses in medical education programs. Learners' participation/contributions in an education program are one of the key factors that maximize learning/teaching. With the use of the flipped classroom education method in organ donation courses offered in medical education programs, students' knowledge and skills that enable them to discuss the topic of donation with patients can be improved. Because when awareness develops, a number of new cognitive schemes occur in an individual's mind. The way individuals react to their experiences may be enriched by increasing the awareness on the thoughts and feelings that drive behaviors.

The objective and learning targets should be identified first when designing organ donation courses using the flipped classroom model in medical education programs. Students should then be informed of the model and be explained in detail what is expected of them. Technical equipment and educational materials that will be used out of the classroom and in the classroom should be prepared. It may be ensured that students understand the topic of organ donation by using voiced over PowerPoint presentations as educational materials. It may also be useful to add videos developed by the educator or presently available videos on organ donation as educational materials. In short, students may be asked to come to class prepared after learning about organ donation topic from videos and taking online quizzes before the actual lesson. During class time, students may be given the opportunity to practice what they have learned by the use of active learning methods as well as case scenarios, discussion sessions, question-answer exercises, project development work, and/or patient simulations. Studies emphasize the importance of in-class activities. Therefore, activities which allow students to practice their pre-class learnings and advance their professional competency should be planned for in-class activities, particularly in clinical case analyses. It should, however, be borne in mind that students not rehearsing their pre-class learnings in the class as part of the lesson (double course) and absence of a connection between pre-class learnings and in-class practices will result in failure. Testing of the students at the end of the class should aim to evaluate their higher-order cognitive learnings on organ transplantation topic such as practice, analysis, and assessment. Evaluation and assessment activities may utilize case analyses or simulated patient communications.

11. Conclusion

The flipped classroom approach involves problem-solving and cooperative learning as well as hybrid and blended learning activities and focuses on more active involvement of the learner in the learning process. With the flipped learning approach, learners find the opportunity to practice their learnings with both the educator and their peers through activities in the classroom such as discussion and project work and that the learning process continued out of the class as well. The role of the educator in this approach is to ensure that the contents are prepared before the class in a format that can be viewed online, to answer students' questions during the class, to provide feedback, and to encourage them toward active learning.

The flipped classroom model is preferred especially because it supports student-centered approaches and enriches curriculums. For educators, it seems to be important in being a setting in which students may be taught critical and independent thinking and gives them the opportunity to develop their learning strategies throughout their lives.

It is important to state that the flipped classroom cannot be the only form of education. Medicine is still very hands-on, and nothing can replace that experience. Thus, the flipped classroom and case-based instruction cannot be the only form of instruction. However, this model represents a potential future as a means for improved instructional efficiency [57].

Author details

Nilufer Yılmaz[1*], Sibel Demiral[2] and Taylan Özgür Sezer[3]

*Address all correspondence to: nilufer.demiral@gmail.com

1 Department of Medical Education School of Medicine, Ege University, Izmir, Turkey

2 Health Sciences University Tepecik Education and Research Hospital, Izmir, Turkey

3 Department of General Surgery School of Medicine, Ege University, Izmir, Turkey

References

[1] Almeida RAM, Quireze CJ, de Faria WML, dos Santos DF, Dias RV, Maynarde IG. Organ donation and transplantation from medical students' perspective: Introducing the experience from an academic league in Brazil. Transplantation Proceedings. 2011;**43**(4):1311-1312

[2] Bardell T, Hunter DJW, Kent WDT, Jain MK. Do medical students have the knowledge needed to maximize organ donation rates? Canadian Journal of Surgery. 2003;**46**(6):453-457

[3] Lage MJ, Platt GJ, Treglia M. Inverting the classroom: A gateway to creating an inclusive learning environment. The Journal of Economic Education. 2000;**31**(1):30-43

[4] Bergmann J, Sams A. The Flipped Classroom? Flip your Classroom: Reach every Student in every Class every Day. 1st ed. Washington, DC: ISTE; 2012

[5] Staker H, Horn MB. Classifying K-12 Blended Learning. 2012. Retrieved from https://www.christenseninstitute.org/wp-content/uploads/2013/04/Classifying-K-12-blended-learning.pdf

[6] Love B, Hodge A, Grandgenett N, Swift AW. Student learning and perceptions in a flipped linear algebra course. International Journal of Mathematical Education in Science and Technology. 2014;**45**:317-324

[7] Fulton K. Upside down and inside out: Flip your classroom to improve student learning. Learning and Leading with Technology. 2012;**39**(8):12-17

[8] Youngkin CA. The flipped classroom: Practices and opportunities for health sciences librarians. Medical Reference Services Quarterly. 2014;**33**(4):367-374

[9] Kurtz G, Tsimerman A, Steiner-Lavi O. The flipped-classroom approach, an answer to future learning. European Journal of Open, Distance and E-Learning. 2014;**17**:171-173

[10] Saint Louis University. 2012. Retrieved from https://www.slu.edu/cttl/resources/teaching-tips-and-resources/flipped-classroom-resources

[11] O'Flaherty J, Phillips C. The use of flipped classrooms in higher education: A scoping review. Internet and Higher Education. 2015;**25**:85-95

[12] Roehl A, Reddy SL, Shannon GJ. The flipped classroom: An opportunity to engage millennial students through active learning strategies. Journal of Family & Consumer Sciences. 2013;**105**(2):44-49

[13] Bishop JL, Verleger MA. The flipped classroom: A survey of the research. Paper presented at the ASEE National Conference Proceedings; Atlanta; 2013

[14] Sage M, Sele P. Reflective journaling as a flipped classroom technique to increase reading and participation with social work students. Journal of Social Work Education. 2015;**51**(4):668-681

[15] Sams A, Bergmann J. Flip your students' learning. Educational Leadership. 2013;**70**(6):16-20

[16] Arshad K, Imran MA. Increasing the interaction time in a lecture by integrating flipped classroom and just-in-time teaching concepts. Compass: Journal of Learning and Teaching. 2013;**4**(7):1-13

[17] Davies RS, Dean DL, Ball N. Flipping the classroom and instructional technology integration in a college-level information systems spreadsheet course. Education Technology Research Development. 2013;**61**:563-580

[18] McLaughlin JE, Gharkholonarehe N, Esserman DA. The flipped classroom: A course redesign to foster learning and engagement in a health professions school. Academic Medicine. 2014;**89**(2):236-243

[19] Halili SH, Zainuddin Z. Flipping the classroom: What we know and what we do not. The Online Journal of Distance Education and e-Learning (TOJDEL). 2015;**3**(1):28-35

[20] Mason GS, Shuman TR, Cook KE. Comparing the effectiveness of an ınverted classroom to a traditional classroom in an upper-division engineering course. IEEE Transactıons on Education. 2013;**56**(4):430-435

[21] Flipped Learning Network – FLN. The four pillars of F-L-I-P. 2014. Retrieved from http://www.flippedlearning.org

[22] Bergmann J, Overmyer J, Wilie B. The flipped class: Myths versus reality. 2012. The Daily Riff. Retrieved from http://www.thedailyriff.com/articles/the-flipped-class-conversation-689

[23] Enfield J. Looking at the impact of the flipped classroom model of instruction on undergraduate multimedia students at CSUN. Techtrends: Linking Research & Practice to Improve Learning. 2013;**57**(6):14-27

[24] Morgan H. Focus on technology: Flip your classroom to ıncrease academic achievement. Childhood Education. 2014;**90**(3):239-241

[25] McCarthy J. Reflections on a flipped classroom in first year higher education. Issues in Educational Research. 2016;**26**(2):332-350

[26] Ornstein AC, Levine DU. Foundation of Education. 10th ed. Boston: Houghton Mifflin; 2008

[27] Ornstein AC, Hunkins FP. Curriculum Foundations: Principles and Theory. Boston: Allynand Bacon; 2004

[28] Wilson BG. Reflections on Constructivism and Lnstructional Design. Denver: Educational Technology Publications; 1997

[29] Persky MA, McLaughlin JE. The flipped classroom – From theory to practice in health professional education. American Journal of Pharmaceutical Education. 2017;**81**(6):118

[30] Belfi LM, Bartolotta RJ, Giambrone AE, Davi C, Min RJ. Flipping the introductory clerkship in radiology impact on medical student performance and perceptions. Academic Radiology. 2015;**22**(6):795-801

[31] Tune JD, Sturek M, Basile DP. Flipped classroom model improves graduate student performance in cardiovascular, respiratory, and renal physiology. Advances in Physiology Education. 2013;**37**:316-320

[32] Mortensen CJ, Nicholson AM. The flipped classroom stimulates greater learning and is a modern 21st century approach to teaching today's undergraduates. Journal of Animal Science. 2015;**93**:3722-3731

[33] Ouda H, Ahmed K. Flipped learning as a new educational paradigm: An analytical critical study. European Scientific Journal. 2016;**12**(10):417-444

[34] Herreid CF, Schiller NA. Case studies and the flipped classroom. Journal of College Science Teaching. 2013;**42**(5):62-66

[35] Strayer JF. How learning in an inverted classroom influences cooperation, innovation, and task orientation. Learning Environment Research. 2012;**15**:171-193

[36] LaFee S. Flipped learning. The Education Digest. 2013;**79**:13-18

[37] Findlay-Thompson S, Mombourquette P. Evaluation of a flipped classroom in an undergraduate business course. Business Education & Accreditation. 2014;**6**(1):63-71

[38] Bristol TJ. Educate, excite, engage. Teaching and Learning in Nursing. 2014;**9**:43-46

[39] Khan Academy. Retrieved from https://www.khanacademy.org

[40] Moffett J. Twelve tips for "flipping" the classroom. Medical Teacher. 2015;**37**:331-336

[41] Lo CK, Hew KF. A critical review of flipped classroom challenges in K-12 education: Possible solutions and recommendations for future research. Research and Practice in Technology Enhanced Learning. 2017;**12**:4

[42] Karanicolas S, Snelling C. Making the transition: Achieving content connectivity and student engagement through flexible learning tools. In: Proceedings of the Distance Education Association of New Zealand (DEANZ) Conference Wellington; 2010

[43] Tan E, Brainard A, Larkin GL. Acceptability of the flipped classroom approach for in-house teaching in emergency medicine. Emergency Medicine Australasia. 2015;**27**:453-459

[44] Galway LP, Corbett KK, Takaro TK, Tairyan K, Frank E. A novel integration of online and flipped classroom instructional models in public health higher education. BMC Medical Education. 2014;**14**:181

[45] Critz CM, Knight D. Using the flipped classroom in graduate nursing education. Nurse Educator. 2013;**38**:210-213

[46] Schlairet MC, Green R, Benton MJ. The flipped classroom: Strategies for an undergraduate nursing course. Nurse Educator. 2014;**39**:321-325

[47] Bergmann J, Sams A. Flipped Learning: Gateway to Student Engagement. 1st ed. Washington: ISTE; 2014

[48] Gilboy MB, Heinerichs S, Pazzaglia G. Enhancing student engagement using the flipped classroom. Journal of Nutrition Education and Behavior. 2015;**47**:109-114

[49] Wong TH, Ip EJ, Lopes I, Rajagopalan V. Pharmacy students' performance and perceptions in a flipped teaching pilot on cardiac arrhythmias. American Journal of Pharmaceutical Education. 2014;**78**:185

[50] Moraros J, Islam A, Yu S, Banow R, Schindelka B. Flipping for success: Evaluating the effectiveness of a novel teaching approach in a graduate level setting. BMC Medical Education. 2015;**28**:15-27

[51] Phillips CR, Trainor JE. Millennial students and the flipped classroom. Proceedings of ASBBS. 2014;**21**:519-530

[52] Mok HN. Teaching tip: The flipped classroom. Journal of Information Systems Education. 2014;**25**:7-10

[53] Pierce R, Fox J. Vodcasts and active-learning exercises in a "flipped classroom" model of a renalpharmacotherapy module. American Journal of Pharmaceutical Education. 2012;**76**:196

[54] Marshall LL, Nykamp DL, Momary KM. Impact of abbreviated lecture with interactive mini-cases vs traditional lecture on student performance in the large classroom. American Journal of Pharmaceutical Education. 2014;**78**:189

[55] Street SE, Gilliland KO, McNeil C, Royal K. The flipped classroom improved medical student performance and satisfaction in a pre-clinical physiology course. Medical Science Educator. 2015;**25**:35-43

[56] Joanne CSM, Lateef F. The flipped classroom: Viewpoints in Asian universities. Education in Medicine Journal. 2014;**6**:20-26

[57] Williams DE. The future of medical education: Flipping the classroom and education technology. Ochsner Journal. 2016;**16**:14-15

[58] Prober CG, Khan S. Medical education reimagined: A call to action. Academic Medicine. 2013;**88**:1407-1410

[59] Vincent DS. Out of the wilderness: Flipping the classroom to advance scholarship in an internal medicine residency program. Hawai'i JMPH. 2014;**73**(Supp 2):1-2

[60] Gillois P, Bosson JL, Genty C, Vuillez JP, Romanet JP. The impacts of blended learning design in first year medical studies. Studies in Health Technology and Informatics. 2015;**210**:607-611

[61] Hew KF, Lo CK. Flipped classroom improves student learning in health professions education: A meta-analysis. Medical Education. 2018;**18**:38

Permissions

All chapters in this book were first published in ODTCSFC, by InTech Open; hereby published with permission under the Creative Commons Attribution License or equivalent. Every chapter published in this book has been scrutinized by our experts. Their significance has been extensively debated. The topics covered herein carry significant findings which will fuel the growth of the discipline. They may even be implemented as practical applications or may be referred to as a beginning point for another development.

The contributors of this book come from diverse backgrounds, making this book a truly international effort. This book will bring forth new frontiers with its revolutionizing research information and detailed analysis of the nascent developments around the world.

We would like to thank all the contributing authors for lending their expertise to make the book truly unique. They have played a crucial role in the development of this book. Without their invaluable contributions this book wouldn't have been possible. They have made vital efforts to compile up to date information on the varied aspects of this subject to make this book a valuable addition to the collection of many professionals and students.

This book was conceptualized with the vision of imparting up-to-date information and advanced data in this field. To ensure the same, a matchless editorial board was set up. Every individual on the board went through rigorous rounds of assessment to prove their worth. After which they invested a large part of their time researching and compiling the most relevant data for our readers.

The editorial board has been involved in producing this book since its inception. They have spent rigorous hours researching and exploring the diverse topics which have resulted in the successful publishing of this book. They have passed on their knowledge of decades through this book. To expedite this challenging task, the publisher supported the team at every step. A small team of assistant editors was also appointed to further simplify the editing procedure and attain best results for the readers.

Apart from the editorial board, the designing team has also invested a significant amount of their time in understanding the subject and creating the most relevant covers. They scrutinized every image to scout for the most suitable representation of the subject and create an appropriate cover for the book.

The publishing team has been an ardent support to the editorial, designing and production team. Their endless efforts to recruit the best for this project, has resulted in the accomplishment of this book. They are a veteran in the field of academics and their pool of knowledge is as vast as their experience in printing. Their expertise and guidance has proved useful at every step. Their uncompromising quality standards have made this book an exceptional effort. Their encouragement from time to time has been an inspiration for everyone.

The publisher and the editorial board hope that this book will prove to be a valuable piece of knowledge for researchers, students, practitioners and scholars across the globe.

List of Contributors

Félix Cantarovich
Faculty of Medical Sciences, Catholic University Argentine, Buenos Aires, Argentina

Yingzi Ming, Baoren Tu and Quan Zhuang
Transplantation Center of the third Xiangya Hospital, Central South University, Changsha, Hunan, China
Engineering and Technology Research Center for Transplantation Medicine of National Ministry of Health, Changsha, Hunan, China

Vasishta S. Tatapudi and Bonnie E. Lonze
NYU Langone Health, Transplant Institute, New York, NY, USA

Wayne J. Hawthorne and Ahmer Hameed
Department of Surgery, Westmead Hospital, Sydney, Australia
Centre for Transplant and Renal Research, Westmead Institute for Medical Research, Sydney, Australia
Sydney Medical School, University of Sydney, Sydney, Australia

Henry Pleass
Department of Surgery, Westmead Hospital, Sydney, Australia
Sydney Medical School, University of Sydney, Sydney, Australia

Katalin Monostory
Institute of Enzymology, Research Centre for Natural Sciences, Hungarian Academy of Sciences, Budapest, Hungary

Katarina Tomulić Brusich
Department of Anesthesiology and Intensive Care, The Magdalena Special Hospital for Cardiovascular Surgery and Cardiology, Croatia

Ivana Acan
Department of Anesthesiology and Intensive Care, University Hospital Merkur, Zagreb, Croatia

Jorge Andrade-Sierra
Department of Physiology, University Health Sciences Center, University of Guadalajara, Guadalajara, Jalisco, Mexico
Department of Nephrology and Organ Transplant Unit, Specialties Hospital, National Occidental Medical Centre, Mexican Social Security Institute (CMNO IMSS), Guadalajara, Jalisco, Mexico
Department of Internal Medicine, Civil Hospital of Guadalajara Dr. Juan I. Menchaca, Guadalajara, Jalisco, Mexico

Pedro Alejandro Vazquez-Galvan and Hernesto Hernandez-Reyes
Department of Nephrology and Organ Transplant Unit, Specialties Hospital, National Occidental Medical Centre, Mexican Social Security Institute (CMNO IMSS), Guadalajara, Jalisco, Mexico

Lydia A. Mercado-Jáuregui
Department of Internal Medicine, Civil Hospital of Guadalajara Dr. Juan I. Menchaca, Guadalajara, Jalisco, Mexico

Jonathan S. Chávez-Iñiguez
Department of Nephrology, Civil Hospital of Guadalajara "Fray Antonio Alcalde", Guadalajara, Jalisco, Mexico

Eduardo González-Espinoza, Benjamin Gómez-Navarro and José I. Cerrillos-Gutiérrez
Department of Nephrology and Organ Transplant Unit, Specialties Hospital, National Occidental Medical Centre, Mexican Social Security Institute (CMNO IMSS), Guadalajara, Jalisco, Mexico

Georgios Vrakas
Oxford University Hospitals, Oxford, UK

Nilufer Yılmaz
Department of Medical Education School of Medicine, Ege University, Izmir, Turkey

Sibel Demiral
Health Sciences University Tepecik Education and Research Hospital, Izmir, Turkey

Taylan Özgür Sezer
Department of General Surgery School of Medicine, Ege University, Izmir, Turkey

Index

www.ingramcontent.com/pod-product-compliance
Lightning Source LLC
LaVergne TN
LVHW060535210926
848485LV00005B/1201